OFFBEAT
BUTTERS

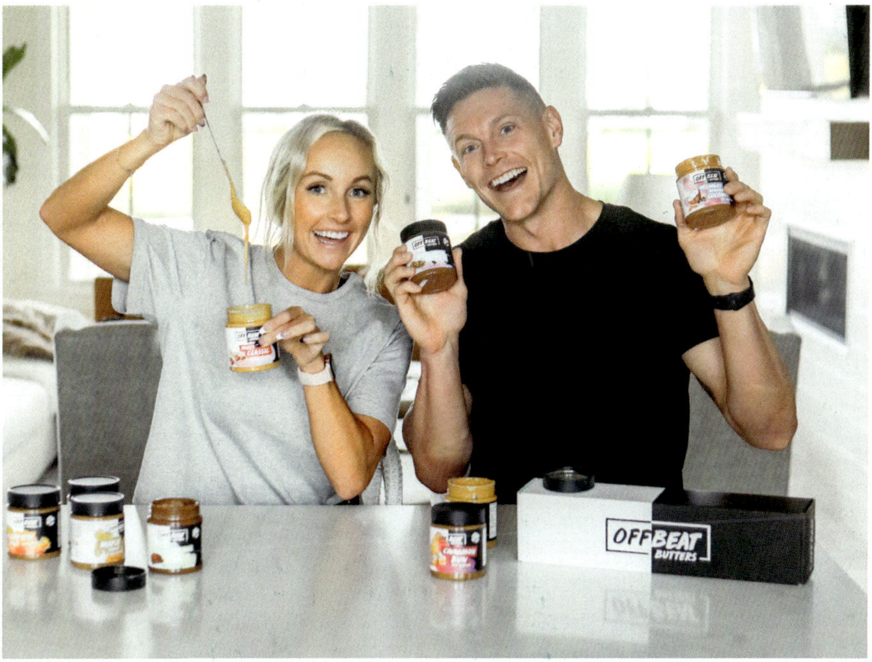

We don't do bland, boring or dull. We have rocked the clean eating scene by mixing healthy and natural ingredients with unique flavor combos! When we say #endlesspossibilities, we mean it! In this book you'll find 100+ recipes: shakes, bites, brownies, bars, cookies, oatmeals, breads, and even entrees! Drizzle, spread or simply enjoy your OffBeat Butter #bythespoonful. We're not drooling, you're drooling!

Enjoy! XO
Erika & JJ

 cleansimpleeats / offbeatbutters

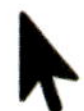 hello@cleansimpleeats.com

cleansimpleeats.com / offbeatbutters.com

RECIPE INDEX

RECIPE INDEX

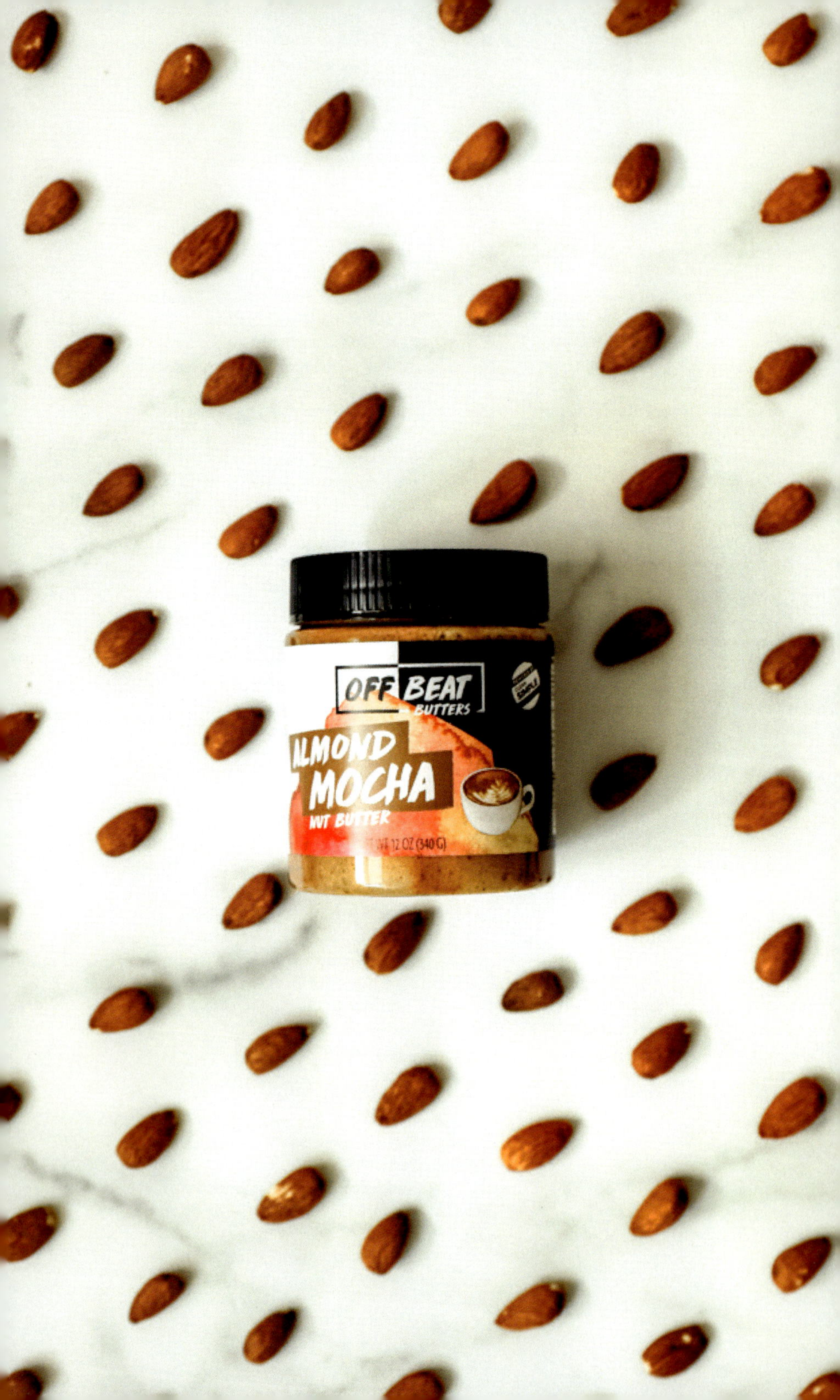

OFF BEAT
BUTTERS
ALMOND
MOCHA
NUT BUTTER
NET 12 OZ (340 G)

YOU MOCHA ME HAPPY

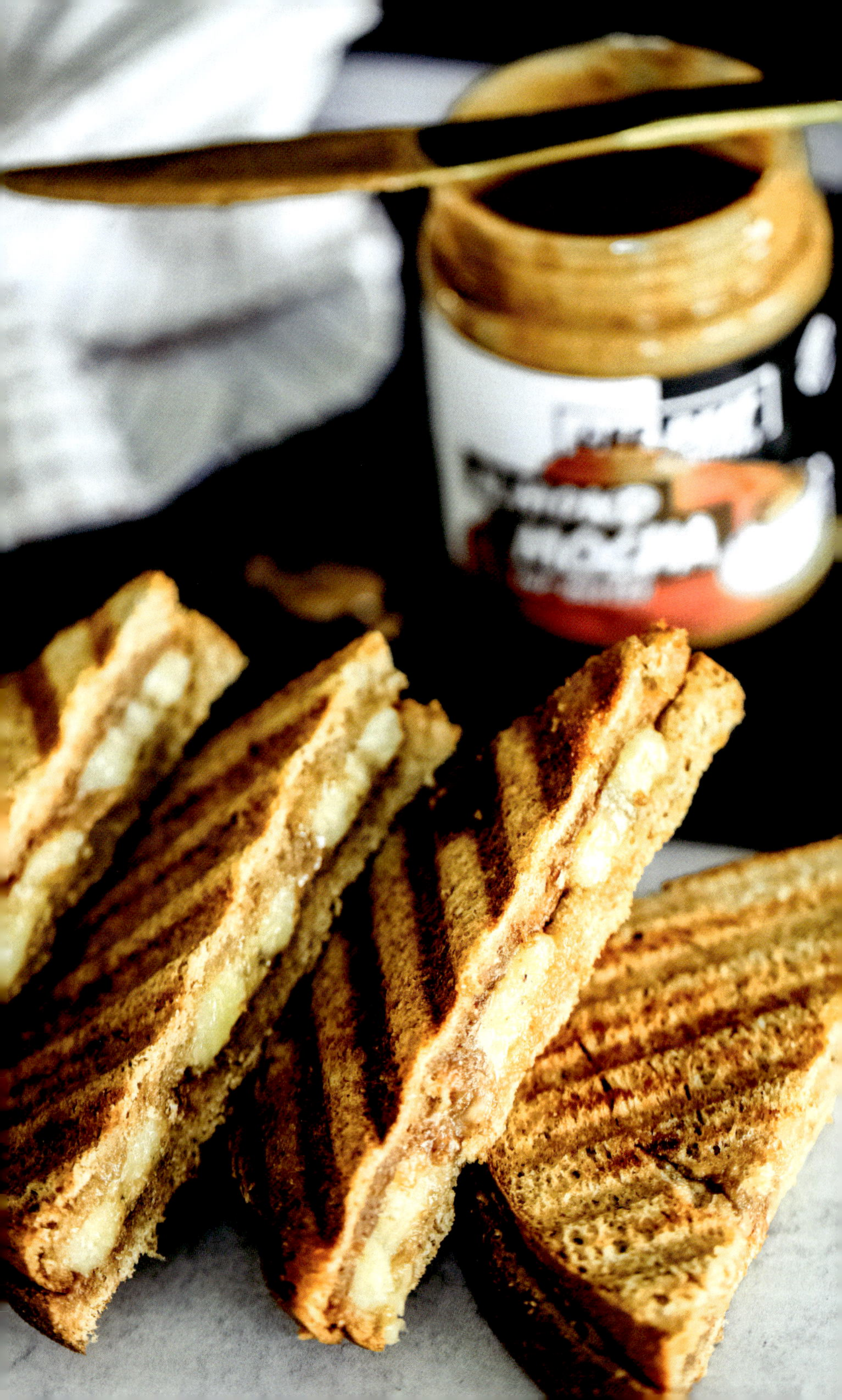

ALMOND MOCHA, BANANA, & HONEY PANINI SAMMY

Makes 1 serving
355 calories / 7F / 63C / 11P

---

2 slices Harper's Bran Bread (or other 80 calorie per slice,
  whole grain bread)
1 Tbs. OffBeat Almond Mocha
  or Midnight Almond Coconut Butter
1 Tbs. raw honey
50g banana slices

1. Heat the panini press or a frying pan to medium heat.

2. Spread the Almond Mocha Butter and honey on the bread.
Add the sliced banana, in a single layer, to one side of the bread.
Sandwich it together.

3. Spray the panini press or pan with cooking spray. Add the
sandwich and cook until the middle is melty and the bread is
golden brown.

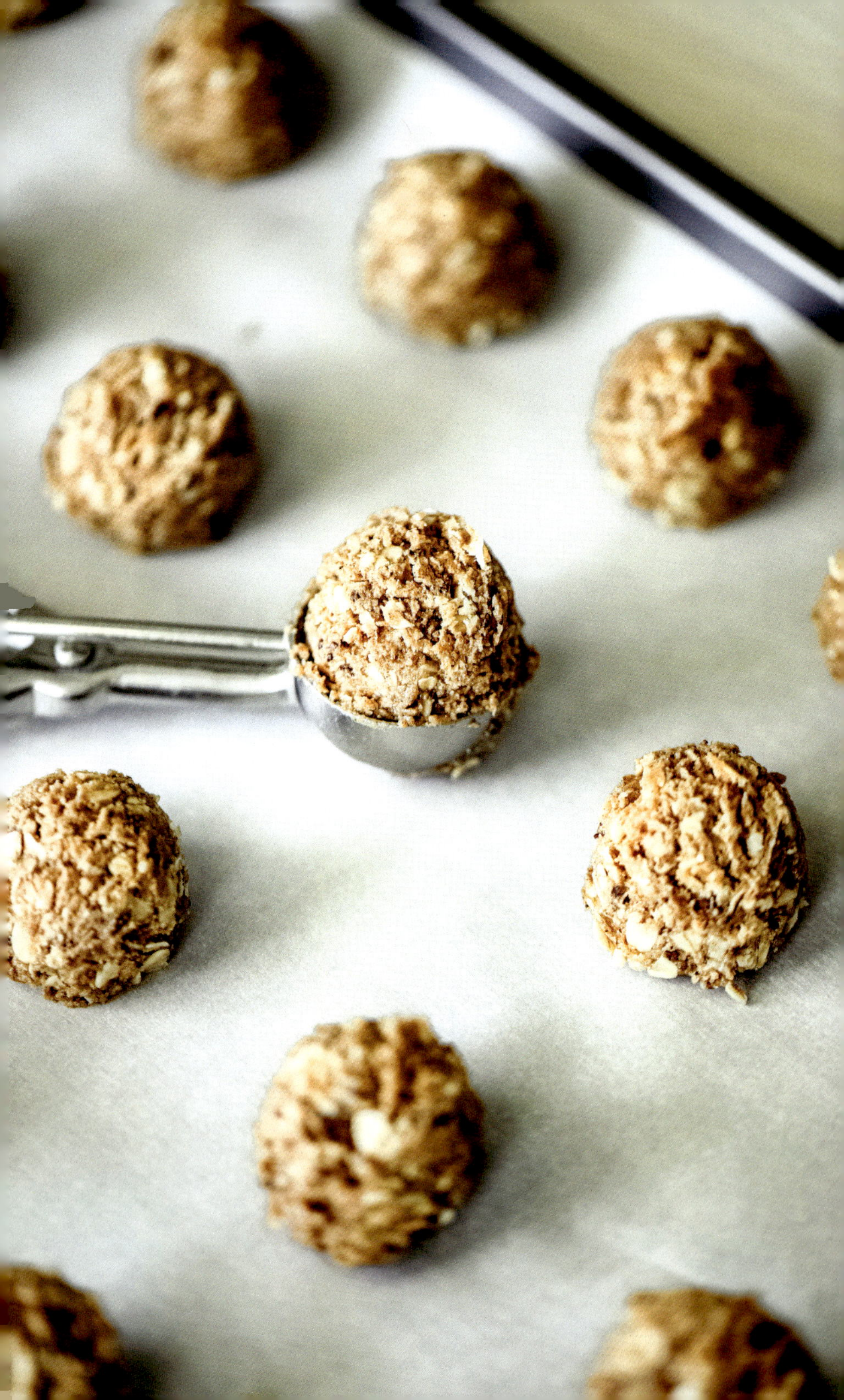

CARAMEL MACCHIATO BITES
Makes 30 servings
90 calories / 4F / 10.5C / 3P / per bite

---

1 cup OffBeat Almond Mocha Butter
½ cup raw honey
2 Tbs. Crio Bru grounds or coffee bean grounds
1 serving CSE Caramel Toffee Protein Powder
½ tsp. vanilla extract
Dash sea salt
1 ½ cups old-fashioned rolled oats

1. Add all the ingredients to a large bowl and mix until well combined.

2. Using a small cookie scoop, scoop into balls and store in the fridge or freezer.

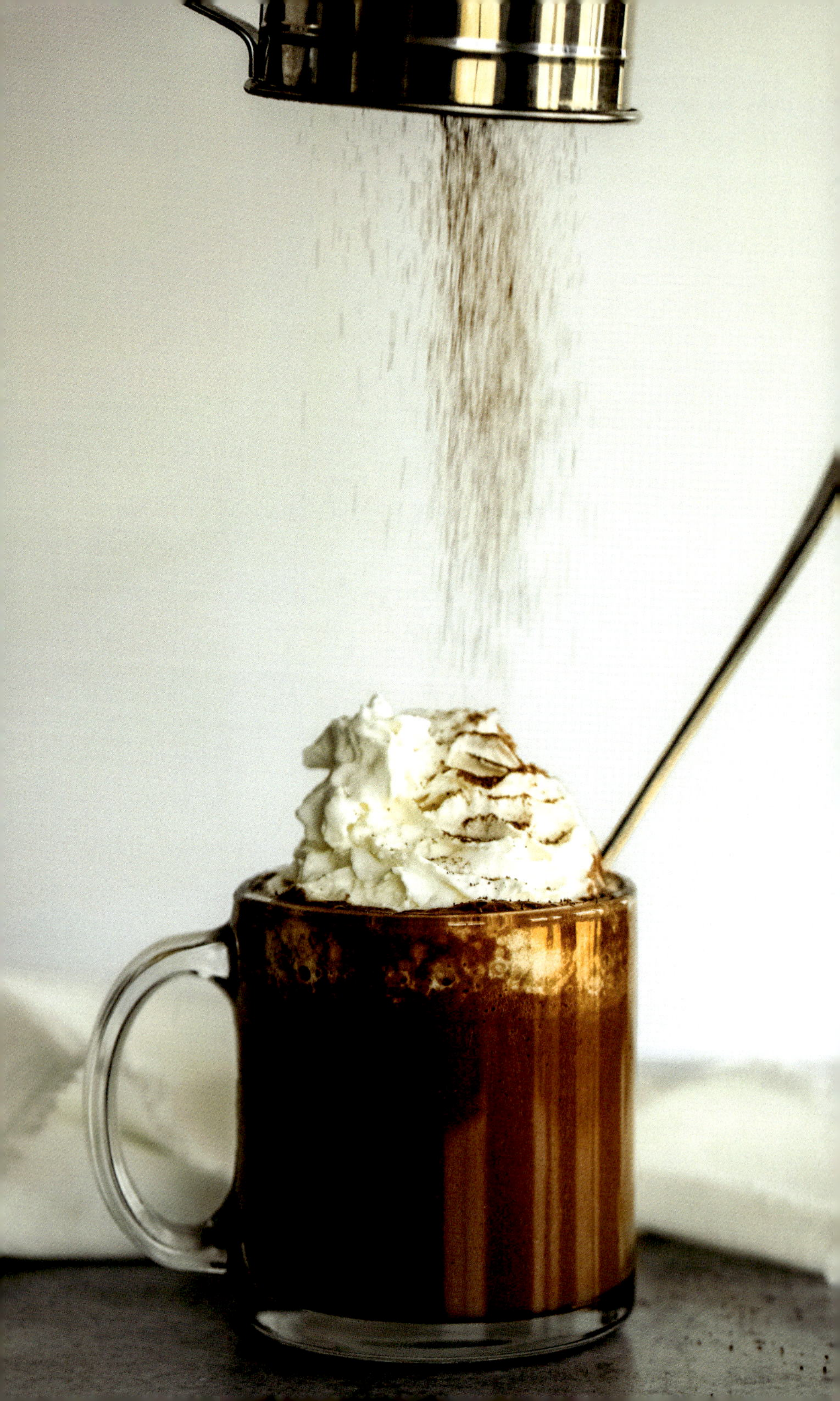

CARAMEL MOCHA PROTEIN HOT CHOCOLATE
Makes 1 serving
225 calories / 11F / 15C / 24.5P

---

1 cup unsweetened vanilla almond milk
1 Tbs. OffBeat Almond Mocha Butter
1 Tbs. cocoa powder
1 serving CSE Caramel Toffee Protein Powder
Topping:
2 Tbs. spray whipped cream topping

1. Pour the almond milk into a mug and microwave for 2 minutes or until hot.

2. Add the Almond Mocha Butter and cocoa powder. Whisk until smooth. Add the protein powder and whisk until smooth and creamy. Top with spray whipped cream, if desired.

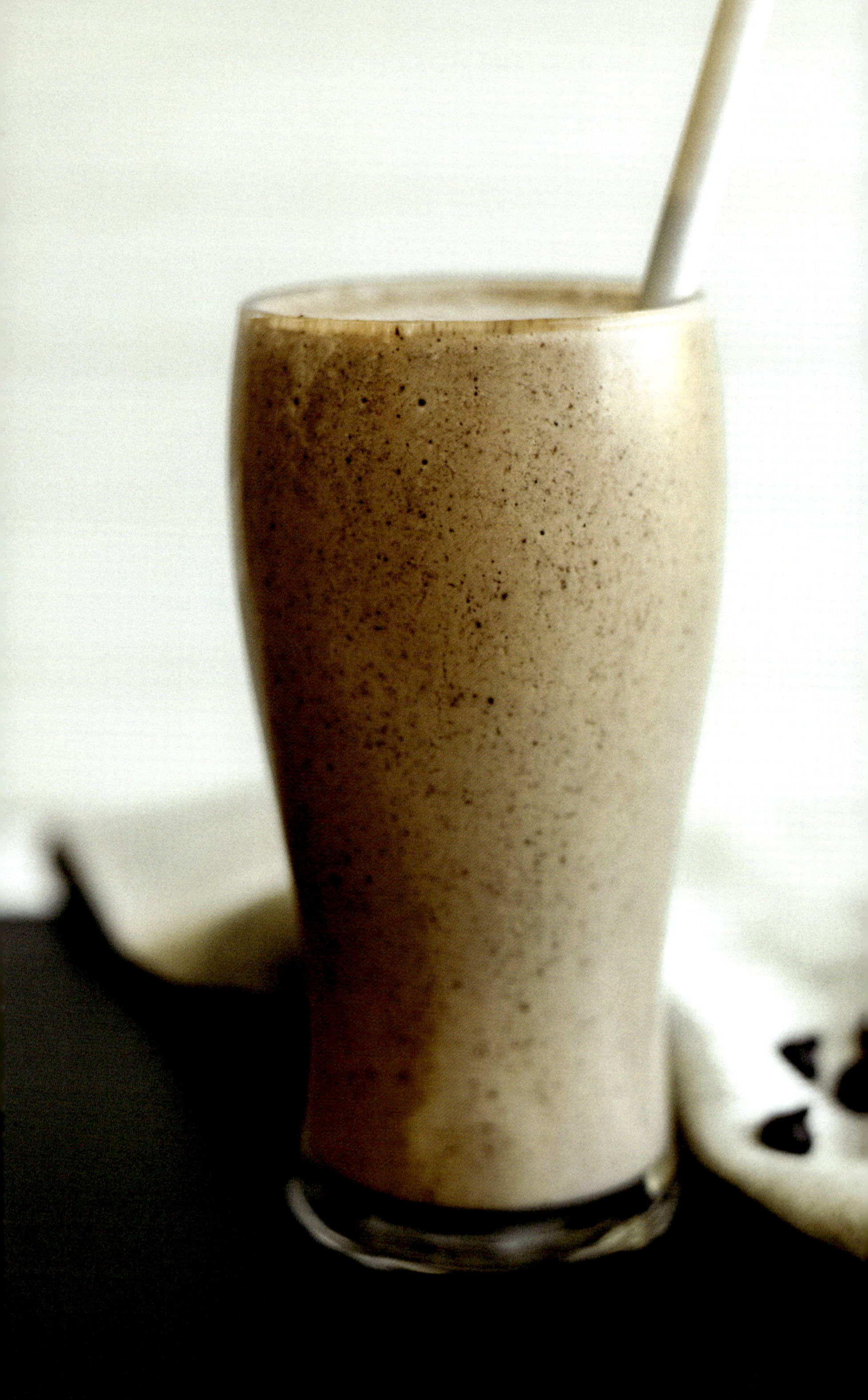

CHOCOLATE CHIP ALMOND MOCHA SHAKE
Makes 1 serving
350 calories / 12F / 33C / 27P

½ cup unsweetened almond milk
½ cup cold brewed coffee or cold brewed Crio Bru
¾ serving CSE Brownie Batter Protein Powder
100g frozen banana slices
2 Tbs. nonfat, plain Greek yogurt
1 Tbs. OffBeat Almond Mocha Butter
15 extra dark chocolate chips
¼ tsp. almond extract, optional
6-8 ice cubes

1. Place all of the ingredients into a high-powered blender. Blend on high until smooth.

2. Pour into a cup and enjoy!

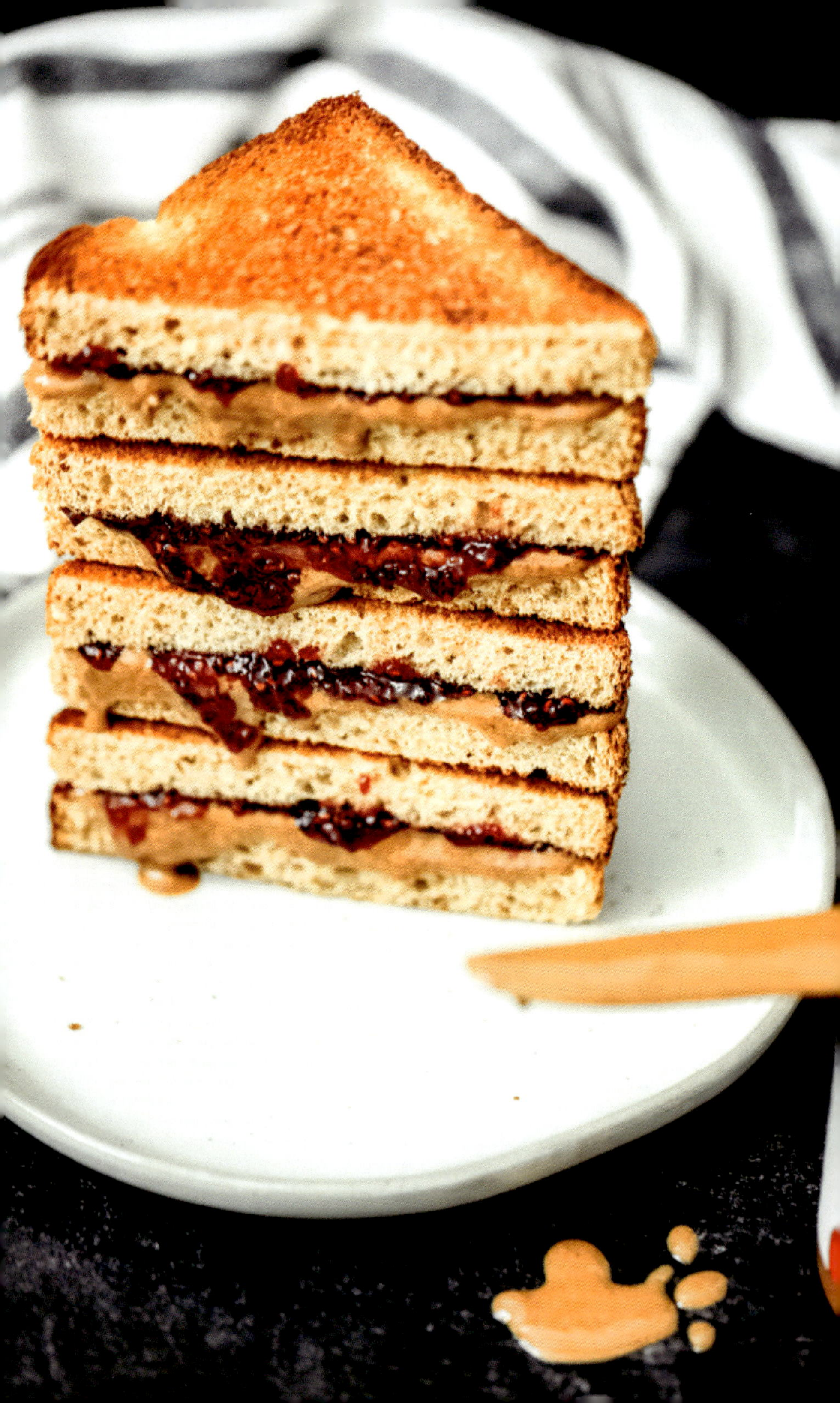

GROWN-UP OFFBEAT BUTTER & JELLY

Makes 1 serving
380 calories / 11F / 37C / 11P

---

2 slices Harper's Bran Bread (or other 80 calorie per slice,
    whole grain bread)
1 Tbs. OffBeat Almond Mocha Butter
2 Tbs. raspberry jam

1. Heat the panini press or a frying pan to medium heat.

2. Spread the Almond Mocha Butter and jam on the bread in a
single layer, to one side of the bread. Sandwich it together.

3. Spray the panini press or pan with cooking spray. Add the
sandwich and cook until the middle is melty and the bread is
golden brown.

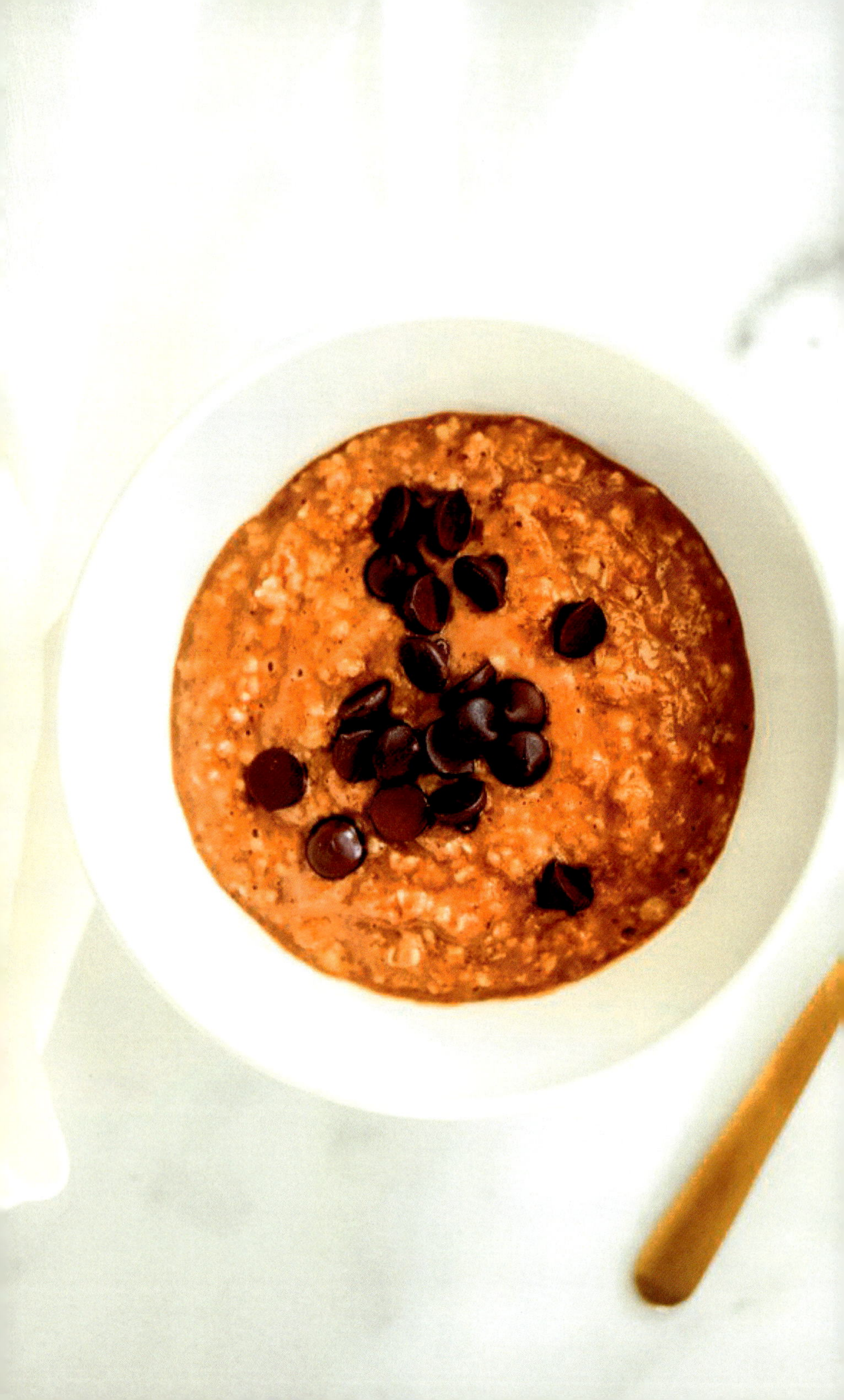

MOCHA CHOCOLATE CHIP OATMEAL

Makes 1 serving
350 calories / 12F / 35C / 26.5P

⅓ cup old-fashioned rolled oats
½ cup water
3 Tbs. (46g) liquid egg whites
1 Tbs. OffBeat Almond Mocha Butter
¾ serving CSE Brownie Batter Protein Powder
Topping:
10g dark chocolate chips

1. Add the oats, water, and egg whites to a microwave-safe bowl. Whisk until the egg whites are well combined. Microwave for 1-2 minutes.

2. Stir in the Almond Mocha Butter. Let cool for a couple minutes, then stir in the protein powder.

3. Top with chocolate chips.

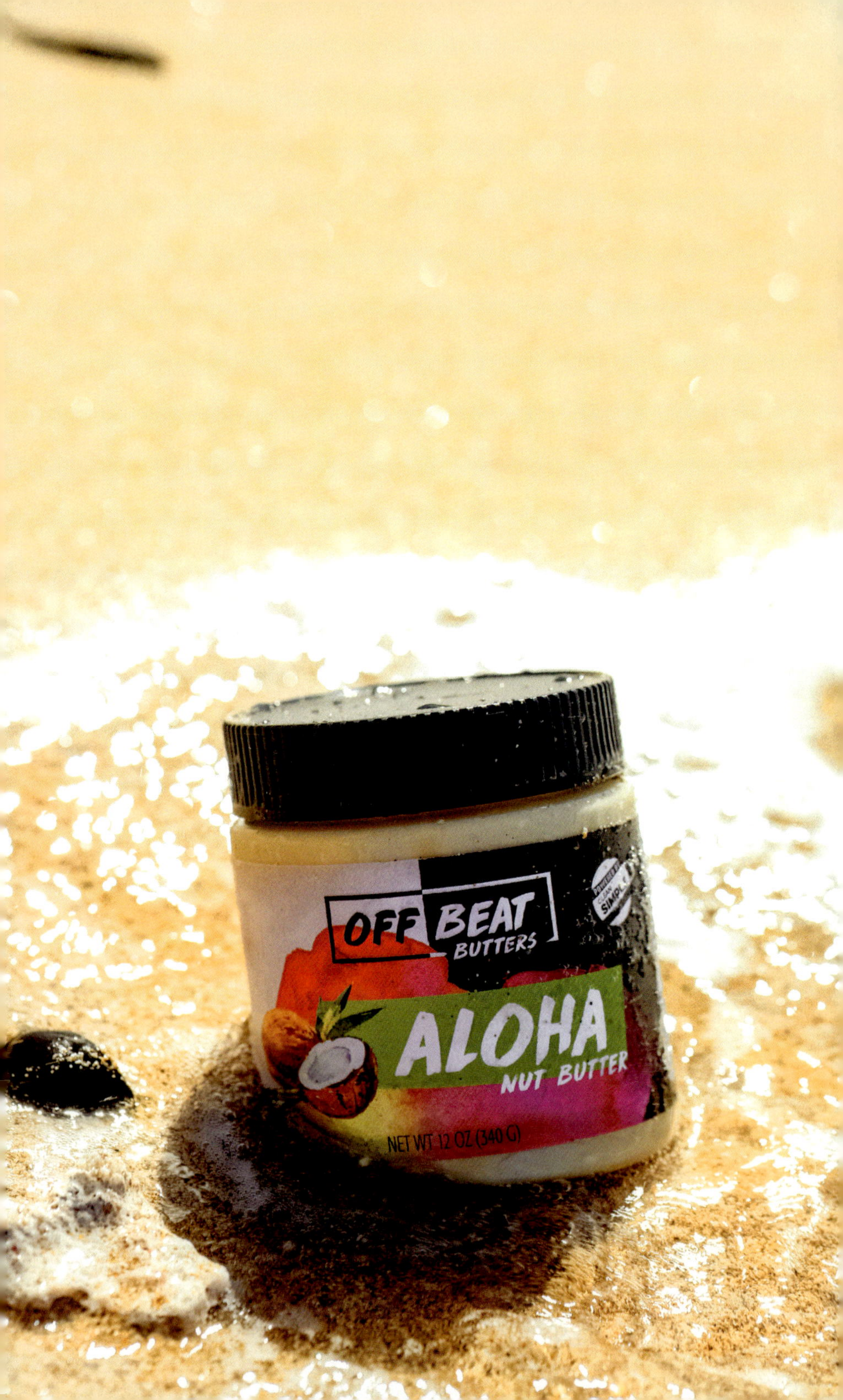

NET WT 12 OZ (340 G)
OFF BEAT
BUTTERS
ALOHA
NUT BUTTER

YOU HAD ME AT 'ALOHA'

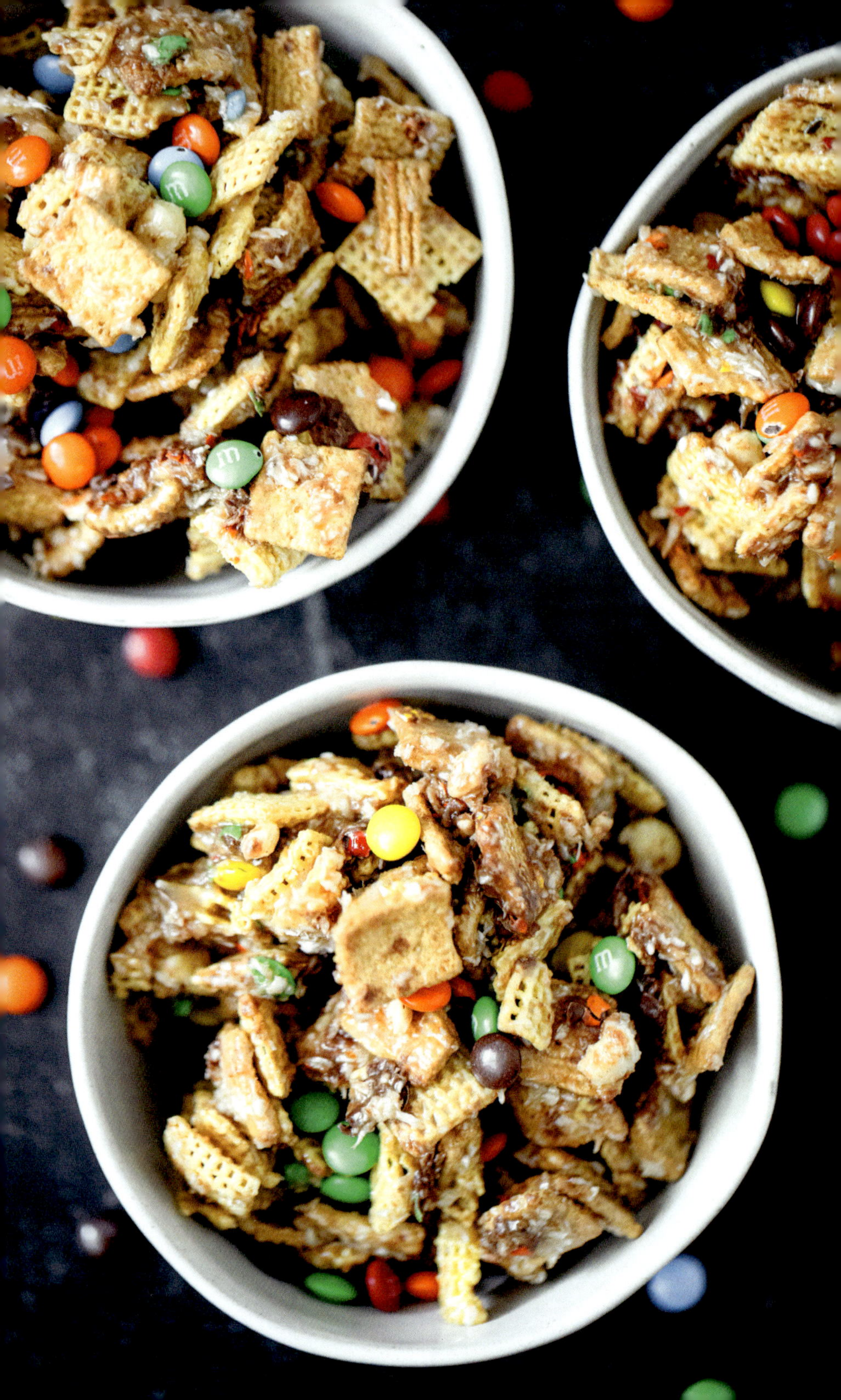

ALOHA ADDICTION*

Makes 16 servings
220 calories / 11F / 30C / 2P / per serving

---

2 ½ cups Chex cereal (corn or rice)
2 ½ cups Golden Graham cereal
¾ cup unsweetened coconut flakes
½ cup Mini M&M's
¼ cup cashews (optional)
½ cup corn syrup
½ cup sugar
¼ cup OffBeat Aloha Butter
¼ cup grass-fed butter

1. Combine cereals, coconut, candies and nuts in a bowl.

2. In a saucepan, bring the corn syrup, sugar, Aloha Butter and butter to a boil.

3. Pour liquid mixture over cereal mixture, stir until well combined, pour out onto wax paper to set for at least 30 mins. Double the recipe for a larger crowd. Enjoy!

**OffBeat Fam Recipe Submitted by Kallie Browne*

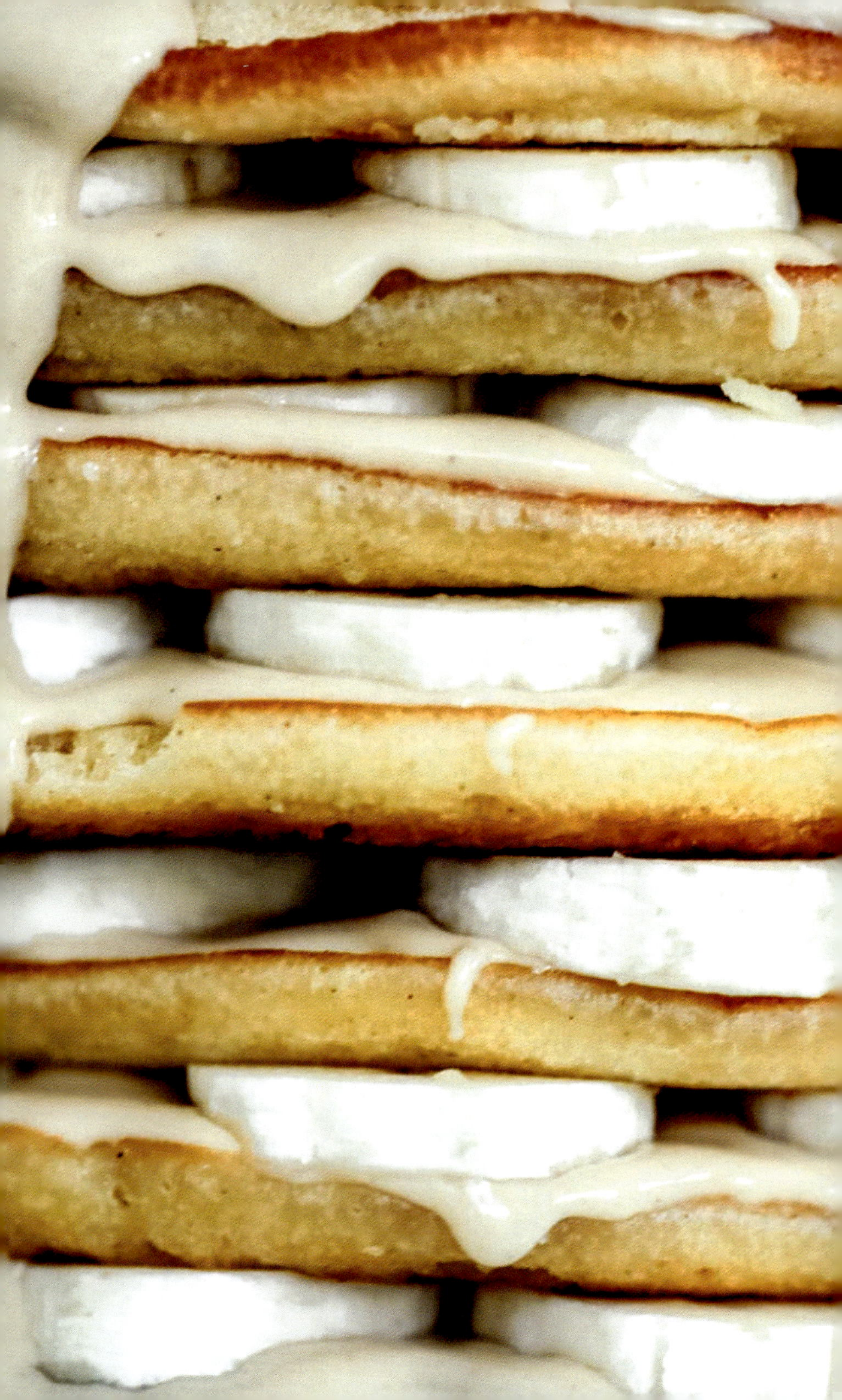

ALOHA BANANA PANCAKES

Makes 1 serving
310 calories / 6F / 49C / 18P

½ cup CSE Vanilla Pancake & Waffle Mix
½ cup water
1 Tbs. OffBeat Aloha Butter
75g banana, sliced

1. Heat griddle to medium heat.

2. Place water and CSE Pancake & Waffle Mix together in a bowl. Mix well.

3. Spray griddle with cooking spray. Using a ¼ measuring cup, pour batter slowly onto the griddle. Once small bubbles form on top of the panckes, flip and cook on the other side.

4. Top the pancakes with Aloha Butter and banana. Enjoy!

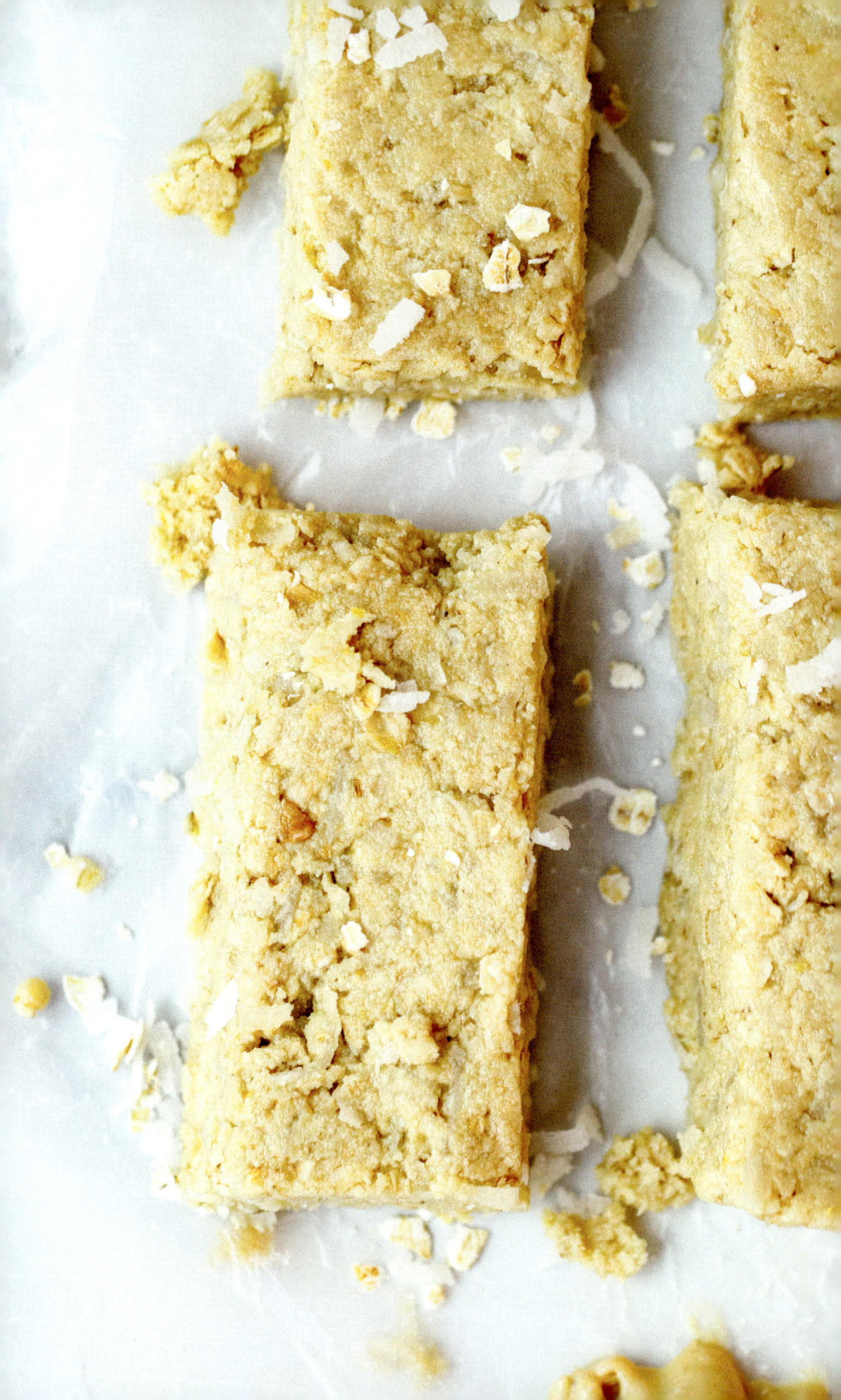

ALOHA BARS*

Makes 12 servings
230 calories / 14F / 18C / 7P / per bar

---

1 cup OffBeat Aloha Butter
1 cup old-fashioned rolled oats
1 cup unsweetened shredded coconut
2 servings CSE Simply Vanilla Protein Powder
¼ cup raw honey
2 Tbs. unsweetened vanilla almond milk

1. Add all of the ingredients to a large bowl. Mix until well combined.

2. Press mixture into an 8x8 baking pan. Refrigerate for 2 hours and then cut into bars. Enjoy!

**OffBeat Fam Recipe Submitted by Amy Newton*

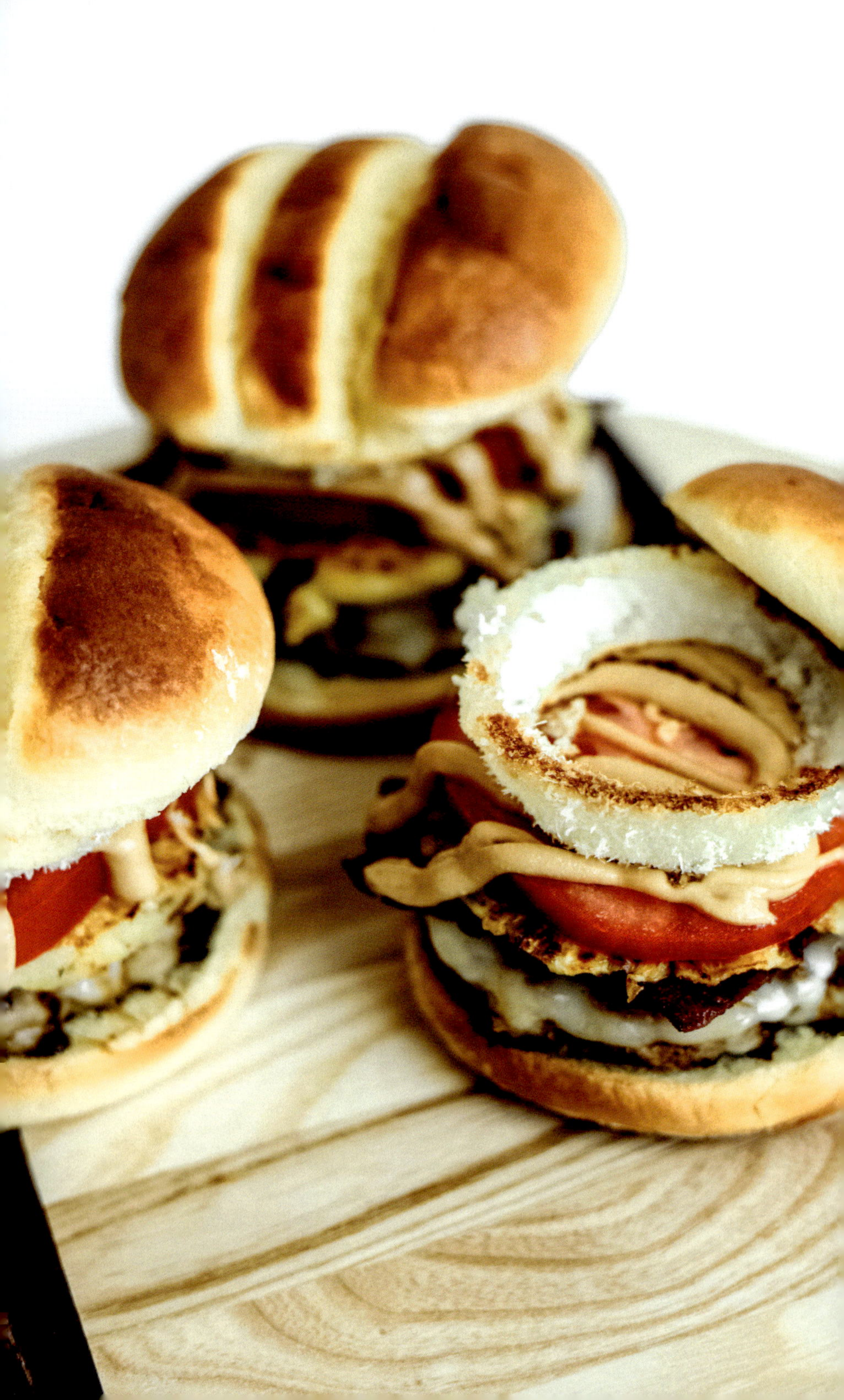

THE ALOHA BURGER
Makes 4 servings
320 calories / 14F / 24C / 25.5P / per serving (½ burger)

---

12 oz. lean ground turkey (raw)
1 Tbs. coconut sugar
2 Tbs. fresh pineapple juice
½ tsp. sea salt
2 fresh pineapple rings
2 slices Swiss cheese
2 tomato slices
2 slices turkey bacon
4 slices yellow onion
4 Tbs. OffBeat Aloha Butter
4 potato hamburger buns

1. Preheat grill or griddle to 350 degrees.

2. Combine the ground turkey, coconut sugar, sea salt, and pineapple juice in a bowl. Mix well. Weigh the mixture and form into two, equal sized burger patties.

3. Place burger patties on the grill or griddle. Cook for 5-7 minutes per side or until fully cooked through. Top each patty with Swiss cheese and allow to fully melt. Remove from heat.

4. Add the turkey bacon, pineapple and onion rings to the grill or griddle. Cook bacon until crispy, and the pineapple and onions until lightly browned.

5. Layer each burger with the bottom bun, patty with melted cheese, tomato slices, pineapple rings, bacon, onion rings, Aloha Butter and top bun. One serving is ½ burger. Enjoy!

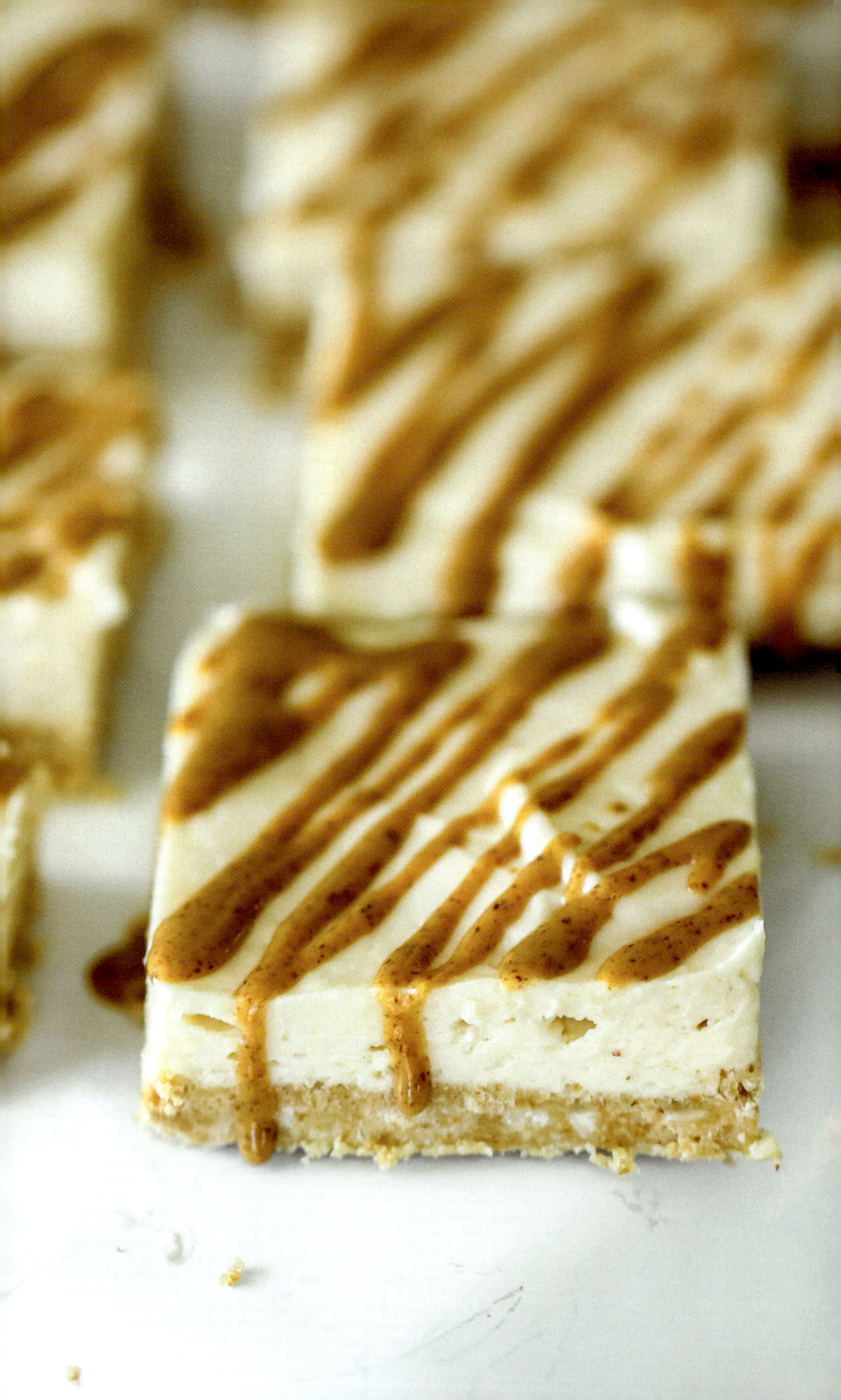

ALOHA CHEESECAKE BARS *
Makes 16 servings
200 calories / 16F / 11C / 3P / per bar

Cheesecake Filling:
8 oz. cream cheese
½ cup powdered sugar
½ cup heavy whipping cream
¼ cup OffBeat Aloha Butter
1 serving CSE Coconut Cream Protein Powder
Crust:
¾ cup graham cracker crumbs
¼ cup slivered almonds, finely ground
¼ cup coconut oil, melted
Topping Per Bar:
½ tsp. OffBeat Aloha Butter
¼ cup unsweetened, shredded coconut

1. Place the slivered almonds in blender and pulse until finely ground. Pour into a bowl.

2. Add the melted coconut oil and graham cracker crumbs to the bowl with the almonds. Mix until well combined.

3. Spray the bottom of an 8x8 inch square pan with cooking spray or line the bottom and sides with parchment paper for easy removal. Press the mixture evenly into the bottom of the pan. Place in fridge.

4. Add the cream cheese, powdered sugar, Aloha Butter, and protein powder to a separate bowl. Beat together until well combined. Set aside.

5. Beat the whipping cream in a separate bowl until stiff peak consistency. Fold the whipped cream into the cream cheese mixture until well combined.

6. Take the crust out of the fridge and pour the cheesecake filling on top. Spread out evenly.

7. Place the pan back into the fridge for about 30 minutes. When ready to serve, cut into 16 squares. Top each square with ½ teaspoon of Aloha Butter and a sprinkle of shredded coconut. Enjoy!

OffBeat Fam Recipe Submitted by Jenn Orr

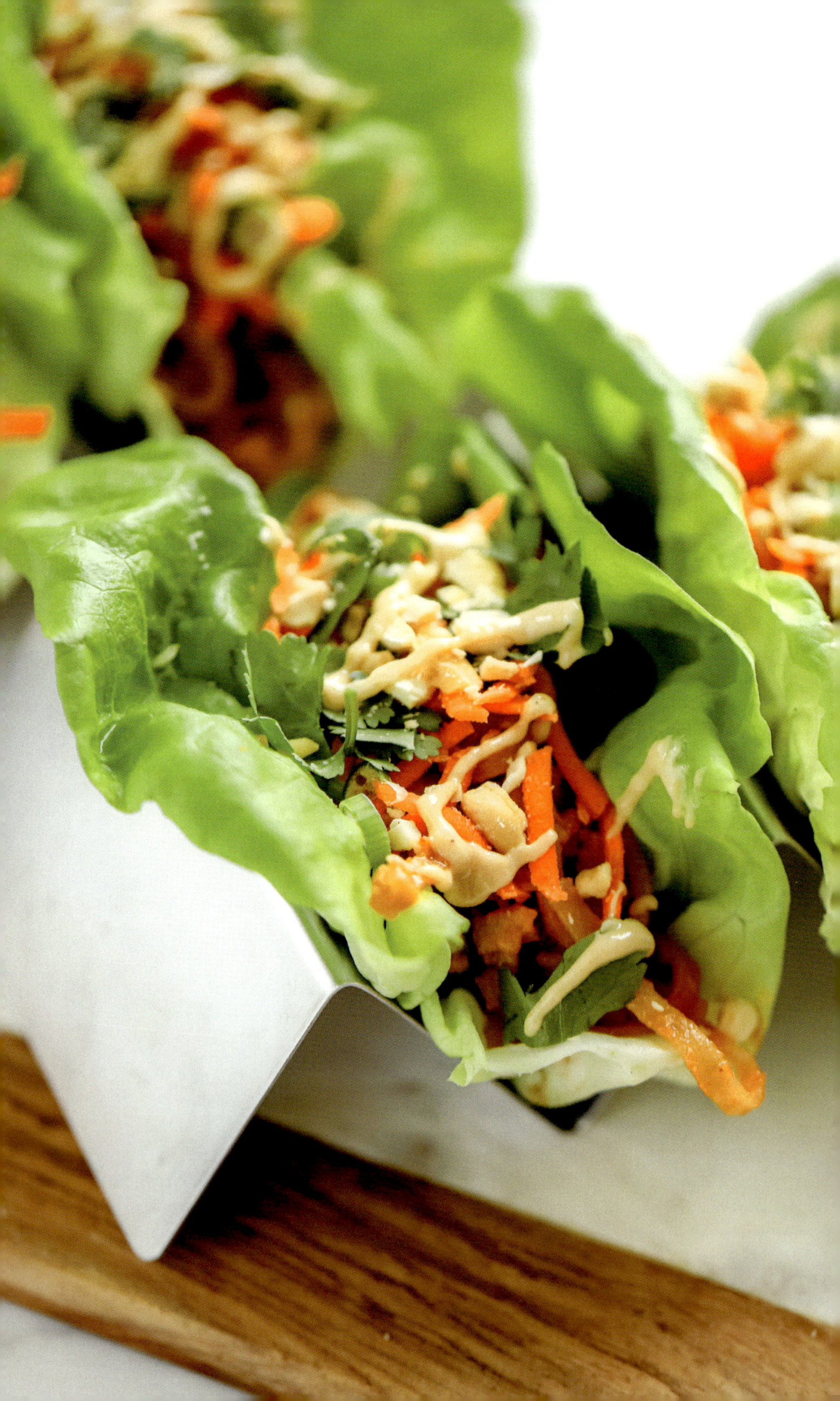

ALOHA CHICKEN LETTUCE WRAPS *
Makes 6 servings
365 calories / 17F / 30.5C / 24P / per wrap

Wraps:
4 oz. brown rice noodles
1 ½ lbs. ground chicken
Sea salt, to taste
Dash crushed red pepper
6 butter lettuce cups
Sauce:
½ cup OffBeat Aloha Butter
⅓ cup coconut aminos
⅓ cup sesame oil
¼ cup rice vinegar
2 Tbs. chili paste
1 Tbs. honey
1 tsp. minced garlic
1-inch piece of ginger, peeled

Toppings Per Serving:
½ tsp. matchstick carrots
¼ tsp. cashews
¼ tsp. green onions
¼ tsp. cilantro
Lime, juice of
OffBeat Aloha Butter (for drizzle)
Sriracha, optional

1. Soak noodles in hot water for 30 minutes.

2. Heat a skillet to medium-high heat. Spray with cooking spray and add the chicken, salt, and crushed red pepper. Cook until chicken is brown and fully cooked through. Transfer to a plate.

3. Add all sauce ingredients in a blender and blend until smooth.

4. Add the drained noodles to the skillet and add in the sauce. Cook and stir for a couple of minutes, then remove from heat and add it to the chicken. Stir to combine.

5. Assemble lettuce wraps. Fill each lettuce cup with chicken noodle mixture and add toppings. Drizzle with Aloha Butter.

OffBeat Fam Recipe Submitted by Maren Ambrose

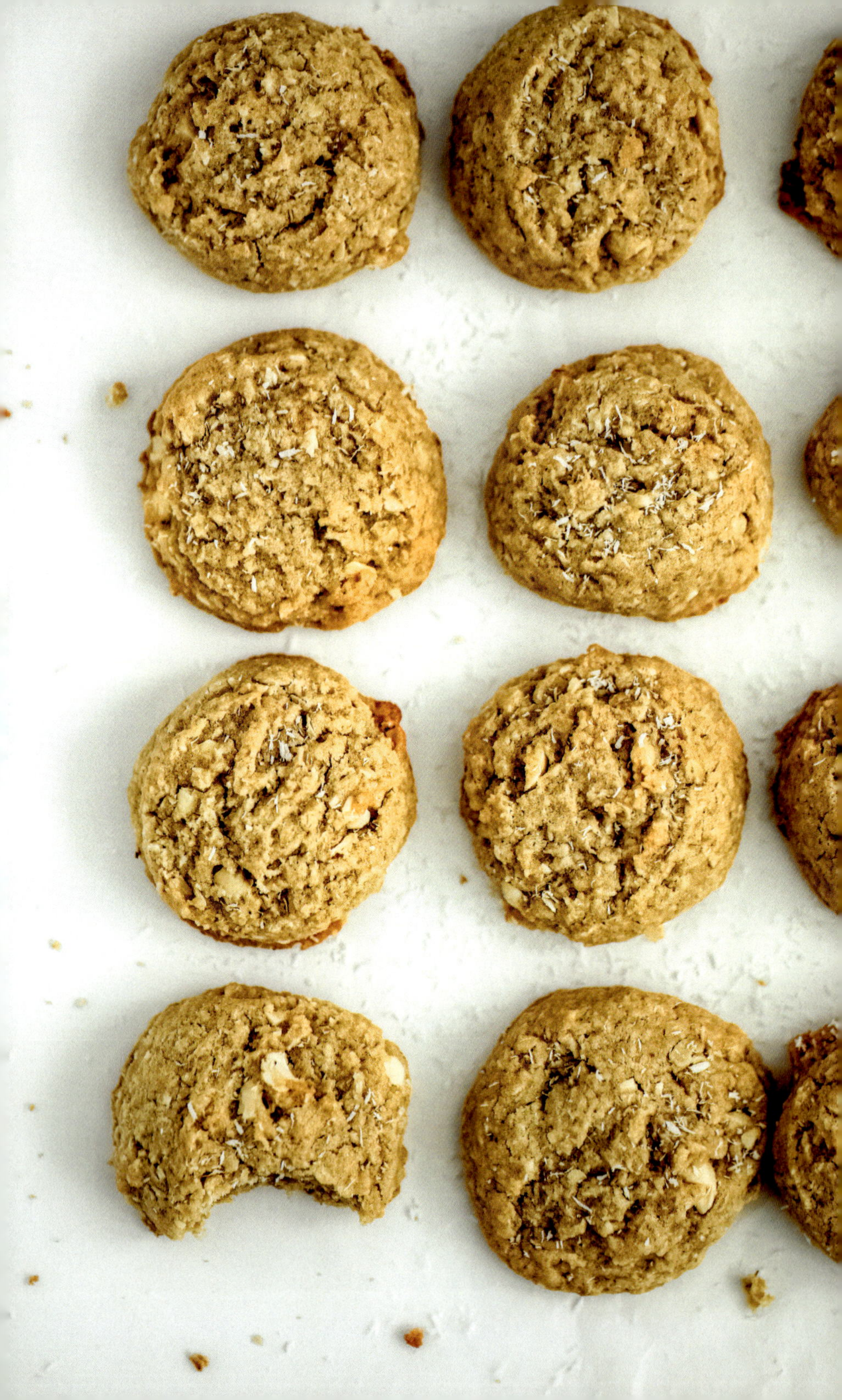

ALOHA ISLAND COOKIES *

Makes 30 cookies
215 calories / 12F / 23C / 3P / per cookie

---

2 cup all-purpose flour
1 tsp. baking powder
1 tsp. salt
½ tsp. baking soda
1 cup butter, softened
1 cup light brown sugar
1 cup granulated sugar
⅔ cup OffBeat Aloha Butter
1 tsp. pure vanilla extract
½ tsp. coconut extract
2 large eggs
2 cups quick cooking oats
1 cup cashews, roughly chopped
1 cup sweetened flaked coconut

1. Preheat the oven to 350. Line two baking sheets with parchment paper.

2. In a medium bowl, stir together the all-purpose flour, baking powder, salt and baking soda. Set aside.

3. In the bowl of a stand mixer (or a large bowl if using a hand mixer), cream together the softened butter, light brown sugar, granulated sugar, Aloha Butter, coconut extract and vanilla. Beat for 3 minutes until smooth, fluffy and light beige in color. Add the eggs, one at a time, beating well after each one. Stop to scrape the bowl every now and then so all of the ingredients fully combine.

4. Add the dry ingredients gradually while beating on low speed, mixing really well between each addition. Repeat until all of the dry ingredients have been added, stopping to scrape the sides of the bowl when needed. After all of the dry ingredients have been added, increase the speed of the mixer and beat for 1 minute.

5. Mix in the oats, cashews, and sweetened flaked coconut by hand with a large non stick spatula. The batter will be stiff.

6. Use a ¼ measuring cup to separate the dough. Place the dough rounds at least 3 inches apart on the baking sheet. Press the centers to flatten slightly for even baking.

7. Bake for 14-16 minutes until barely golden. Cool on the cookie sheet for 5 minutes, then remove to a cooling rack to cool completely. Enjoy!

OffBeat Fam Recipe Submitted by Shae Memmott

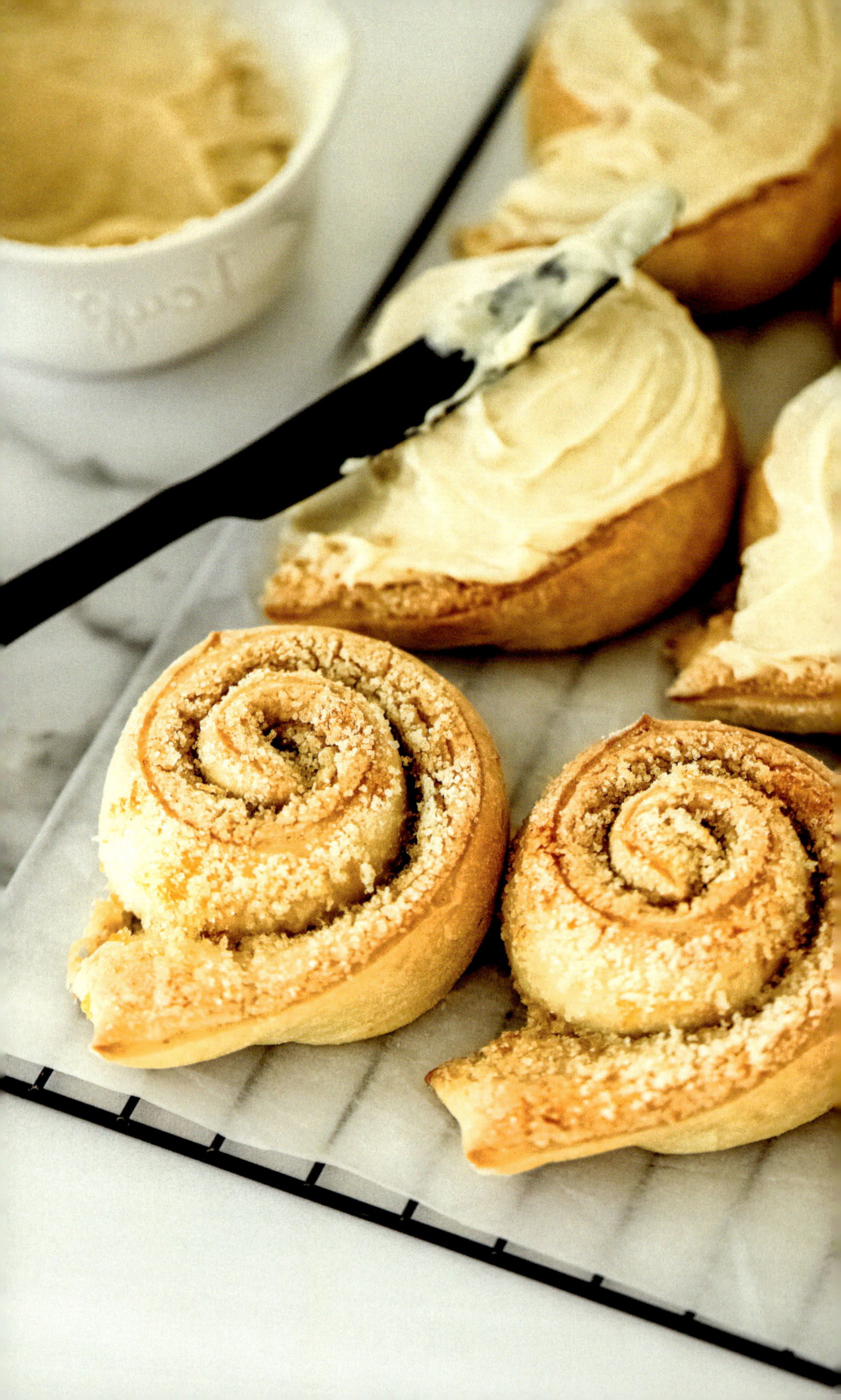

ALOHA ORANGE ROLLS *

Makes 12 servings
560 calories / 22F / 81C / 9P / per roll

Rolls:
1 cup milk
¼ cup granulated white sugar
1 Tbs. active dry yeast
1 tsp. salt
½ cup butter, softened
1 egg
2 tsp. orange zest
¼ cup fresh orange juice
4 cups all-purpose flour (plus extra
   for rolling)

Filling:
1 cup sugar
2 tsp. orange zest
½ tsp. ground ginger
½ cup OffBeat Aloha Butter
4-5 Tbs. all-purpose flour
Frosting:
4 oz. cream cheese, softened
½ cup OffBeat Aloha Butter
½ tsp. vanilla extract
2 Tbs. frozen orange juice concentrate
2 cups powdered sugar

1. In a small bowl, combine warm milk, sugar, and active dry yeast, and let sit 5 minutes or until bloomed.

2. In a mixer, combine salt, butter, egg, orange zest, orange juice, and four cups of flour. Pour yeast mixture in and mix with dough hook on low speed for 5 minutes until elastic. Dough should pull away from sides of bowl.

3. Spray a large bowl with cooking spray and place dough in the greased bowl, covered with plastic wrap. Let the dough rise at room temperature for 1 hour or until doubled in size.

4. In a medium bowl, combine sugar, orange zest and ground ginger. Set aside.

5. On a floured work surface, roll dough to a 24x12 inch shape.

6. Spread Aloha Butter over dough. Sprinkle and spread sugar mixture evenly over nut butter. Sprinkle 4-5 tablespoons of flour evenly over filling. Carefully roll dough long ways to form a long log.

7. Cut the dough into 12 rolls. Place the rolls on a 9x13 inch pan or large baking sheet with enough room for the dough to rise.

8. Put a dish towel over the rolls and allow the dough to double in size. While the rolls are rising, preheat your oven to 350 degrees. Bake for 25 minutes. Cool slightly before icing.

9. Mix together your softened cream cheese and Aloha Butter and mix until smooth. Mix in powdered sugar, vanilla, and orange juice concentrate until everything is incorporated and frosting is thick. Lather the icing on those DELICIOUS rolls and taste the island breeze.

OffBeat Fam Recipe Submitted by Libbie Watterson

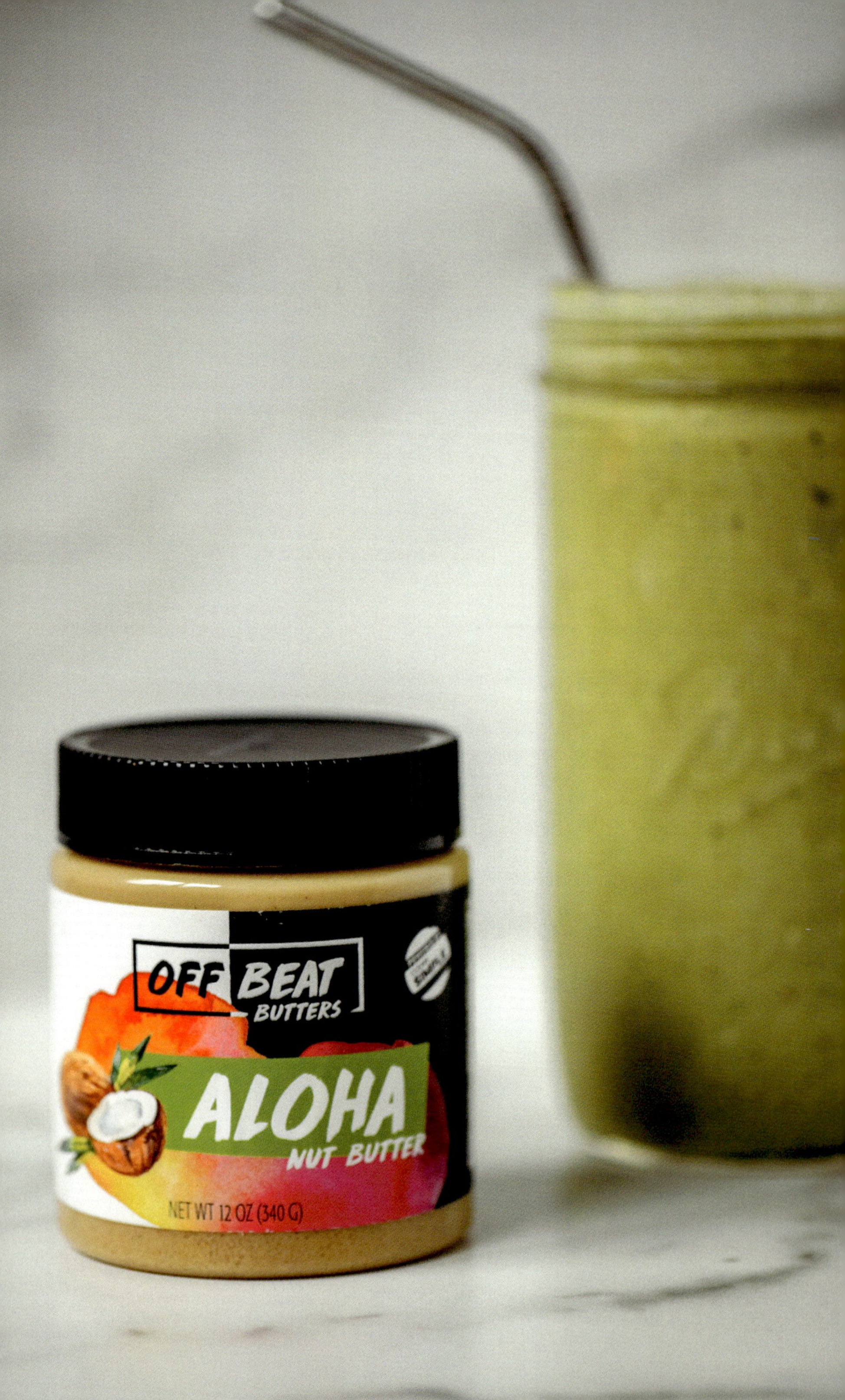

OFF BEAT
BUTTERS
ALOHA
NUT BUTTER
NET WT 12 OZ (340 G)

ALOHA SUNRISE SMOOTHIE*
Makes 1 serving
295 calories / 9F / 32C / 24P

⅔ cup unsweetened almond milk
½ orange, peeled
⅓ cup frozen pineapple
⅓ cup frozen strawberries (about 3-4)
1 cup spinach
½ serving CSE Coconut Cream or Simply Vanilla Protein Powder
1 Tbs. full fat coconut milk, canned
½ Tbs. OffBeat Aloha Butter, plus more for drizzling

1. Add all ingredients into a high-powered blender and blend on high until smooth.

2. Pour into a glass and drizzle with nut butter.

OffBeat Fam Recipe Submitted by Laura Howes

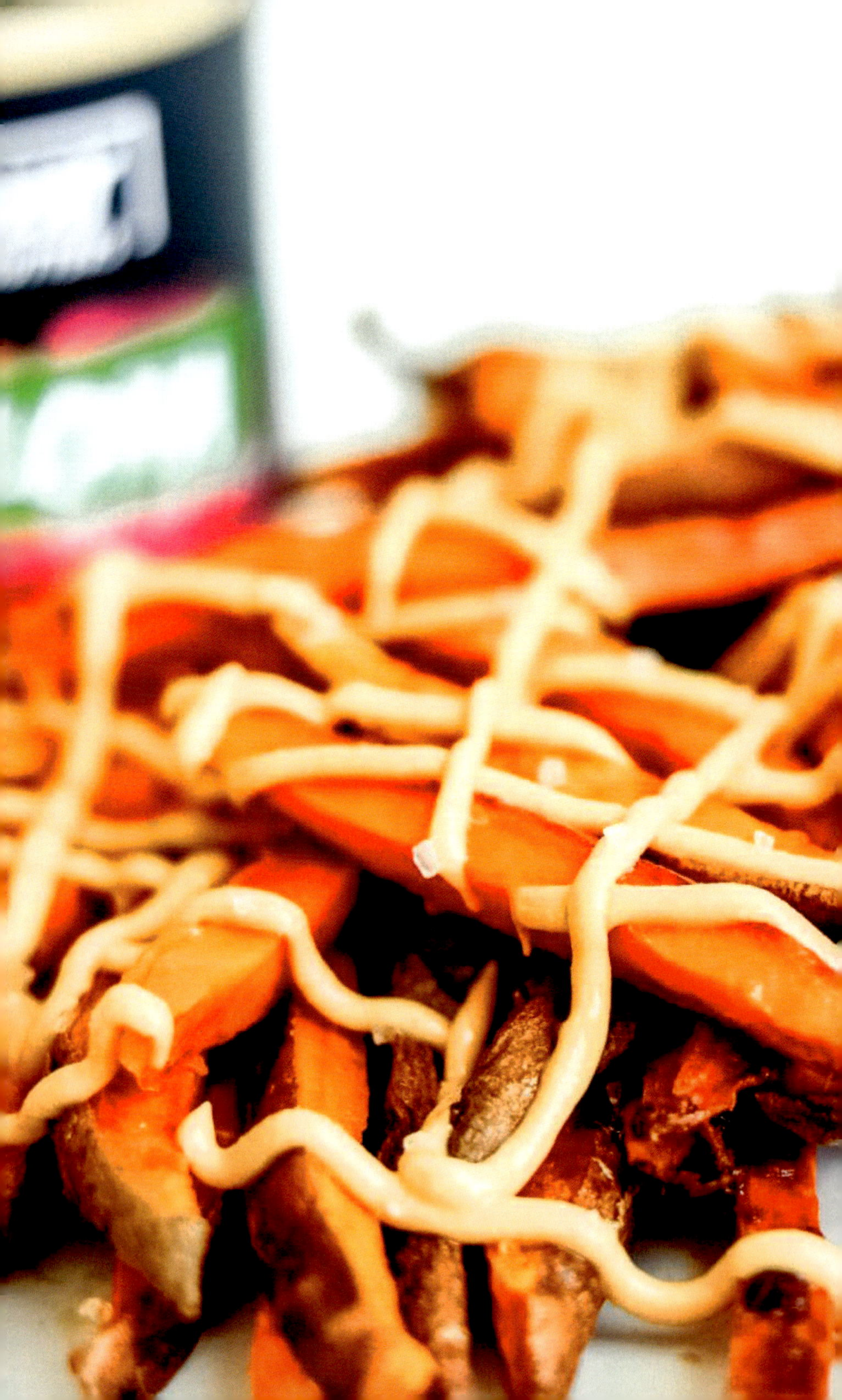

ALOHA SWEET POTATO FRIES
Makes 4 servings
125 calories / 3.5F / 23C / 2P / per serving

2 (250g) sweet potatoes
1 Tbs. coconut sugar
Dash sea salt
2 Tbs. OffBeat Aloha Butter
1 Tbs. raw honey

1. Preheat the oven to 400 degrees.

2. Slice sweet potatoes into fries.

3. Place fries on a baking sheet lined with parchment paper. Spray tops with cooking spray and sprinkle with coconut sugar and sea salt. Bake for 40 minutes, flipping halfway. Optional, place in airfyer for 2-3 minutes at 400 degrees to crisp.

4. Pile the fries up on a plate and drizzle the Aloha Butter and honey over the top. Enjoy warm!

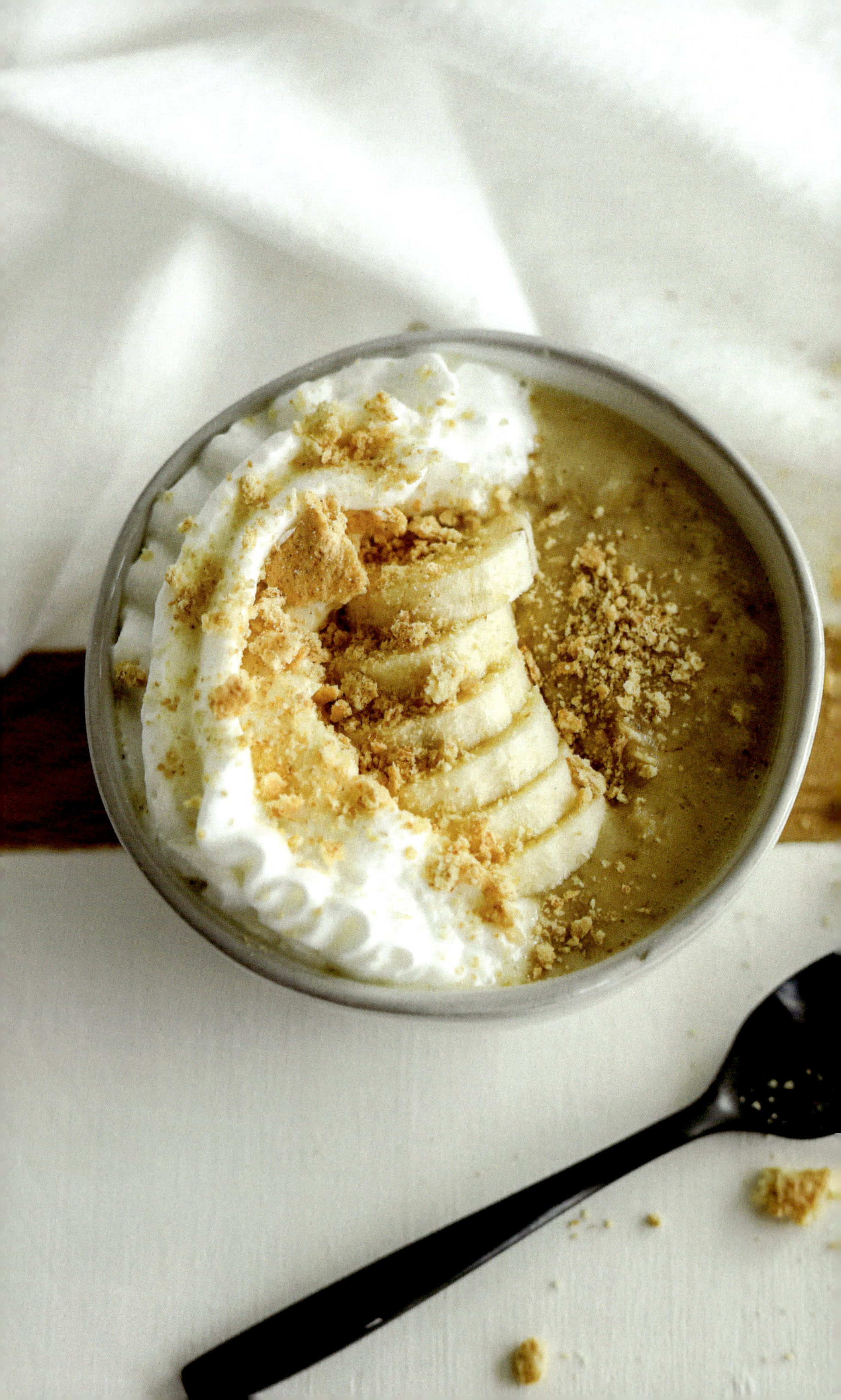

BANANA CREAM PIE OATS
Makes 1 serving
350 calories / 8F / 45C / 25P

⅓ cup old-fashioned rolled oats
½ cup water
2 tsp. OffBeat Aloha
1 serving CSE Simply Vanilla Protein
Toppings:
20g thinly sliced bananas
2 Tbs. spray whipped cream
10g graham crackers crushed
Dash sea salt

1. Add the oats and water to a microwave-safe bowl. Microwave for 1-2 minutes.

2. Stir in the Aloha Butter. Let cool for a couple minutes, then stir in the protein powder.

3. Top with a dash of sea salt, banana slices, crushed graham crackers, and spray whipped cream.

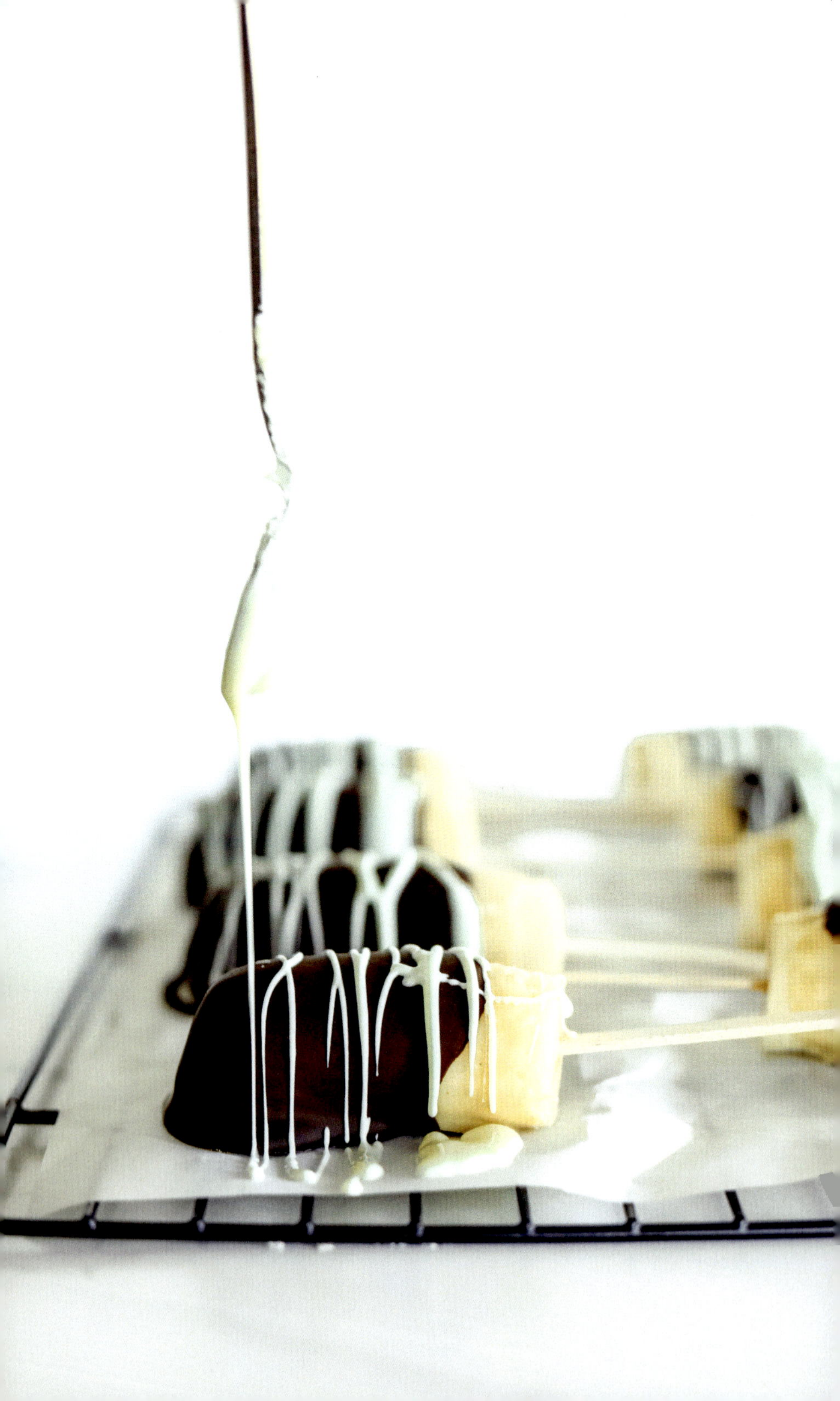

CHOCOLATE ALOHA DIPPED BANANAS

Makes 8 servings
250 calories / 14F / 30C / 3P / per serving (½ banana)

---

4 (120g each) bananas
½ cup OffBeat Aloha Butter
½ cup dark chocolate chips
¼ cup white chocolate chips

1. Slice each banana in half and stick a popsicle stick into the end of each one. Slice off the pointed edge of each half banana. Place on a baking sheet lined with parchment paper. Freeze 2+ hours.

2. Add the Aloha Butter to a cup and stir well. Dip each frozen banana into the butter about ⅞ of the way up. Let the excess drip off, then place back onto the baking sheet. Return the baking sheet to the freezer until ready to dip into the chocolate.

3. Add the dark chocolate chips to a tall cup. Microwave for 30 seconds at a time, stirring in between, until completely melted and smooth.

4. Dip each banana into the melted chocolate. Let the excess drip off, then place back onto the baking sheet.

5. Melt the white chocolate chips in a small bowl in the microwave. Drizzle over the double dipped bananas.

6. Return all the dipped bananas to the freezer. Let the chocolate harden and enjoy!

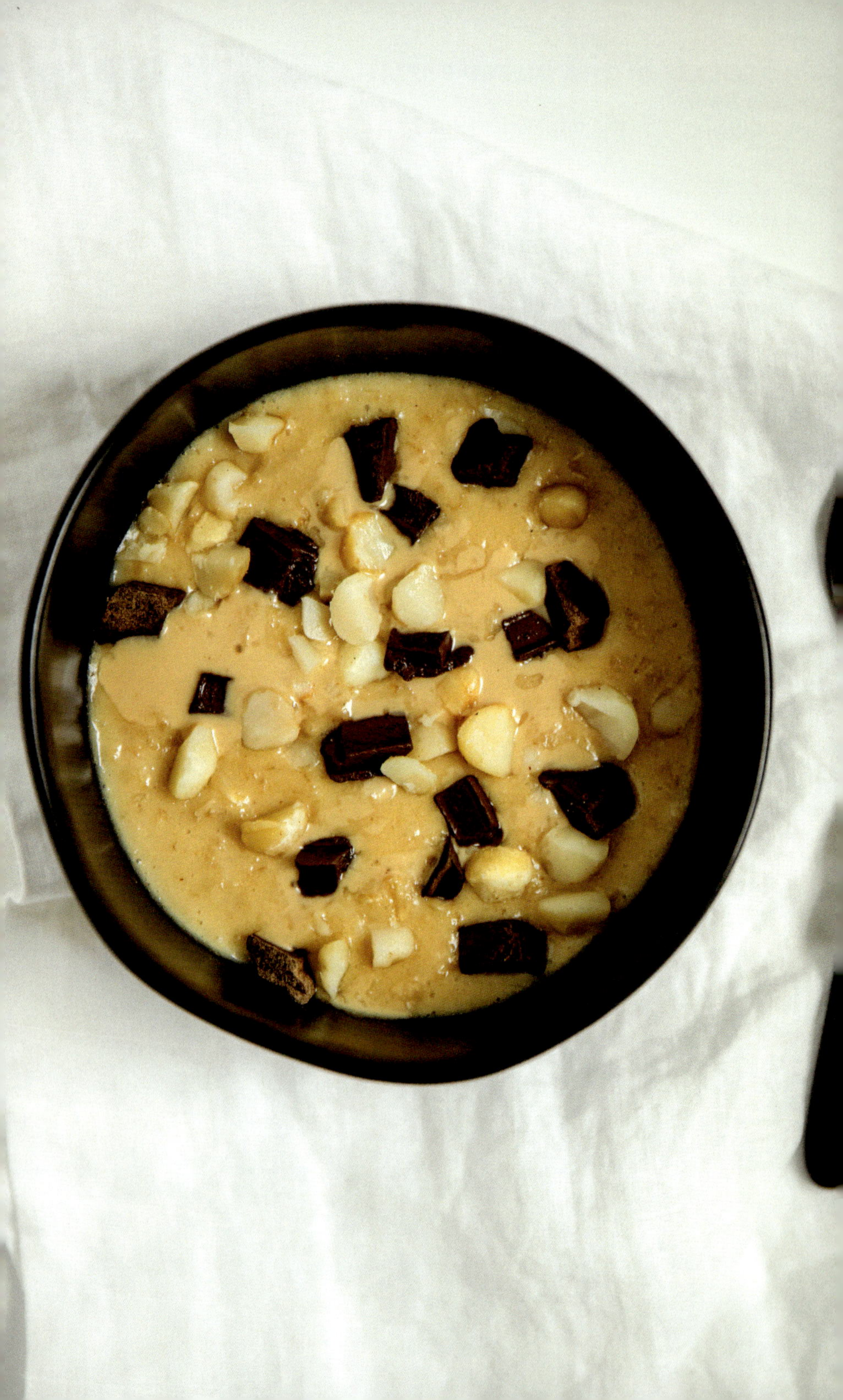

CHOCOLATE COVERED MAC NUT OATMEAL
Makes 1 serving
375 calories / 14F / 39C / 25.5P

⅓ cup old-fashioned rolled oats
⅔ cup water
½ Tbs. OffBeat Aloha Butter
1 serving CSE Simply Vanilla Protein Powder
Toppings:
8g crushed macadamia nuts
8g chocolate chips

1. Add the oats, water, and egg whites to a microwave-safe bowl. Whisk until the egg whites are well combined. Microwave for 1-2 minutes.

2. Stir in the Aloha Butter. Let cool for a couple minutes, then stir in the protein powder.

3. Top with macadamia nuts and chocolate chips.

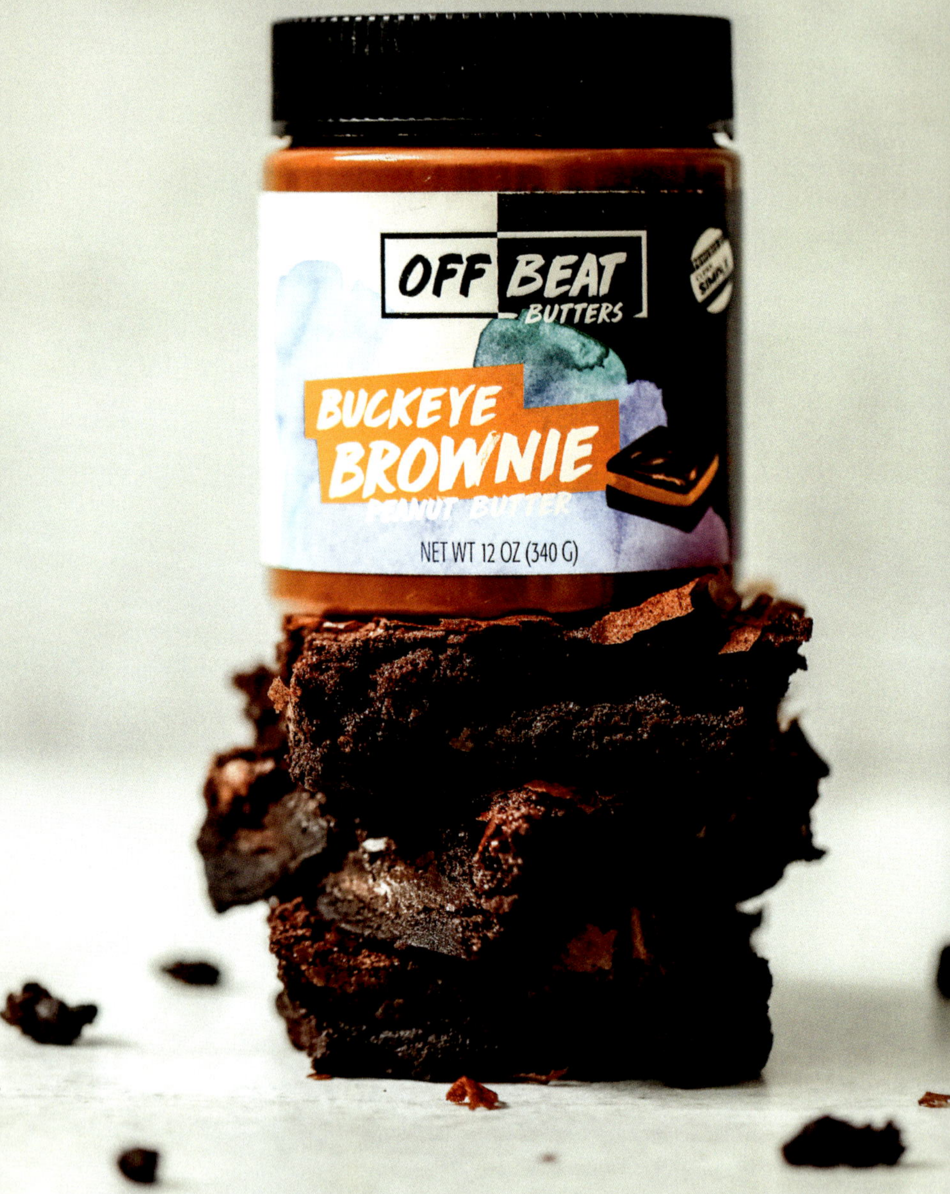

OFF BEAT
BUTTERS
BUCKEYE
BROWNIE
PEANUT BUTTER
NET WT 12 OZ (340 G)

CHOCOLATE AND PEANUT BUTTER... NAME A BETTER DUO

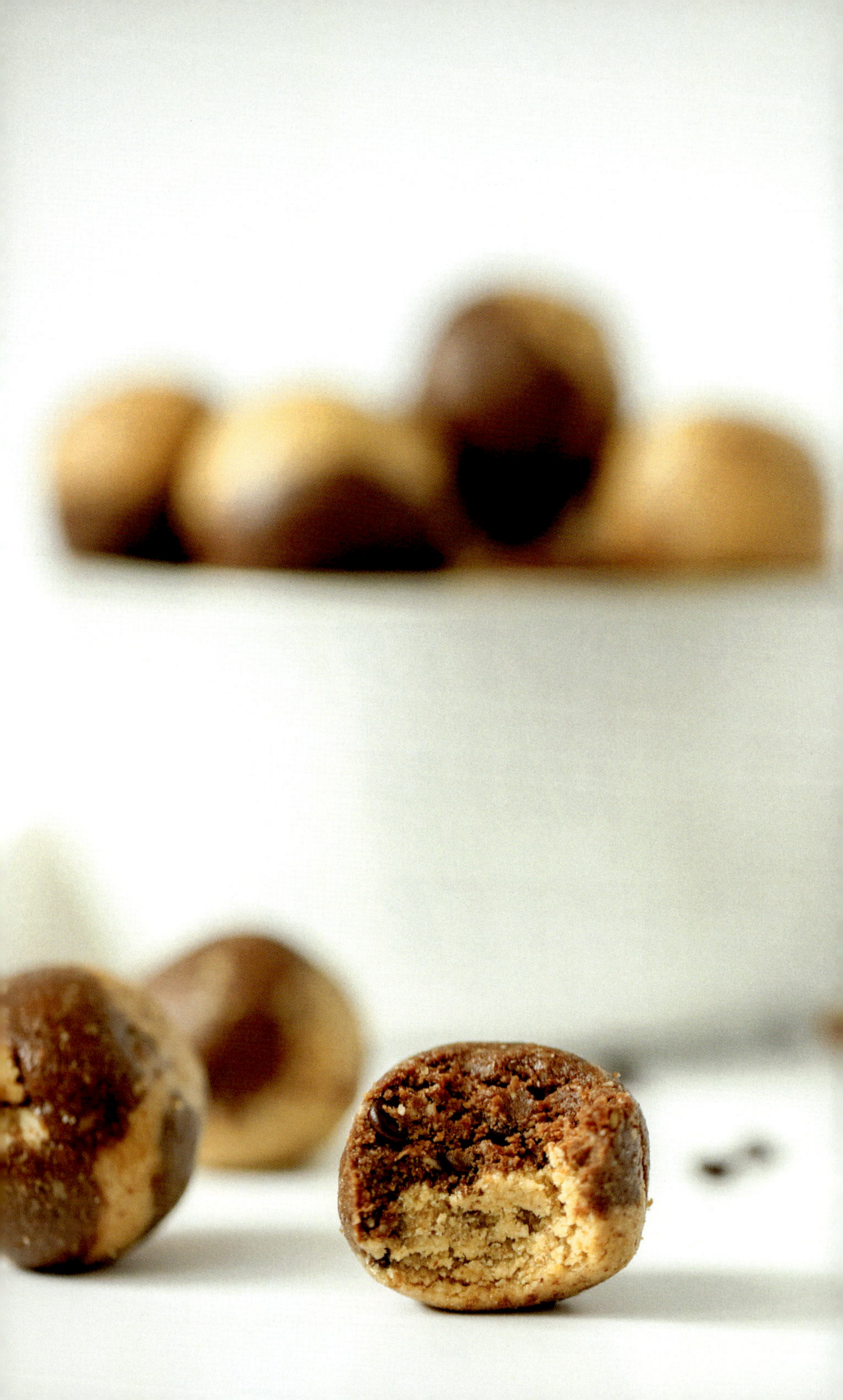

BROOKIE PROTEIN BALLS*
Makes 24 servings
95 calories / 3F / 15C / 2P / per bite

Chocolate Brownie Dough:
1 cup old-fashioned rolled oats
½ cup OffBeat Buckeye Brownie Peanut Butter
⅓ cup honey
1 serving CSE Brownie Batter Protein Powder
1 tsp. vanilla extract
1 Tbs. unsweetened almond milk
1 Tbs. cocoa powder
2 Tbs. mini chocolate chips
Cookie Dough:
1 cup old-fashioned rolled oats
½ cup OffBeat Salted Caramel Butter
⅓ cup honey
1 serving CSE Simply Vanilla Protein Powder
1 tsp. vanilla extract
¼ tsp. salt
2 Tbs. mini chocolate chips

*Easily prepared in a Kitchen Aid Mixer.

1. Place 2 cups of oats in a blender or food processor and pulse until broken down into a flour. Set aside.

2. Make the two different dough recipes in separate bowls by adding all of the ingredients and mixing until well combined.

3. Using your hands, roll together about 2 teaspoons of the Chocolate Brownie Dough with 2 teaspoons of Cookie Dough. Store in the fridge or freezer. Enjoy!

OffBeat Fam Recipe Submitted by Rachel Morgan

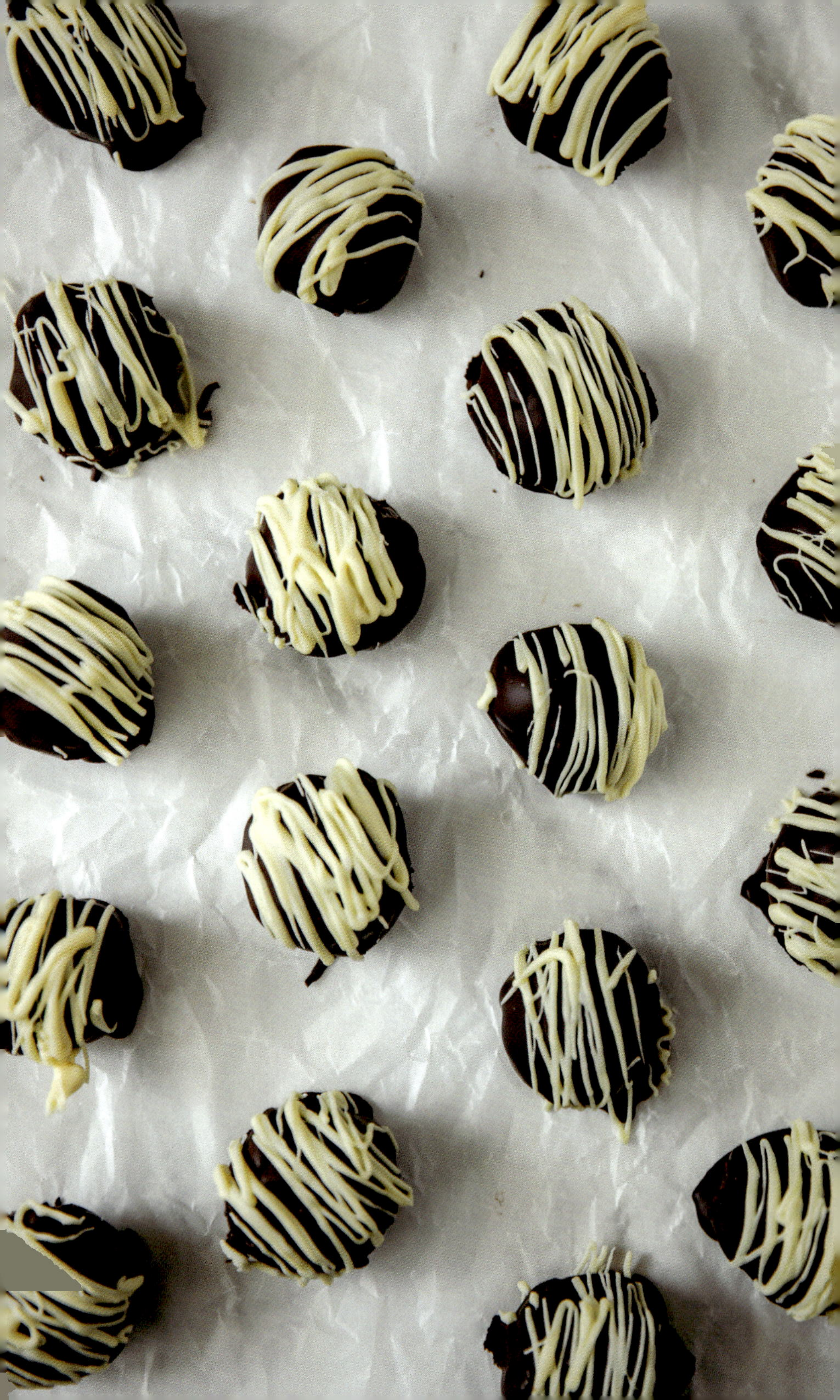

THE BRUCIE BITES *

Makes 28 servings
110 calories / 7F / 16C / 2P / per bite

---

1 cup oat flour
1 cup Swerve granulated sugar
¾ cup cocoa powder
½ tsp. salt
1 ½ tsp. baking powder
¼ cup avocado oil
1 cup unsweetened almond milk
2 tsp. Stevia Vanilla Crème drops
2 large eggs, beaten
⅓ cup OffBeat Buckeye Brownie Peanut Butter
½ cup hot water

Chocolate Coating:
1 ½ Tbs. coconut oil, melted
1 cup dark chocolate chips, melted
¼ cup white chocolate, melted

1. Preheat the oven to 350 degrees. Line a baking sheet with parchment paper.

2. Mix all dry ingredients until well combined. In a separate bowl, beat together the wet ingredients until thoroughly combined, adding the hot water last.

3. Add the wet ingredients to the dry ingredients; mix until well combined. Pour the entire mixture onto the prepared baking sheet, spreading evenly.

4. Bake for 18-20 minutes. Remove from the oven, then lift from the baking sheet using the parchment paper. Allow to cool on the counter until easy to handle.

5. Line the baking sheet with a new sheet of parchment paper.

6. Using your hands, remove enough of the baked mixture to make a firm 1-inch ball, and place on the baking sheet (should feel a little doughy).

7. Place a toothpick through the center of each ball, then freeze for 30 minutes to 1 hour.

8. Melt the dark chocolate with the coconut oil, microwaving in 30 second intervals, until smooth.

9. Remove bites from the freezer, individually submerging into the melted dark chocolate to fully coat. Use a spoon to assist. Place back onto the parchment paper, allowing the chocolate to harden.

10. In a separate bowl, microwave the white chocolate and stir until smooth.

11. Once the dark chocolate has hardened, remove the toothpicks and drizzle the melted white chocolate over the tops. Store in the fridge or freezer. Enjoy!

OffBeat Fam Recipe Submitted by Jamie Eddy

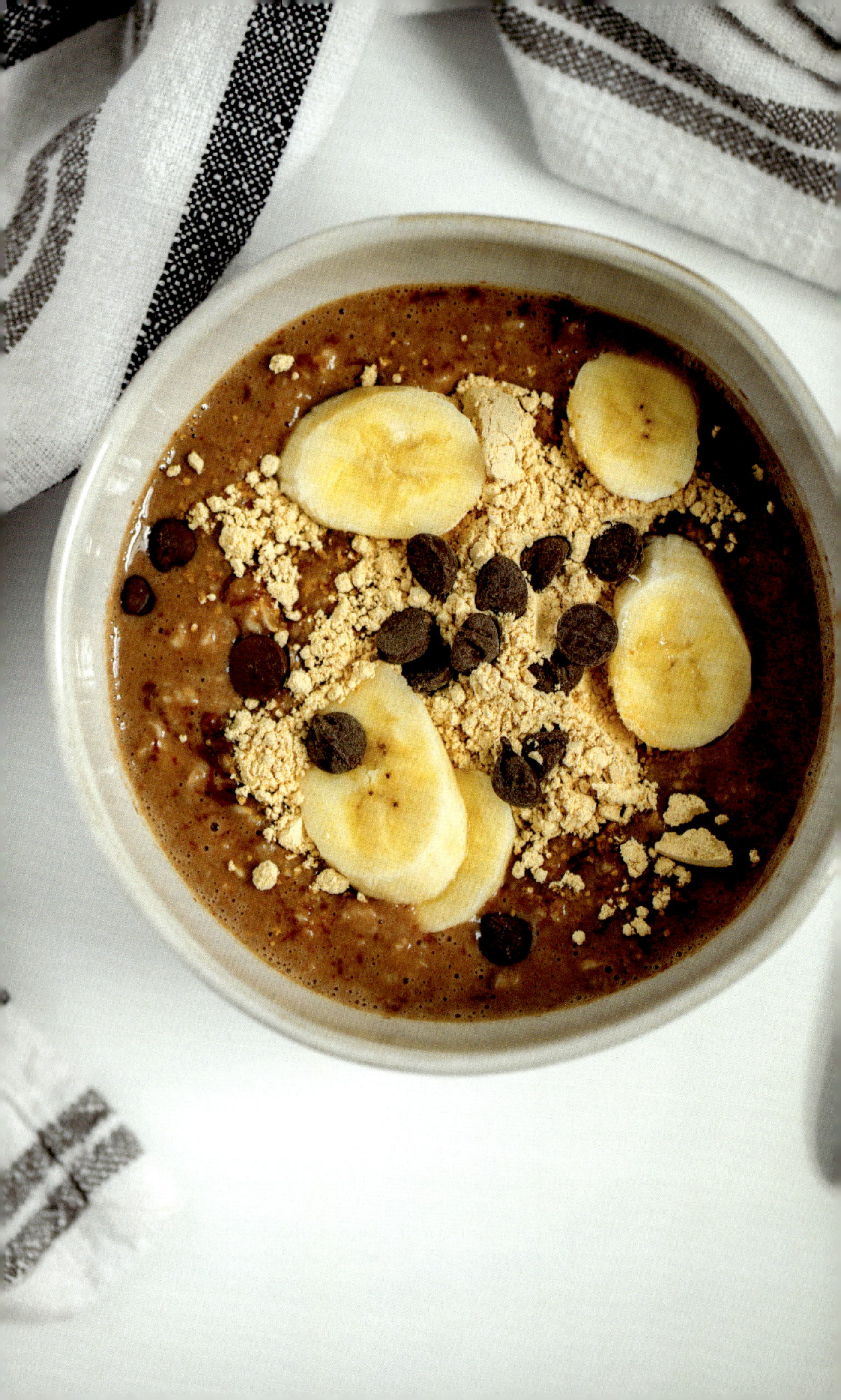

BUCKEYE BROWNIE BOWL
Makes 1 serving
367 calories / 11.5F / 38.7C / 29.8P

⅓ cup old-fashioned rolled oats
½ cup water
3 Tbs. egg whites
14g OffBeat Buckeye Brownie Peanut Butter
¾ serving CSE Brownie Batter Protein Powder
Toppings:
1 Tbs. powdered peanut butter
1 banana
5g extra dark chocolate chips

1. Add the oats, water, egg whites, and chopped apples to a microwave-safe bowl. Whisk until the egg whites are well combined. Microwave for 1-2 minutes.

2. Stir in the Buckeye Brownie Peanut Butter. Let cool for a couple minutes, then stir in the protein powder.

3. Top with powdered peanut butter, banana slices, and chocolate chips.

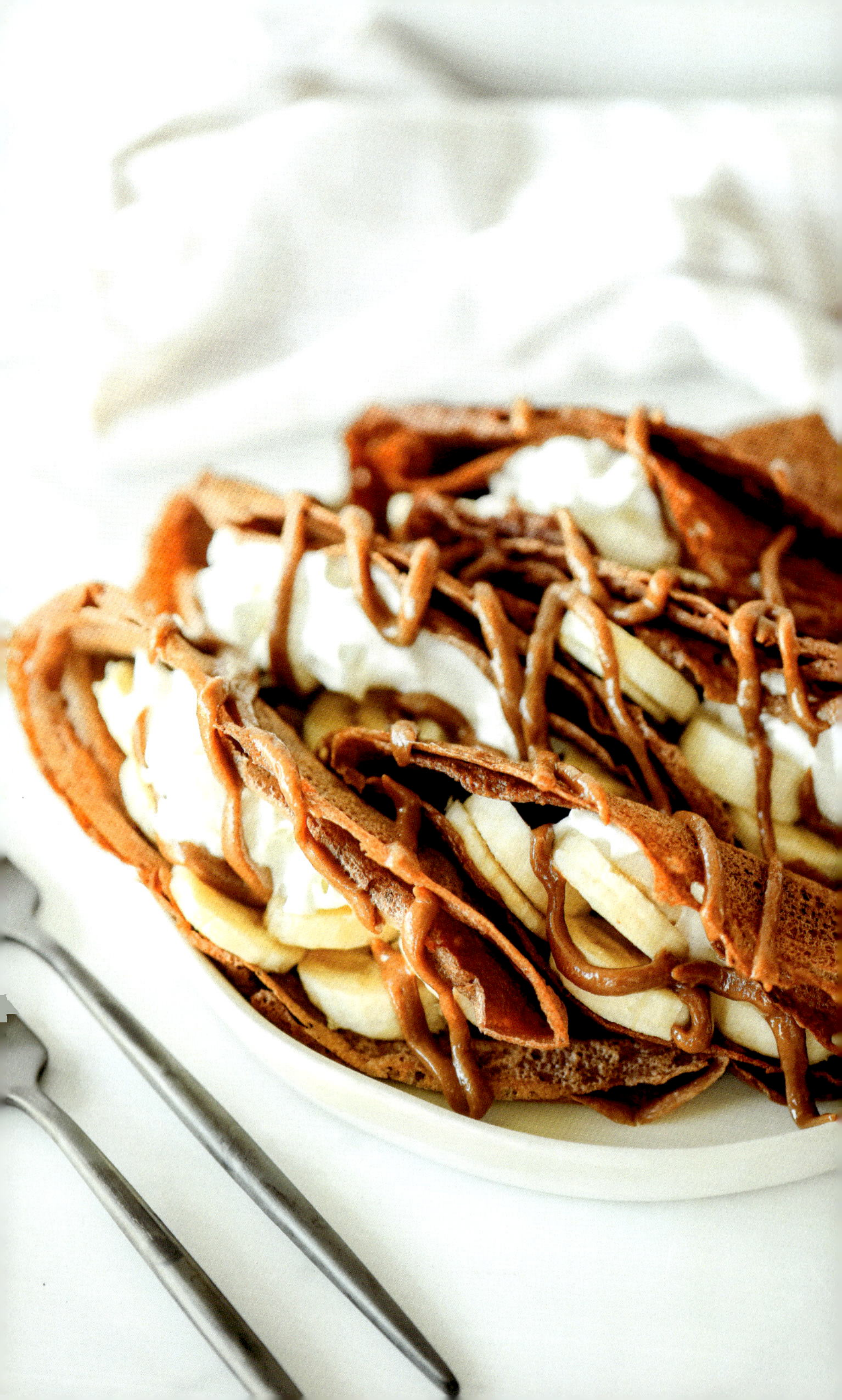

BUCKEYE BROWNIE CHOCOLATE CREPES*

Makes 4 servings
280 calories / 8.5F / 34.5C / 17P / per serving (2 crepes)

Crepes:
½ cup Kodiak Cakes Dark Chocolate Power Cakes mix
1 serving CSE Brownie Batter Protein Powder
¾ cup fat-free milk
½ cup liquid egg whites
1 Tbs. non-fat plain Greek yogurt
1 tsp. vanilla
Dash sea salt
Filling:
480g sliced bananas
Toppings:
2 Tbs. OffBeat Buckeye Brownie Peanut Butter
2 Tbs. OffBeat Sweet Classic Peanut Butter
1 Tbs. raw honey
Spray whipped cream (optional)

1. Add all crepe ingredients to a blender. Blend on low for about 30 seconds, scraping down sides as necessary. Heat a medium-sized frying pan over medium heat.

2. Spray pan with cooking spray and pour about ¼ cup batter into the pan. Swirl around to make a thin circle. Cook about 1-2 minutes until it looks set and most bubbles have popped, then flip and cook for an additional minute. Transfer to a plate and repeat with remaining batter, spraying pan as necessary. Should make about 8 crepes.

3. In a small bowl, mix together honey, and OffBeat Butters. If desired, heat in the microwave for 10 second increments, stirring in between, until thin enough to drizzle.

4. Fill each crepe with 60g sliced bananas, roll up and drizzle or spread topping. Add spray whipped cream, if desired.

OffBeat Fam Recipe Submitted by Markie Farmer

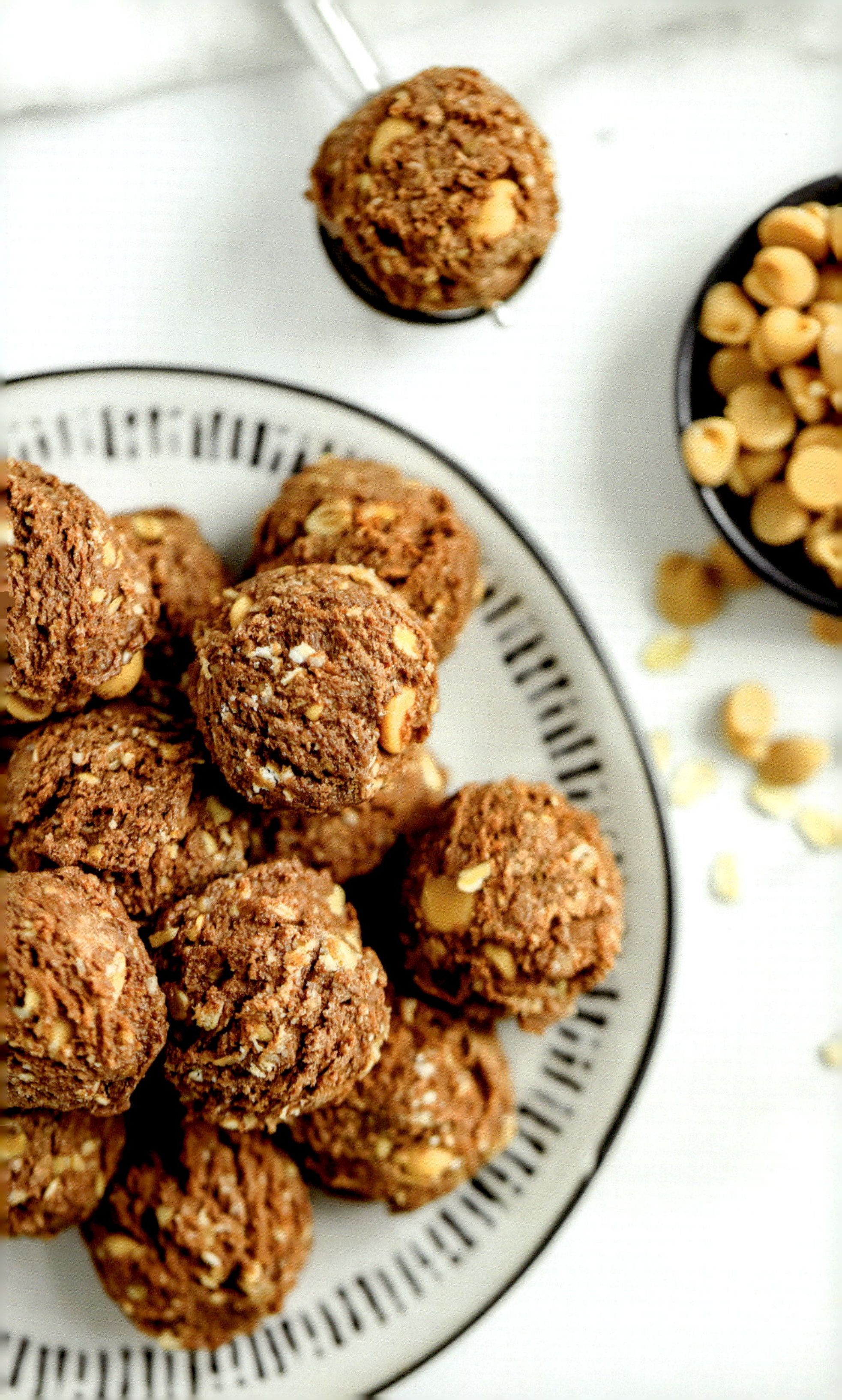

BUCKEYE BROWNIE POWER BITES
Makes 28 servings
110 calories / 5.5F / 12C / 4P / per bite

1 cup OffBeat Buckeye Brownie Peanut Butter
½ cup raw honey
2 servings CSE Brownie Batter Protein Powder
1 cup old-fashioned rolled oats
¼ cup peanut butter chips

*Easily prepared in Kitchen Aid Mixer.

1. Add all of the ingredients to a bowl and mix until well combined.

2. Using a small cookie scoop, scoop into balls. Place in a container and store in the fridge or freezer.

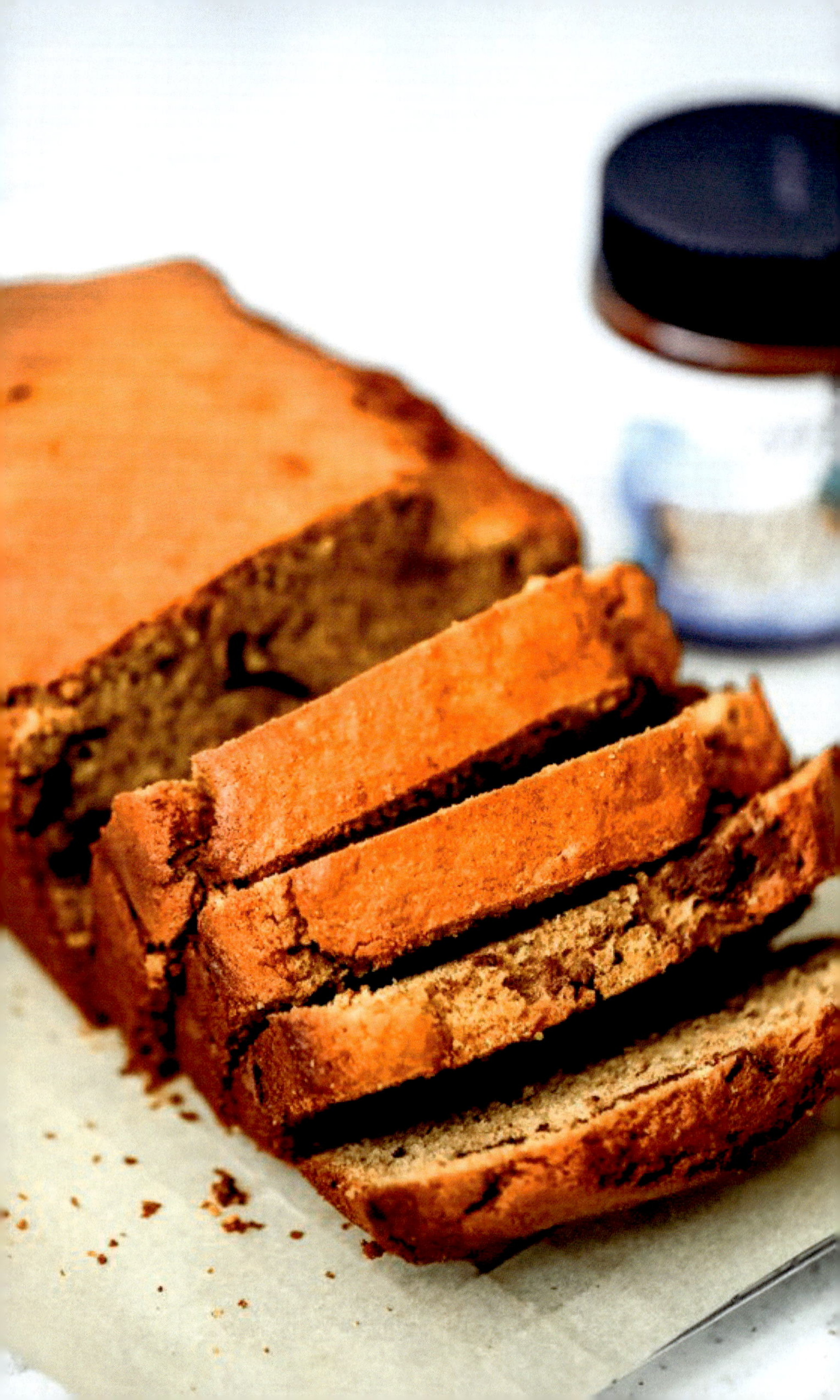

BUCKEYE BROWNIE SWIRLED BANANA BREAD*

Makes 1 loaf / 12 slices
290 calories / 16F / 27C / 5P / per slice

½ cup butter
¾ cup brown sugar, packed
2 eggs, large
1 tsp. vanilla extract
3 large bananas, ripe, mashed
1 cup all-purpose flour
1 cup whole wheat flour
1 tsp. baking soda
1 tsp. baking powder
½ tsp. salt
½ cup milk
½ cup OffBeat Buckeye Brownie Peanut Butter

1. Preheat the oven to 350 degrees. Grease a 9x5 loaf pan.

2. In a large mixing bowl, cream together the butter and sugar until light and fluffy. Beat in the eggs one at a time, mixing well between additions. Beat in the vanilla extract and mashed bananas until fully incorporated. Mix in the flours, baking soda, baking powder, and salt. Stir in the milk. Set aside.

3. Microwave the nut butter until drizzle-consistency.

4. In a greased loaf pan, transfer ⅓ of the bread batter. Drizzle ⅓ of the Buckeye Brownie Peanut Butter over the top and using a butter knife, lightly swirl into the batter. Complete this step two more times, creating three layers.

5. Bake for 55-65 minutes, or until a toothpick inserted into the center comes out clean. Cool loaf in pan for 10 minutes before removing and transferring to a cooling rack to cool completely.

OffBeat Fam Recipe Submitted by Jasmine Burton

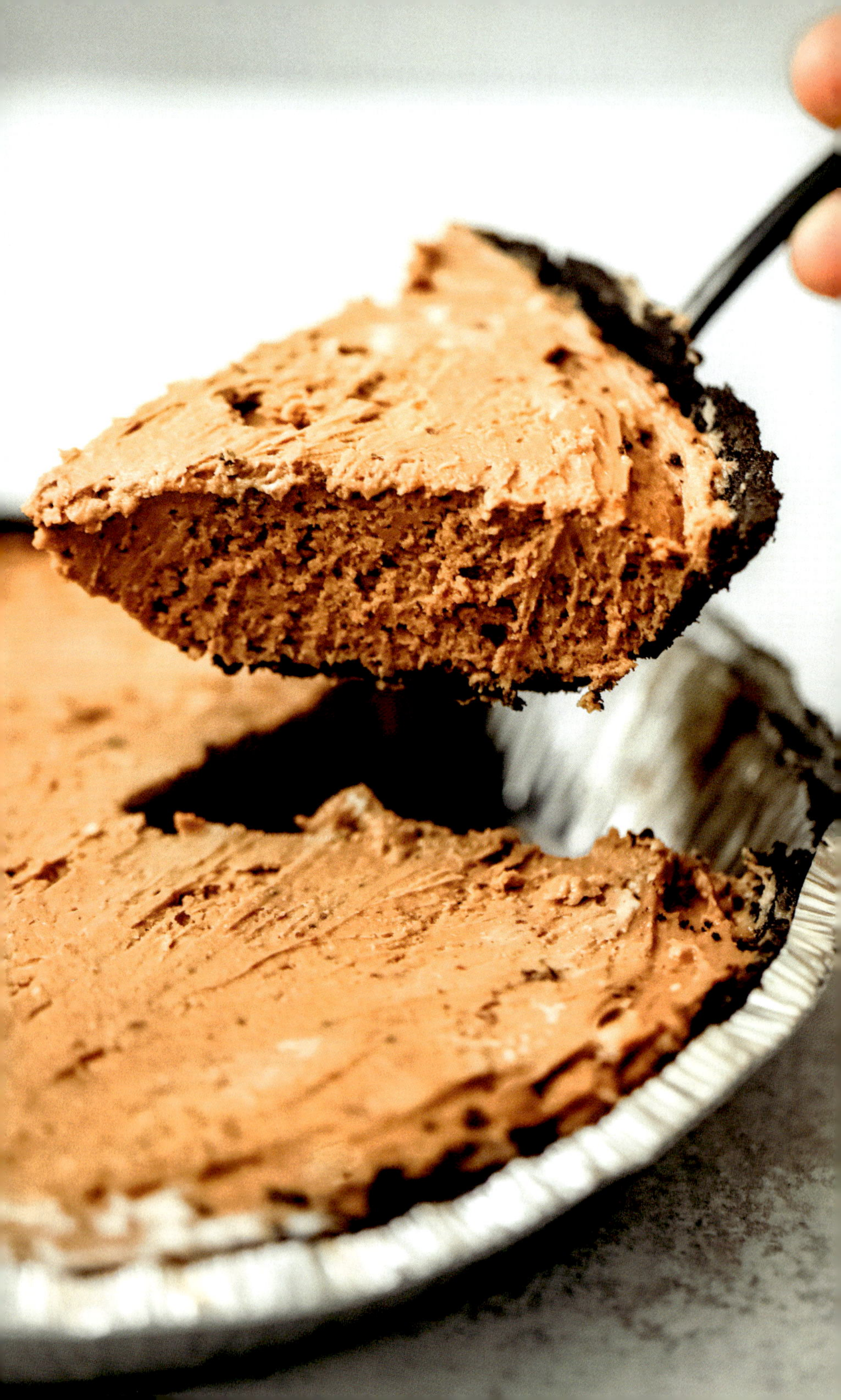

BUCKEYE PIE*
Makes 12 servings
380 calories / 27.5F / 31C / 6P / per serving

Filling:
1 cup heavy whipping cream
1 ⅓ cup powdered sugar
1 tsp. vanilla extract
1 cup OffBeat Buckeye Brownie Peanut Butter
1 8-ounce package of cream cheese, softened
Crust:
1 pre-made Oreo pie crust

1. With an electric mixer, beat whipping cream, ¼ cup powdered sugar and vanilla on medium-high until peaks form. Set aside.

2. In a separate bowl, beat the Buckeye Brownie Peanut Butter with the softened cream cheese until smooth. Add the remaining powdered sugar and beat until smooth.

3. Fold in the whipped cream with the peanut butter mixture.

4. Pour the mixture into the pre-made crust. Chill in the fridge for 1 hour before serving.

OffBeat Fam Recipe Submitted by Kat Robinson

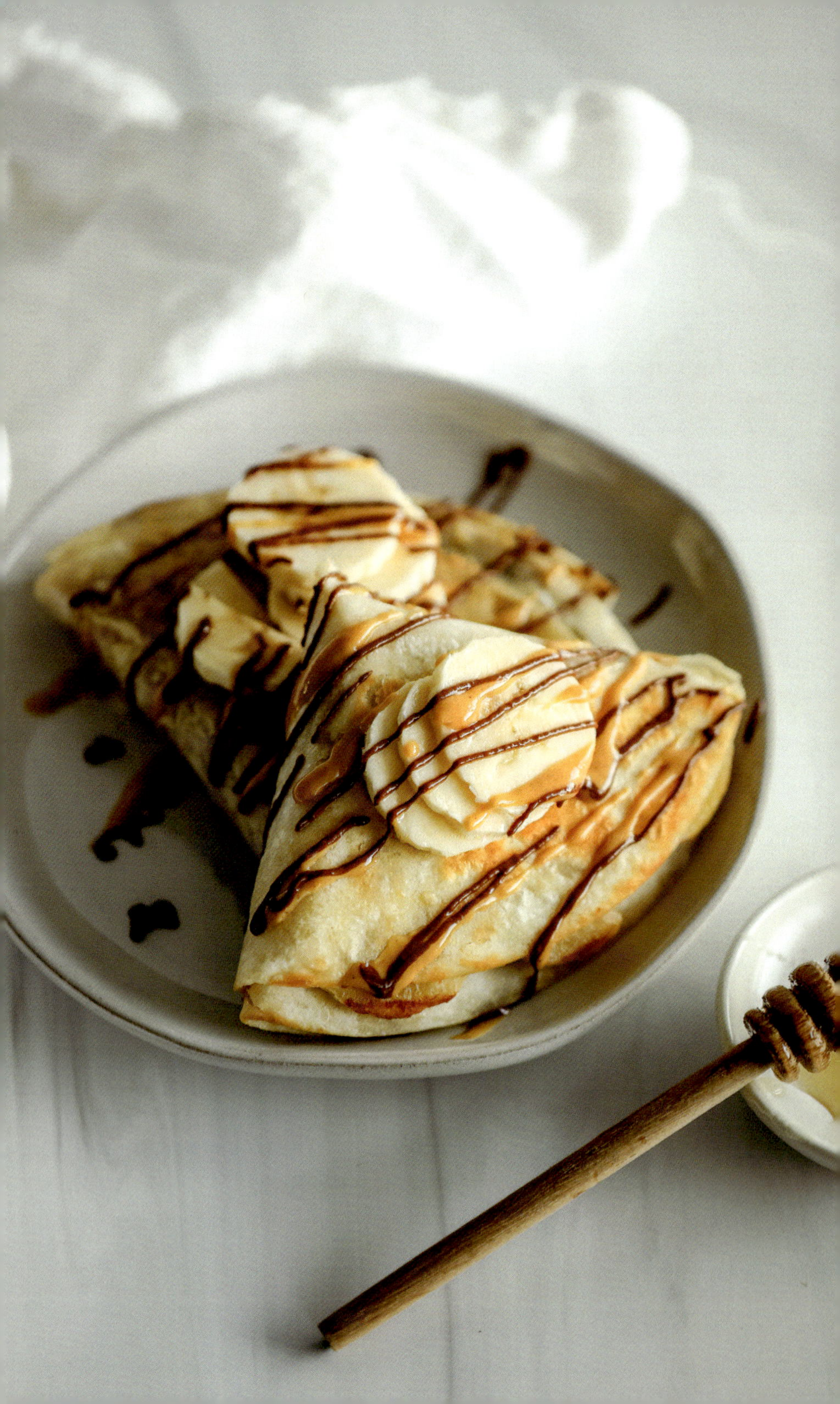

CHOCOLATE PEANUT BUTTER BANANA QUESADILLA

Makes 1 serving

260 calories / 41C / 9F / 7P

---

1 La Tortilla Factory, 100 calorie tortilla
½ Tbs. OffBeat Buckeye Brownie Peanut Butter
½ Tbs. OffBeat Sweet Classic Peanut Butter
60g banana slices
1 tsp. raw honey

1. Lay the tortilla flat on a cutting board. Place a knife in the center and make one slice in the tortilla down to the bottom edge.

2. Spread the Buckeye Brownie Peanut Butter in the bottom left corner of the tortilla, taking up ¼ of the entire tortilla. Place ½ of the the sliced bananas in the top left corner of the tortilla, and the other half in the top right. Spread the Sweet Classic Peanut Butter in the bottom right corner.

3. Fold the bottom left corner up over the the top left. Fold over toward the right and then down over the Sweet Classic Peanut Butter.

4. Place the stuffed tortilla in a greased frying pan over medium heat. Once browned on one side, flip and brown on the other side.

5. Drizzle the honey over the top. Enjoy!

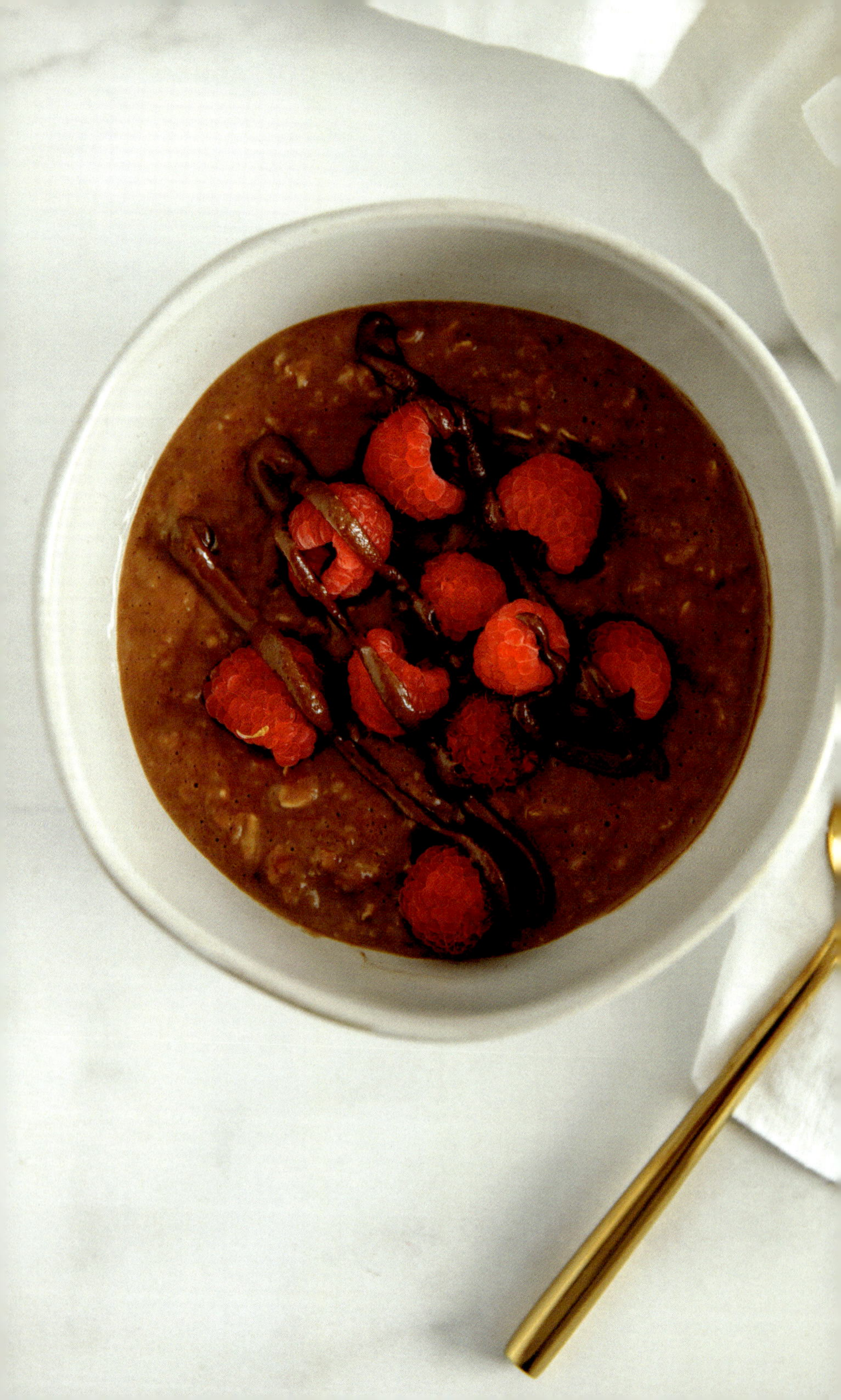

DARK CHOCOLATE RASPBERRY OATS

Makes 1 serving
330 calories 9F / 34C / 28P

⅓ cup old-fashioned rolled oats
½ cup cold water
46g liquid egg whites
10g OffBeat Buckeye Brownie Peanut Butter
¾ serving CSE Brownie Batter Protein
Toppings:
50g fresh raspberries
4g OffBeat Buckeye Brownie Peanut Butter

1. Add the oats, water, and egg whites to a microwave-safe bowl. Whisk until the egg whites are well combined. Microwave for 1-2 minutes.

2. Stir in the Buckeye Brownie Peanut Butter (10g. Let cool for a couple minutes, then stir in the protein powder.

3. Top with fresh raspberries and drizzle the remaining nut butter over the top.

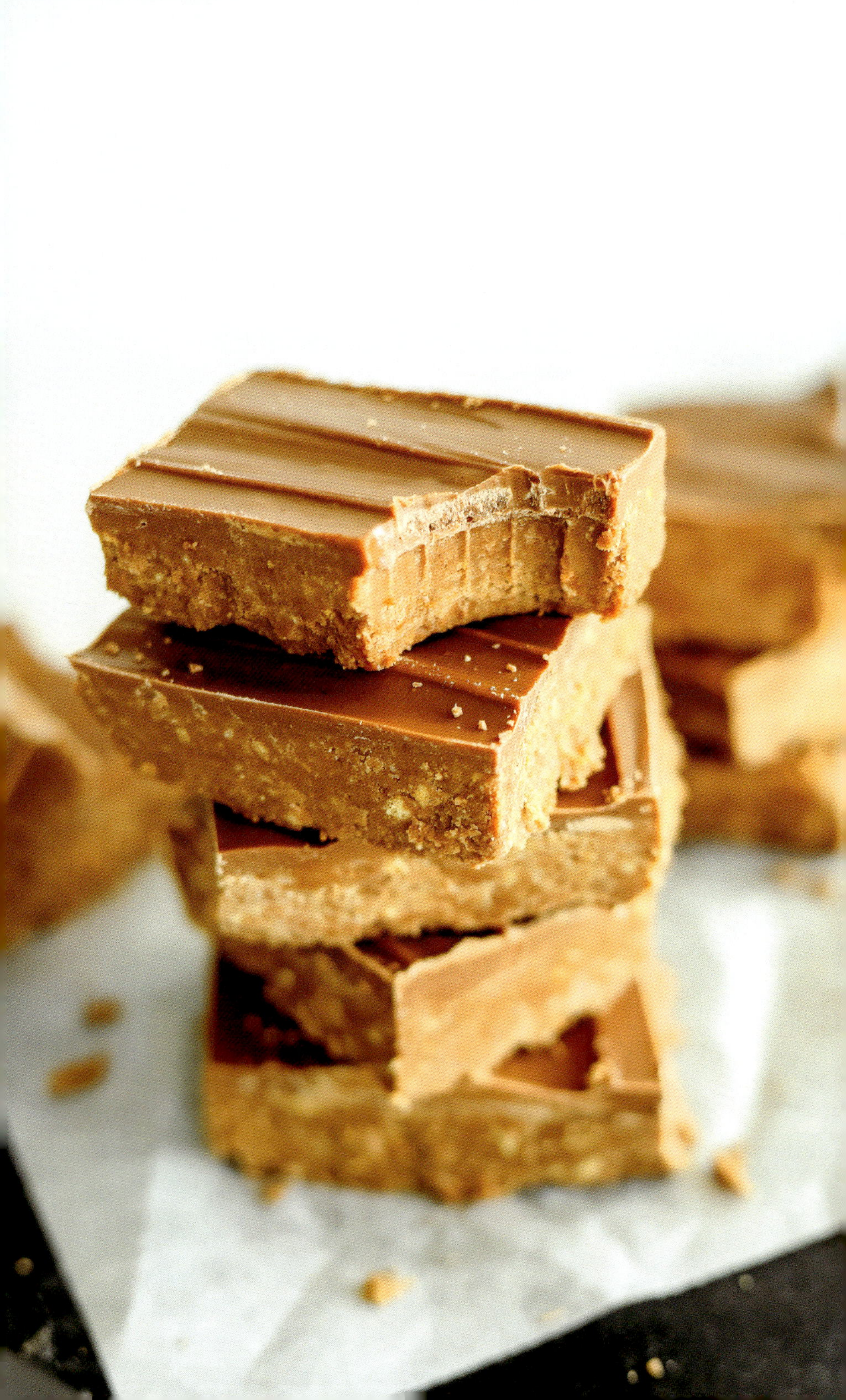

INSIDE OUT BARS*
Makes 16 serving
305 calories / 17F / 33C / 5P / per bar

---

1 cup OffBeat Buckeye Brownie Peanut Butter
½ cup butter, melted
1 cup graham crackers, finely crushed
2 cups powdered sugar
½ cup peanut butter baking chips
½ cup milk chocolate chips

1. In a medium bowl, mix the Buckeye Brownie Peanut Butter and melted butter together until smooth.

2. Add the crushed graham crackers and powdered sugar; mix until fully incorporated. Press into the bottom of a 9x9 inch baking pan.

3. Melt the peanut butter chips and chocolate chips together in the microwave. Heat for 30 seconds at a time, stirring in between, until completely melted and smooth.

4. Pour the melted chocolate over the top of the bars and spread out evenly. Chill in the refrigerator for 30+ minutes.

5. When ready to serve, let sit at room temperature for 5 minutes and then slice into bars.

*OffBeat Fam Recipe Submitted by Camille Easton

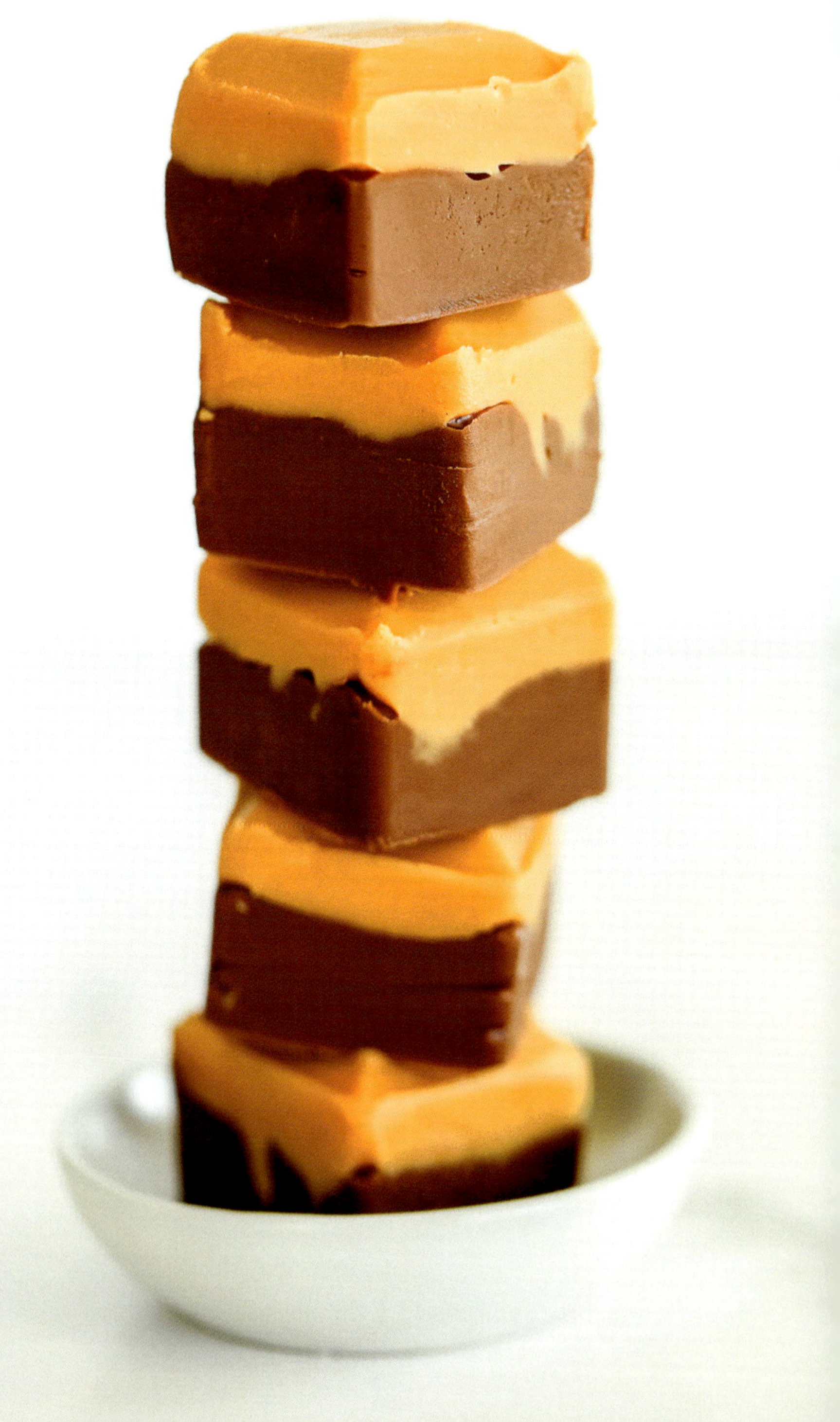

PEANUT BUTTER CUP FREEZER FUDGE
Makes 6 servings
155 calories / 12.5F / 6C / 5P / per serving

¼ cup OffBeat Sweet Classic Peanut Butter
1 Tbs. pure maple syrup
¼ tsp. vanilla extract
¼ cup OffBeat Buckeye Brownie Peanut Butter
1 Tbs. grass-fed butter or coconut oil

1. Mix the Sweet Classic Peanut Butter with the maple syrup and vanilla. Spoon ½ tablespoon of the mixture into an ice cube tray, making six servings. Freeze for 30+ minutes.

2. Add the Buckeye Brownie Peanut Butter and the butter or coconut oil into a bowl. Microwave for 10-20 seconds or until the butter/coconut oil is melted. Whisk together until smooth. Spoon ½ tablespoon of the chocolate mixture on top of the peanut butter mixture in the ice cube tray. Freeze 4+ hours.

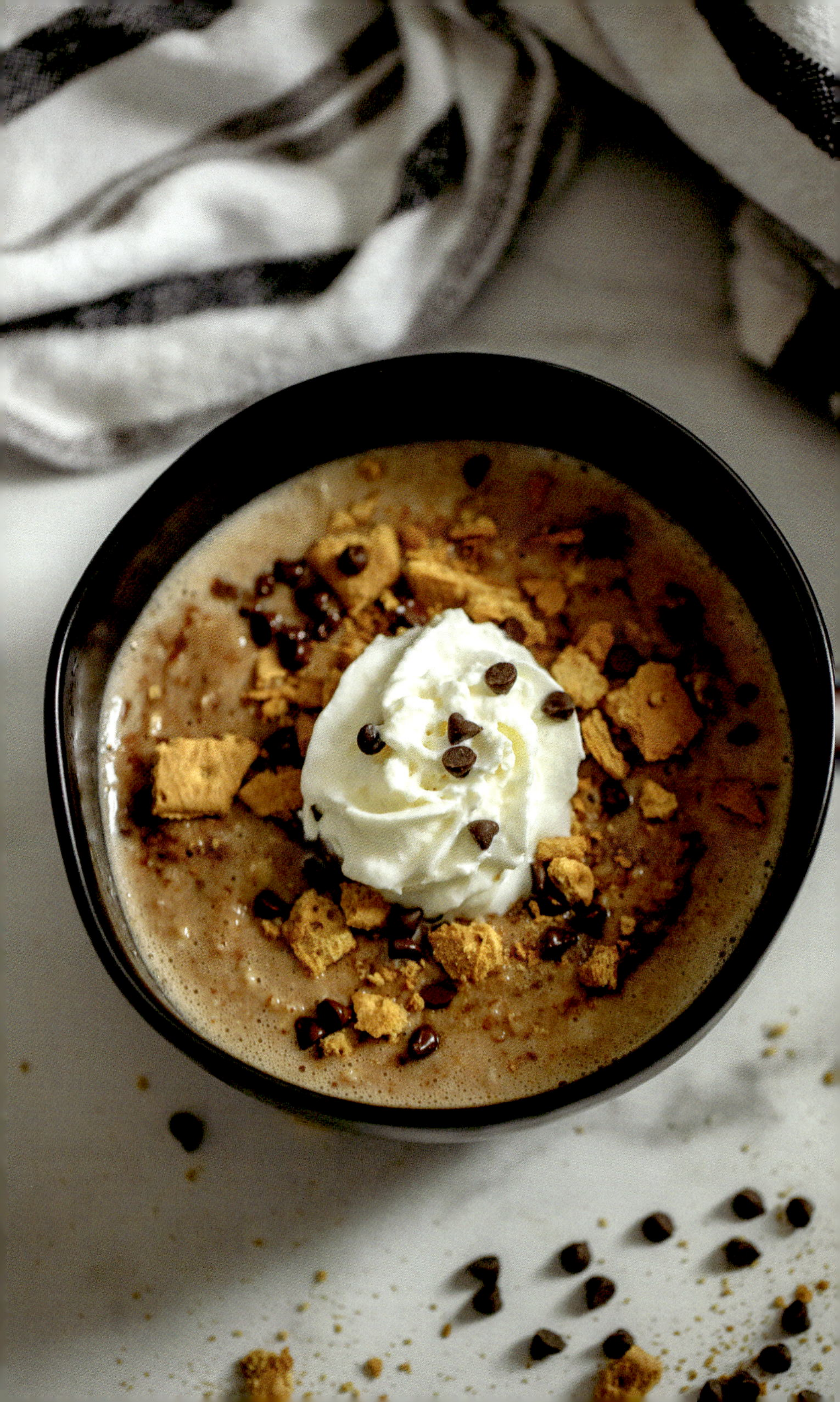

PEANUT BUTTER CUP S'MORES OATMEAL*

Makes 1 serving
320 calories / 33F / 10C / 26P

½ cup old-fashioned rolled oats
⅔ cup water
3 Tbs. egg whites
1 Tbs. OffBeat Buckeye Brownie Peanut Butter
1 serving vanilla stevia
¾ serving CSE Simply Vanilla protein powder
Toppings:
¼ sheet of a graham cracker
2 Tbs. spray whipped cream
1 tsp. mini chocolate chips

1. Combine water, egg whites, and oats in large microwave-safe bowl and microwave for 2-3 minutes.

2. Stir in the Buckeye Brownie Peanut Butter. Let cool for a couple minutes, then stir in the protein powder and stevia.

3. Top with crushed graham sheet, whipped cream, and chocolate chips. Enjoy!

OffBeat Fam Recipe Submitted by Bethany Happy

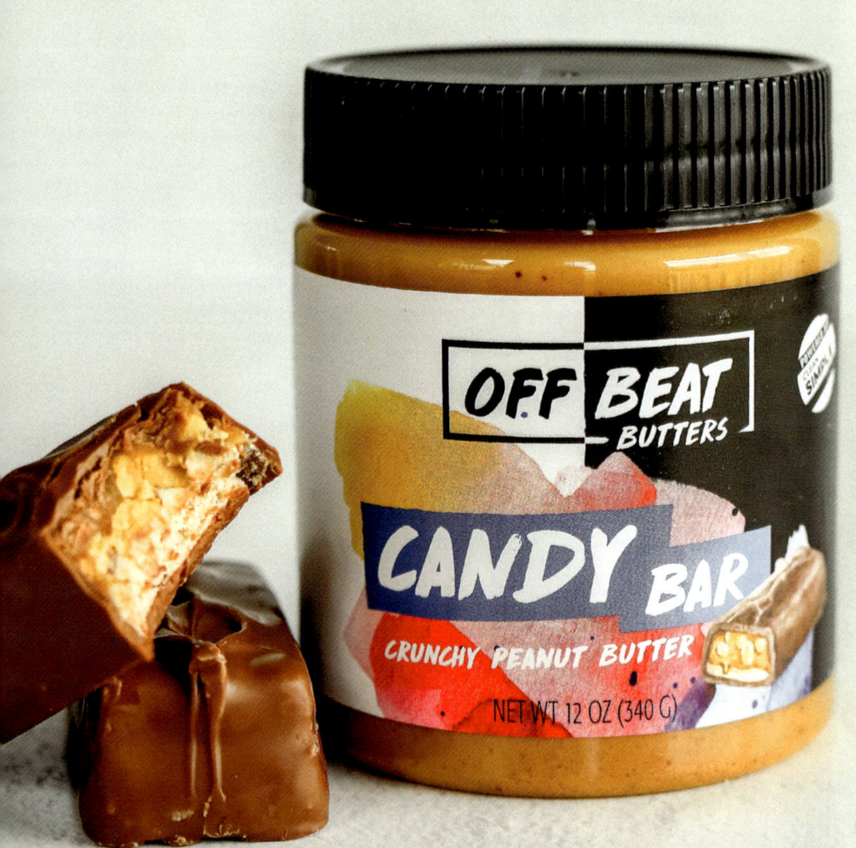
O.F.F BEAT
BUTTERS
CANDY BAR
CRUNCHY PEANUT BUTTER
NET WT 12 OZ (340 G)

LIFE IS SHORT; MAKE IT SWEET

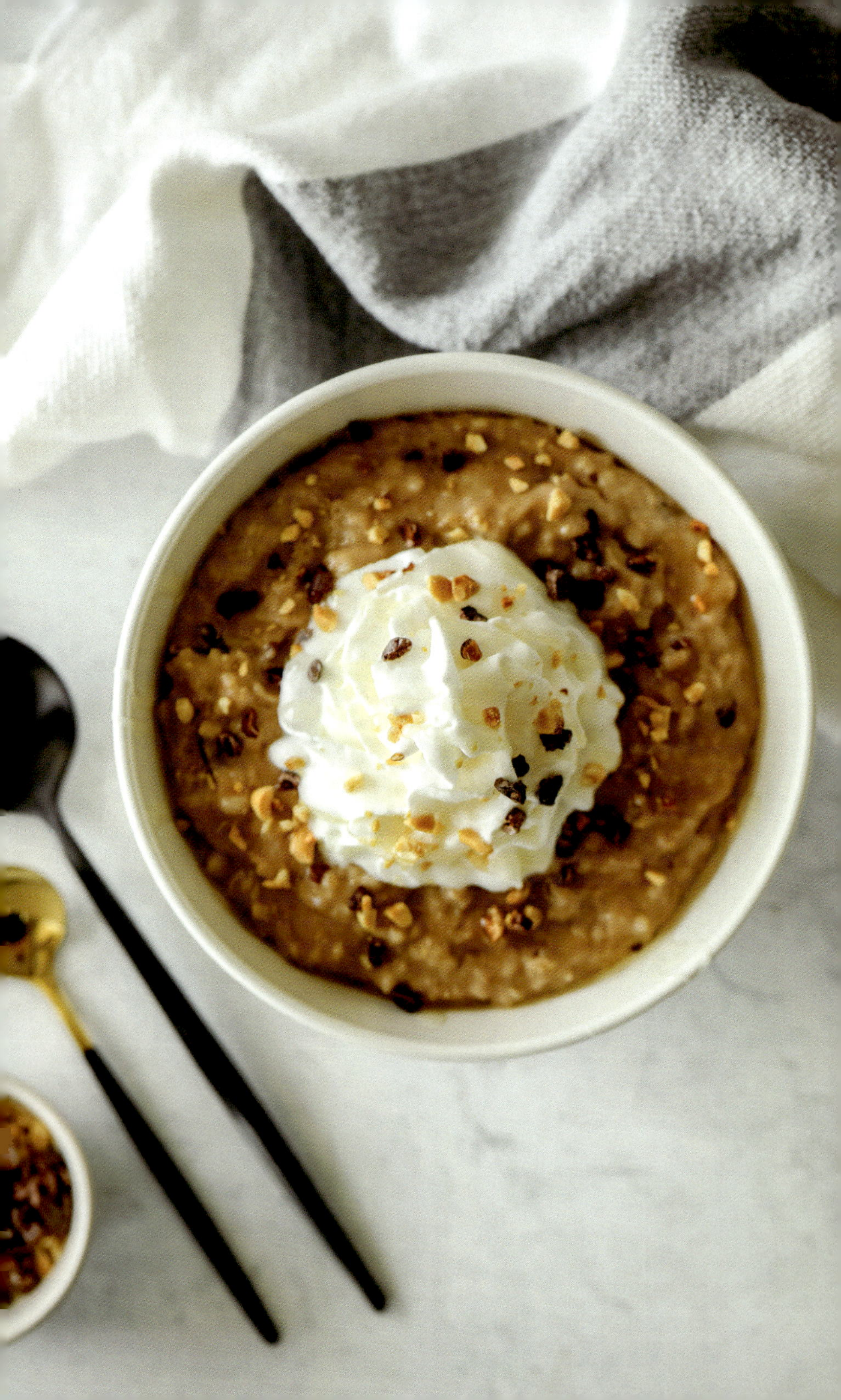

CANDY BAR OATS
Makes 1 serving
355 calories / 13F / 32C / 28P

⅓ cup old-fashioned rolled oats
½ cup water
1 Tbs. OffBeat Candy Bar Peanut Butter
1 serving CSE Chocolate Peanut Butter Protein Powder
Toppings:
1 Tbs. spray whipped cream
½ (4g) Tbs. cacao nibs or dark chocolate chips
½ (4g) Tbs. chopped peanuts
½ tsp. honey

1. Add the rolled oats and water to a microwave-safe bowl. Microwave for 1-2 minutes.

2. Stir in the Candy Bar Peanut Butter. Let cool for a couple minutes, then stir in the protein powder.

3. Top with whipped cream, nibs, chopped peanuts and honey. Enjoy!

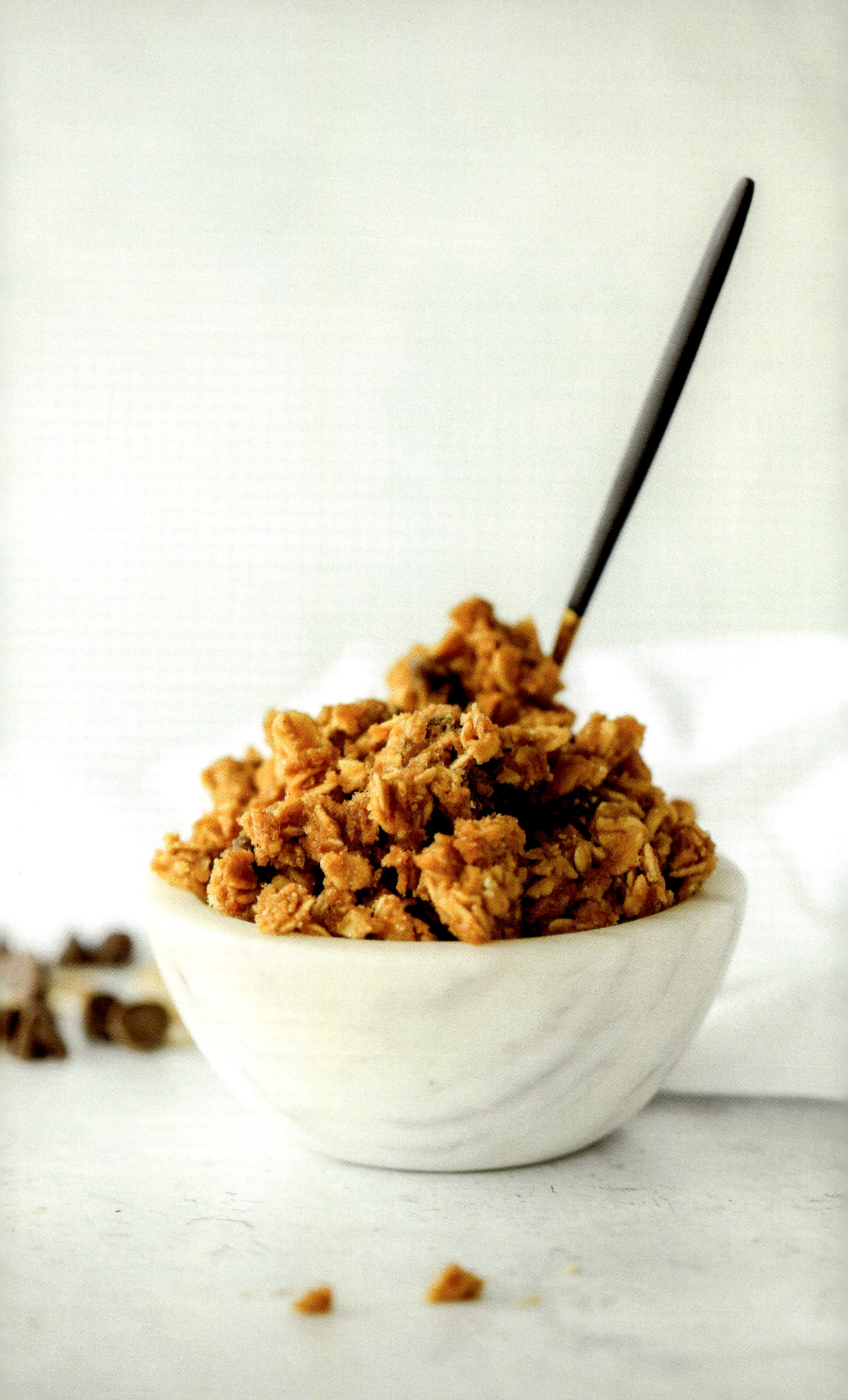

PB OATMEAL CHOCOLATE CHIP COOKIE DOUGH

Makes 16 servings
125 calories / 5F / 18C / 3P / per serving

½ cup OffBeat Candy Bar Peanut Butter
   or Sweet Classic Peanut Butter
½ cup coconut sugar
¼ cup organic sugar in the raw
¼ cup pasteurized egg whites
1 tsp. vanilla extract
1½ cups old-fashioned rolled oats
¼ tsp. sea salt
¼ cup dark chocolate chips

1. Add the Candy Bar Peanut Butter, coconut sugar and raw sugar to a bowl. Beat until smooth. Add in the egg whites and vanilla. Beat until well combined.

2. Add in the rolled oats, sea salt and chocolate chips. Mix on low or stir together with a wooden spoon.

3. Using a cookie scoop, scoop into balls and enjoy! Store in the fridge for up to 2 weeks or 3 months in the freezer.

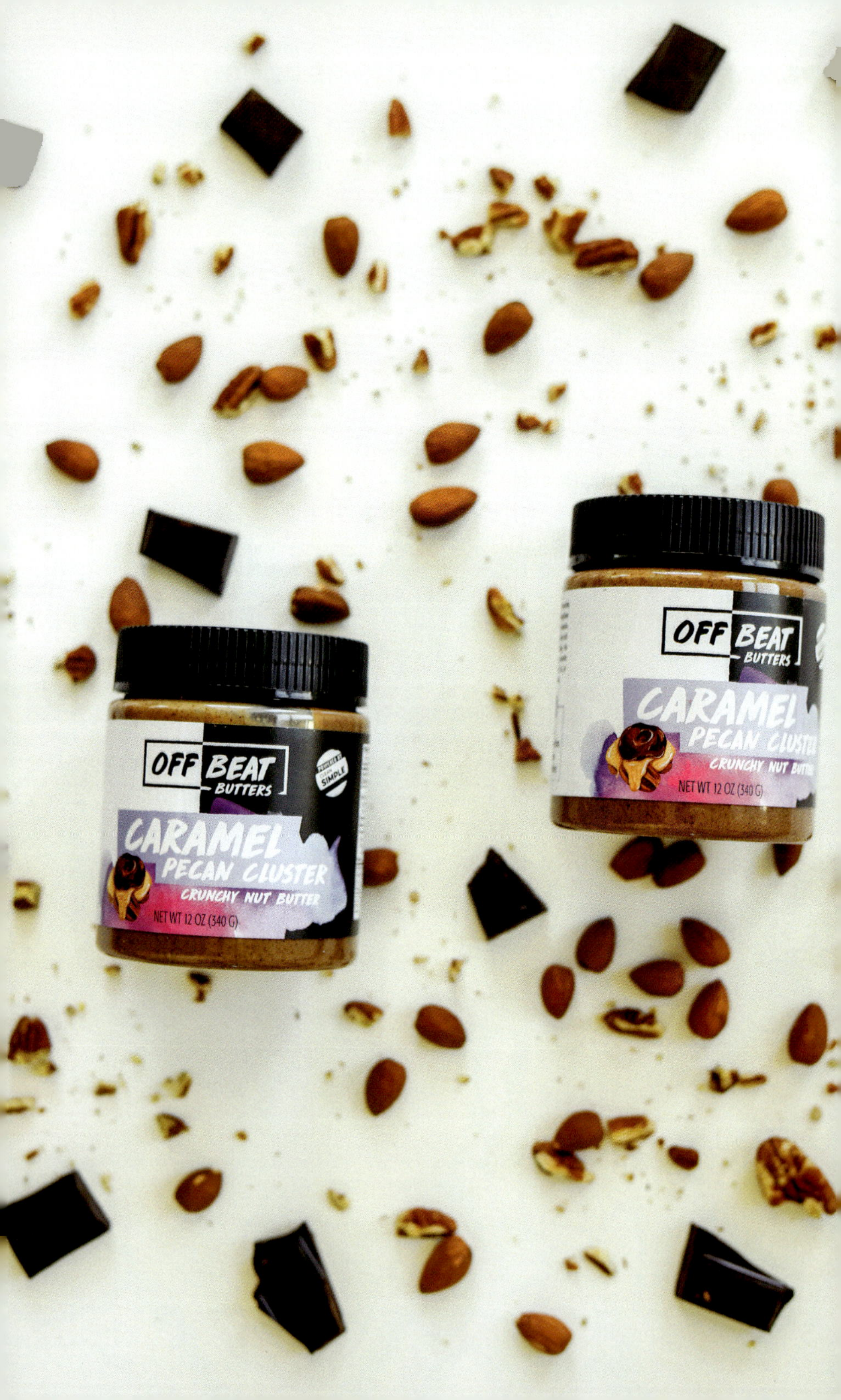
OFF BEAT
BUTTERS
CARAMEL
PECAN CLUSTER
CRUNCHY NUT BUTTER
NET WT 12 OZ (340 G)
OFF BEAT
BUTTERS
CARAMEL
PECAN CLUSTER
CRUNCHY NUT BUTTER
NET WT 12 OZ (340 G)

I'M LIKE THE BEST KIND OF ALMOND BUTTER... HALF SWEET, HALF NUTS!

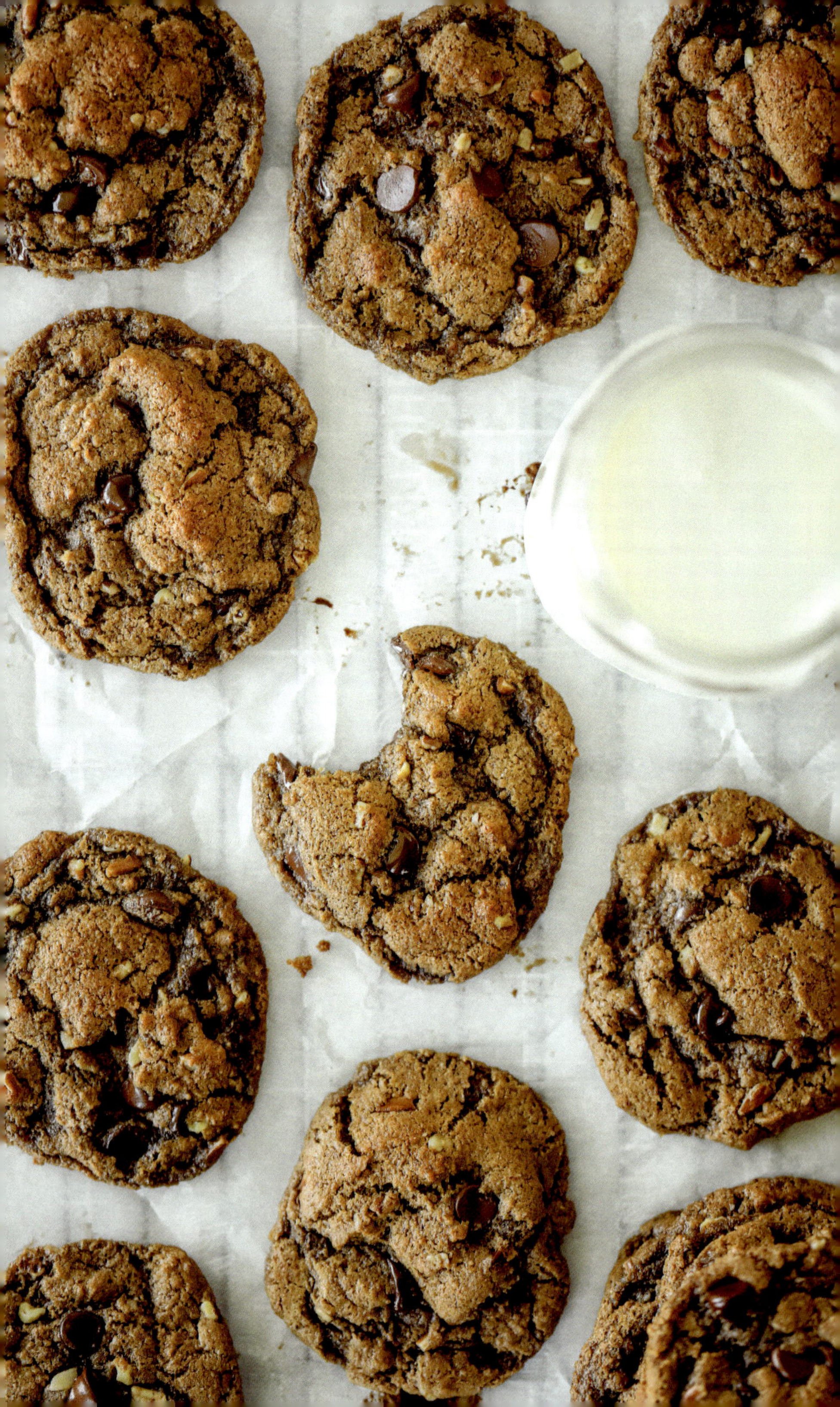

CPC MELTAWAYS
Makes 16 cookies
150 calories / 8.5F / 18C / 2.5P / per cookie

1 cup (225g) OffBeat Caramel Pecan Cluster Butter
1 cup firmly packed brown sugar or coconut sugar
1 large egg
1 tsp. baking soda
⅓ cup (65g) dark chocolate chips

1. Preheat the oven to 350 degrees.

2. Add all of the ingredients, except the chocolate chips, to a mixing bowl. Mix together with a wooden spoon until blended. Stir in chocolate chips.

3. Using a small cookie scoop, scoop cookie dough onto a baking sheet lined with parchment paper. Bake for 8-9 minutes. Let cool for 5 minutes on the pan and then transfer to a cooling rack. Enjoy!

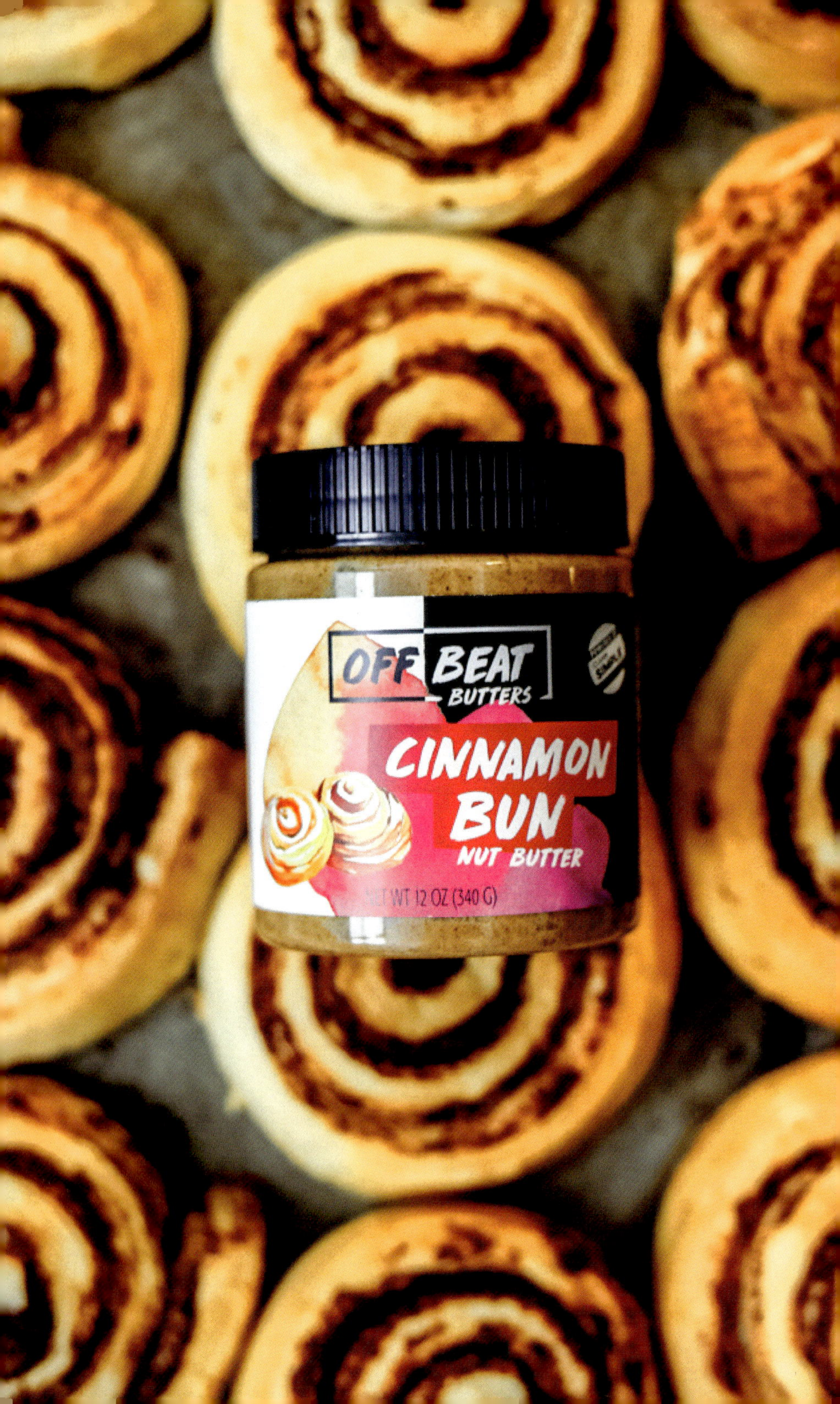

OFF BEAT
BUTTERS
CINNAMON
BUN
NUT BUTTER
NET WT 12 OZ (340 G)

YOU CAN'T PLEASE 'EM ALL... YOU AREN'T CINNAMON BUN BUTTER

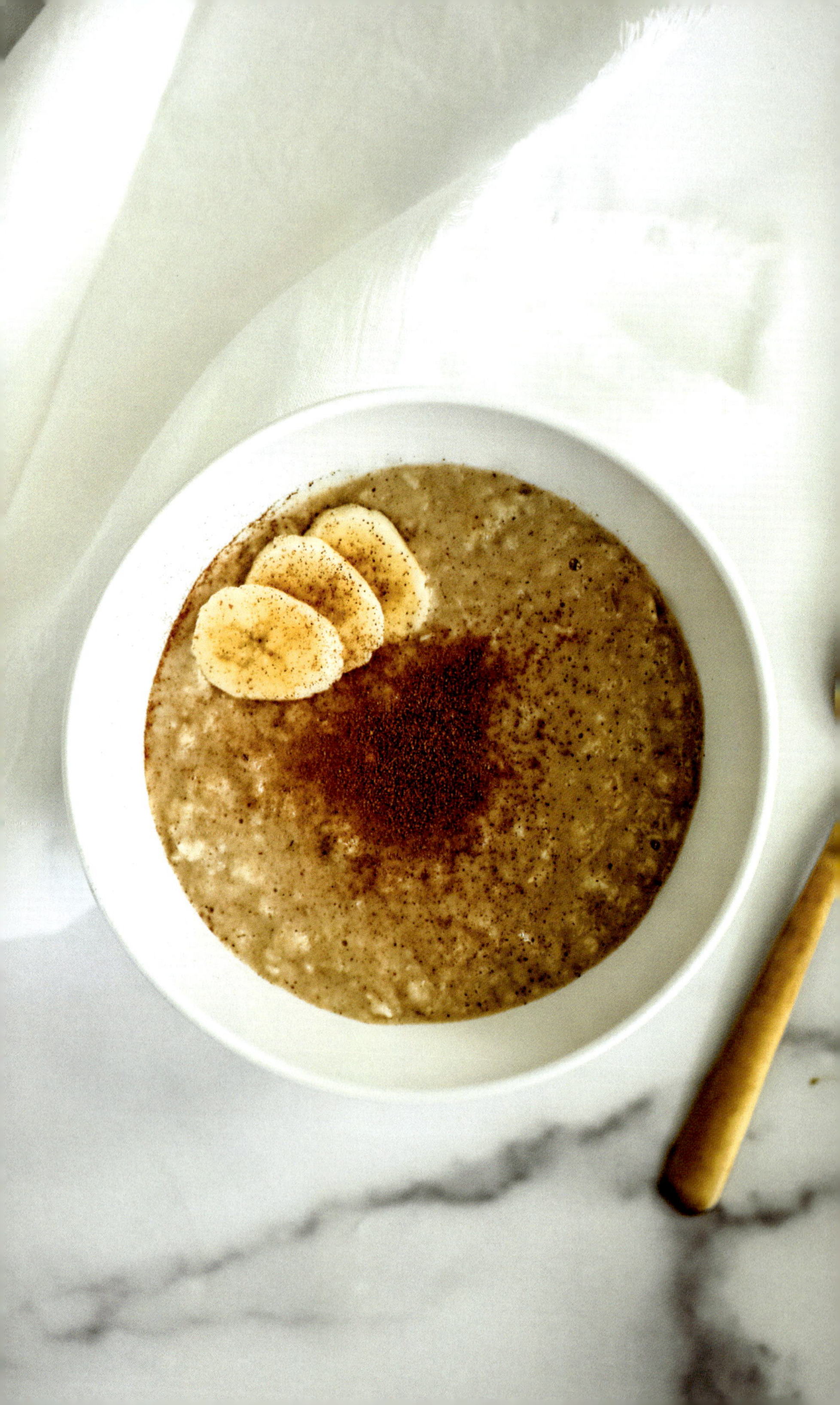

BANANAS FOSTER OATMEAL
Makes 1 serving
335 calories / 8.5F / 38C / 26P

⅓ cup old-fashioned rolled oats
½ cup water
3 Tbs. (46g) liquid egg whites
40g mashed banana
1 Tbs. (14g) OffBeat Cinnamon Bun Butter
¾ serving (27g) CSE Bananas Foster Protein Powder
Topping:
Dash cinnamon

1. Add the oats, water, egg whites, and mashed banana to a microwave-safe bowl. Whisk until the egg whites are well combined. Microwave for 1-2 minutes.

2. Stir in the Cinnamon Bun Butter. Let cool for a couple minutes, then stir in the protein powder.

3. Top with cinnamon. Enjoy!

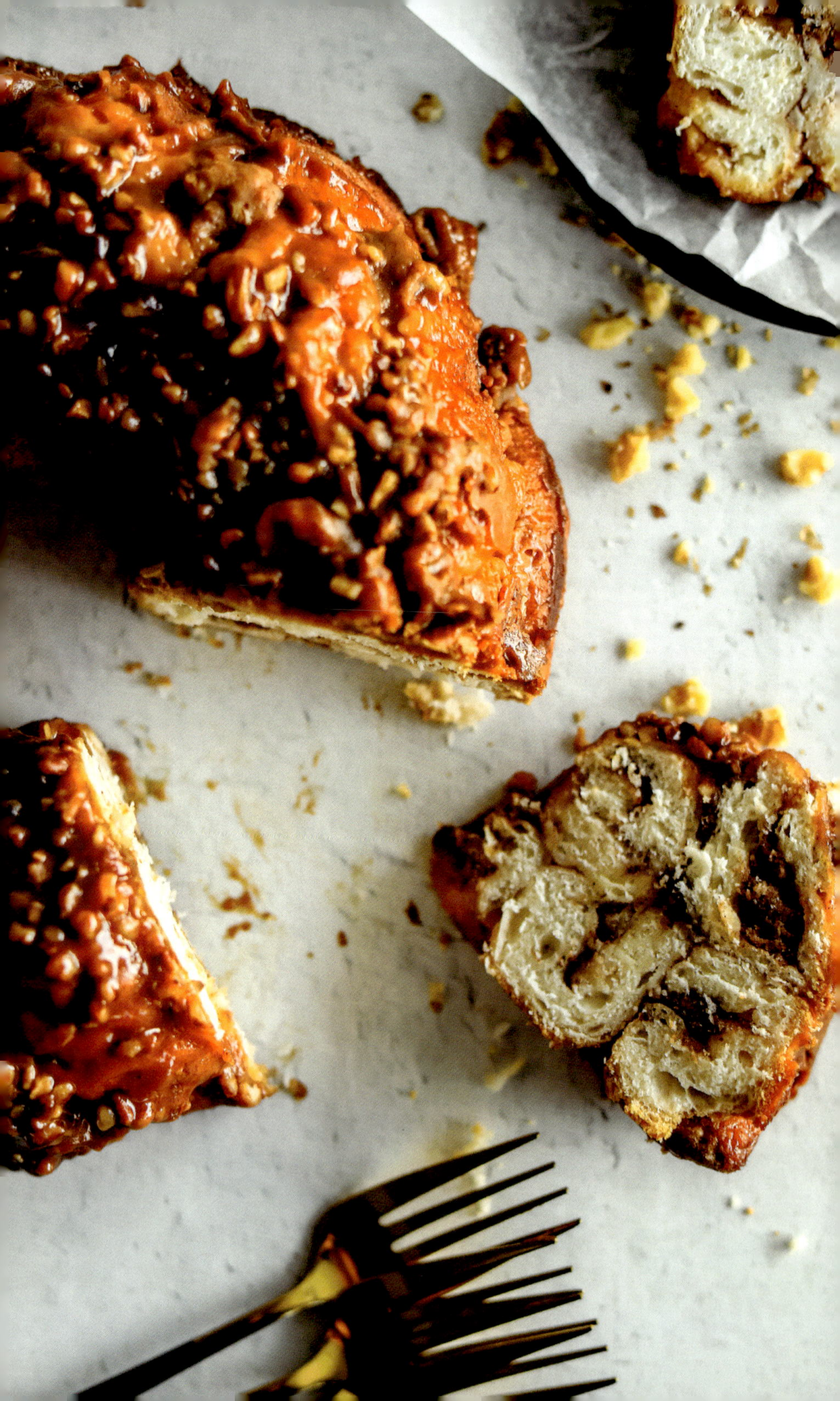

CINNAMON BUN FILLED MONKEY BREAD *
Makes 16 servings
320 calories / 16F / 37C / 7P / per serving

1½ cups OffBeat Cinnamon Bun Butter, divided
2 cans non-flaky buttermilk biscuits
½ package Cook & Serve butterscotch pudding mix
½ cup finely chopped pecans
¾ cup granulated sugar
2-3 tsp. ground cinnamon
¼ cup grass-fed butter
¼ cup OffBeat Cinnamon Bun Butter
½ cup brown sugar
2 Tbs. unsweetened almond milk
1 tsp. vanilla extract

1. Heat oven to 350 degrees. Spray a Bundt pan with nonstick cooking spray (do not use a tube pan). Pour in chopped pecans and sprinkle with butterscotch pudding mix.

2. In a gallon zip top bag, combine ¾ cup of sugar with two to three teaspoons of cinnamon.

3. Separate the biscuit dough into 16 biscuits (eight per can). Cut each biscuit into quarters, making 64 pieces. Flatten each quarter into a circle shape. Place one teaspoon of Cinnamon Bun Butter in the center of the dough. Close edges over the filling and pinch shut, encasing the filling completely. Repeat with all remaining dough circles. Add filled dough balls, a few at a time, to the bag of cinnamon sugar. Shake in the bag to coat the dough.

4. In a small saucepan, melt the butter with ¼ cup Cinnamon Bun Butter, brown sugar, vanilla and milk over medium heat, stirring constantly. Let boil for 30 seconds.

5. Arrange ½ of the filled, coated biscuit balls in the Bundt pan. Pour ½ of the butter mixture over the biscuits. Repeat with remaining biscuit balls and butter mixture. The pan should be ½ - ⅔ full.

6. Bake for about 40 minutes, or until the crust is a deep brown on top. Flip over on a large plate while still hot and drizzle with the remaining Cinnamon Bun Butter. Enjoy!

OffBeat Fam Recipe Submitted by Jasmine Burton

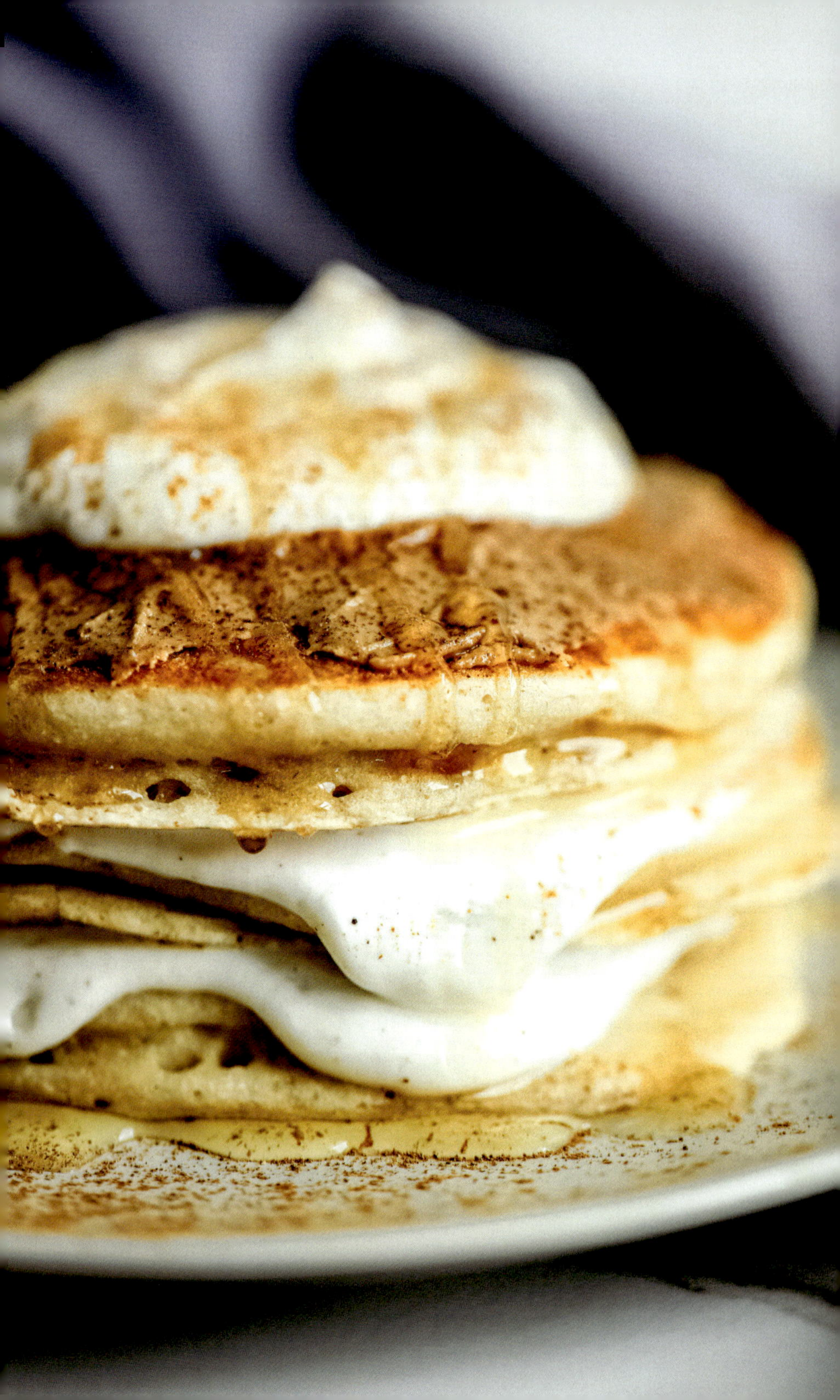

CINNAMON BUN PANCAKES
Makes 1 serving
250 calories / 8F / 26C / 19P

⅓ cup CSE Vanilla Pancake & Waffle Mix
¼ cup water
2 Tbs. egg whites
1 Tbs. OffBeat Cinnamon Bun Butter
¼ cup nonfat, plain Greek yogurt
2 Tbs. zero calorie syrup of choice

1. Heat griddle to medium heat or 300 degrees.

2. Combine the CSE Pancake & Waffle Mix, water and egg whites together in a bowl. Spray griddle with cooking spray and pour the pancake batter onto the griddle. Once browned on one side, flip and let cook on the other side.

3. Spread the Cinnamon Bun Butter on the warm pancakes.

4. In a small bowl, whisk together the Greek yogurt and pancake syrup. Pour over the pancakes.

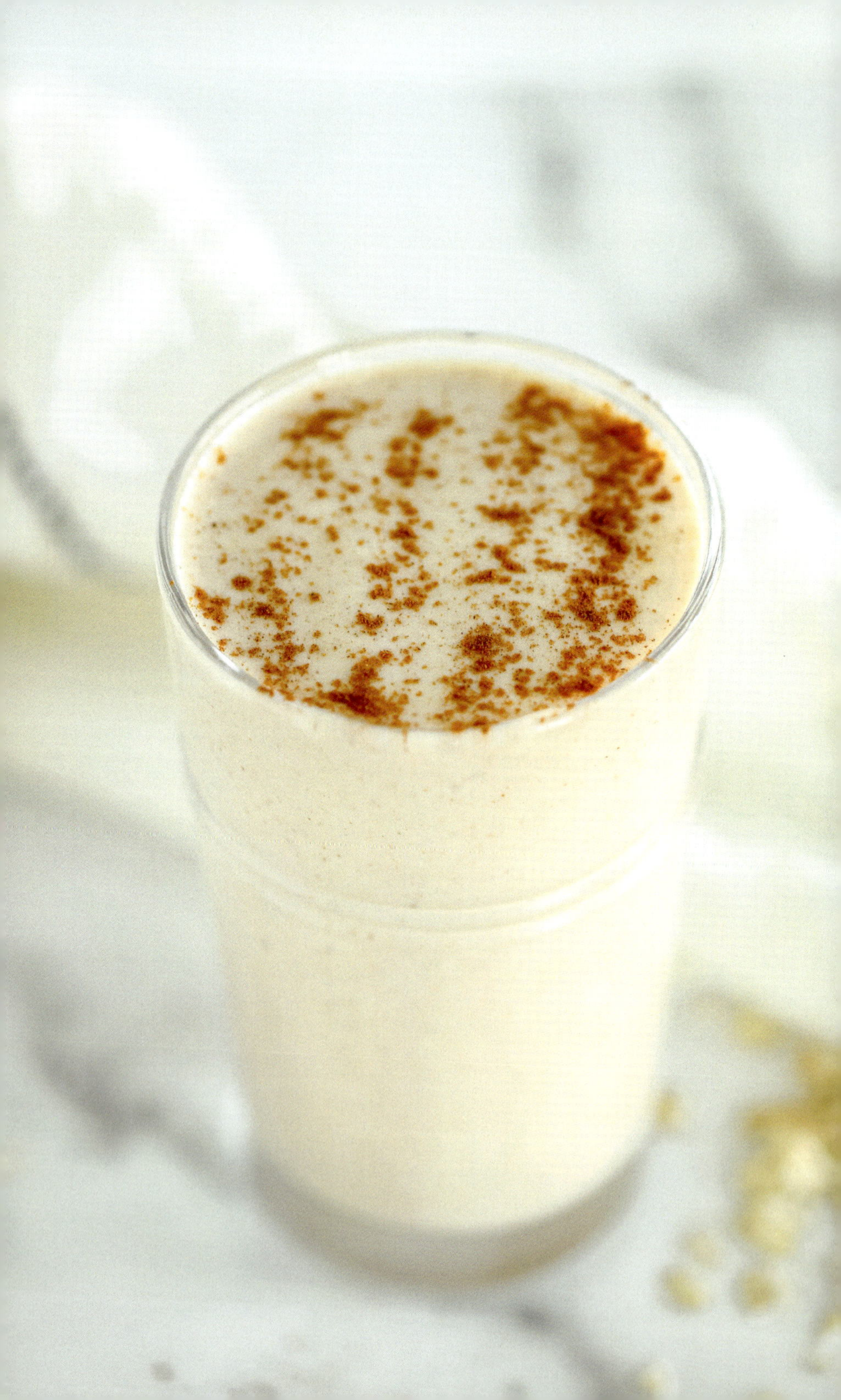

CINNAMON BUN SHAKE
Makes 1 serving
335 calories / 13F / 34.5C / 27P

---

1 cup unsweetened almond milk
¼ cup low-fat cottage cheese
¾ serving (25g) CSE Cinnamon Roll Protein Powder
50g frozen bananas slices
2 Tbs. old-fashioned rolled oats
1 Tbs. OffBeat Cinnamon Bun Butter
½ tsp. cinnamon
6-8 (120g) ice cubes

1. Add all of the ingredients to a high-powered blender. Blend on high until smooth.

2. Pour into a cup. Enjoy!

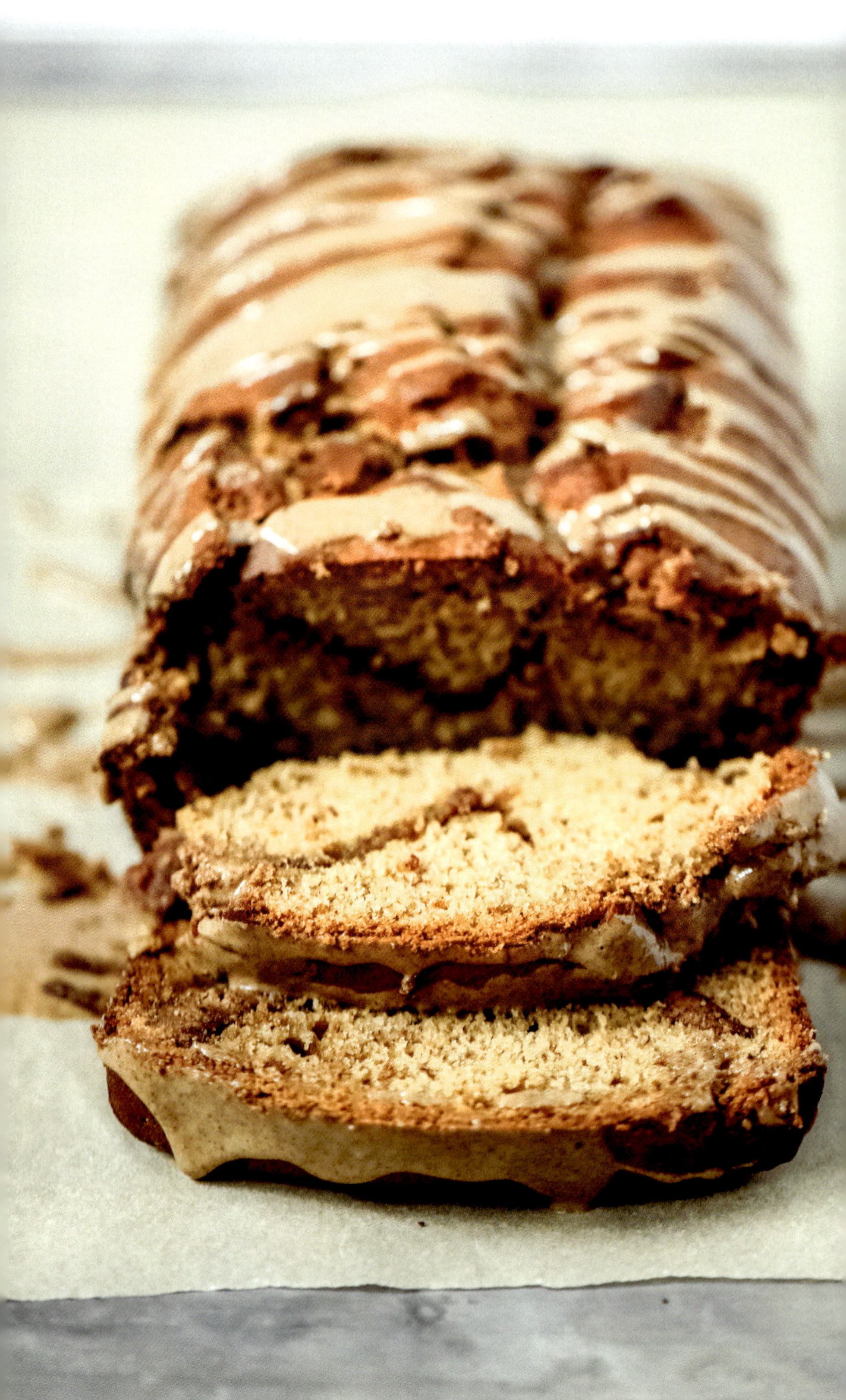

CINNAMON BUN-ANA BREAD
Makes 12 servings
274 calories / 11F / 39C / 5P / per serving

½ cup grass-fed butter
¾ cup brown sugar, packed
2 eggs, large
1 tsp. vanilla extract
3 large bananas, ripe, mashed
1 cup all-purpose flour
1 cup whole wheat flour
1 tsp. baking soda
1 tsp. baking powder
½ tsp. salt
½ cup milk
½ cup OffBeat Cinnamon Bun Butter

1. Preheat oven to 350 degrees. Grease a 9x5 loaf pan.

2. In a large mixing bowl, cream together the butter and sugar until light and fluffy. Beat in the eggs one at a time, mixing well between additions. Beat in the vanilla extract and mashed bananas until fully incorporated. Mix in the flours, baking soda, baking powder, and salt. Stir in the milk. Set aside.

3. Microwave the Cinnamon Bun Butter until drizzle-consistency.

4. In the loaf pan, transfer ⅓ of the bread batter. Drizzle ⅓ of the Cinnamon Bun Butter over the top and using a butter knife, lightly swirl into the batter. Complete this step two more times, creating three layers.

5. Bake for 55 to 65 minutes, or until a toothpick inserted into the center comes out clean. Cool loaf in pan for 10 minutes before removing and transferring to a cooling rack to cool completely. Enjoy!

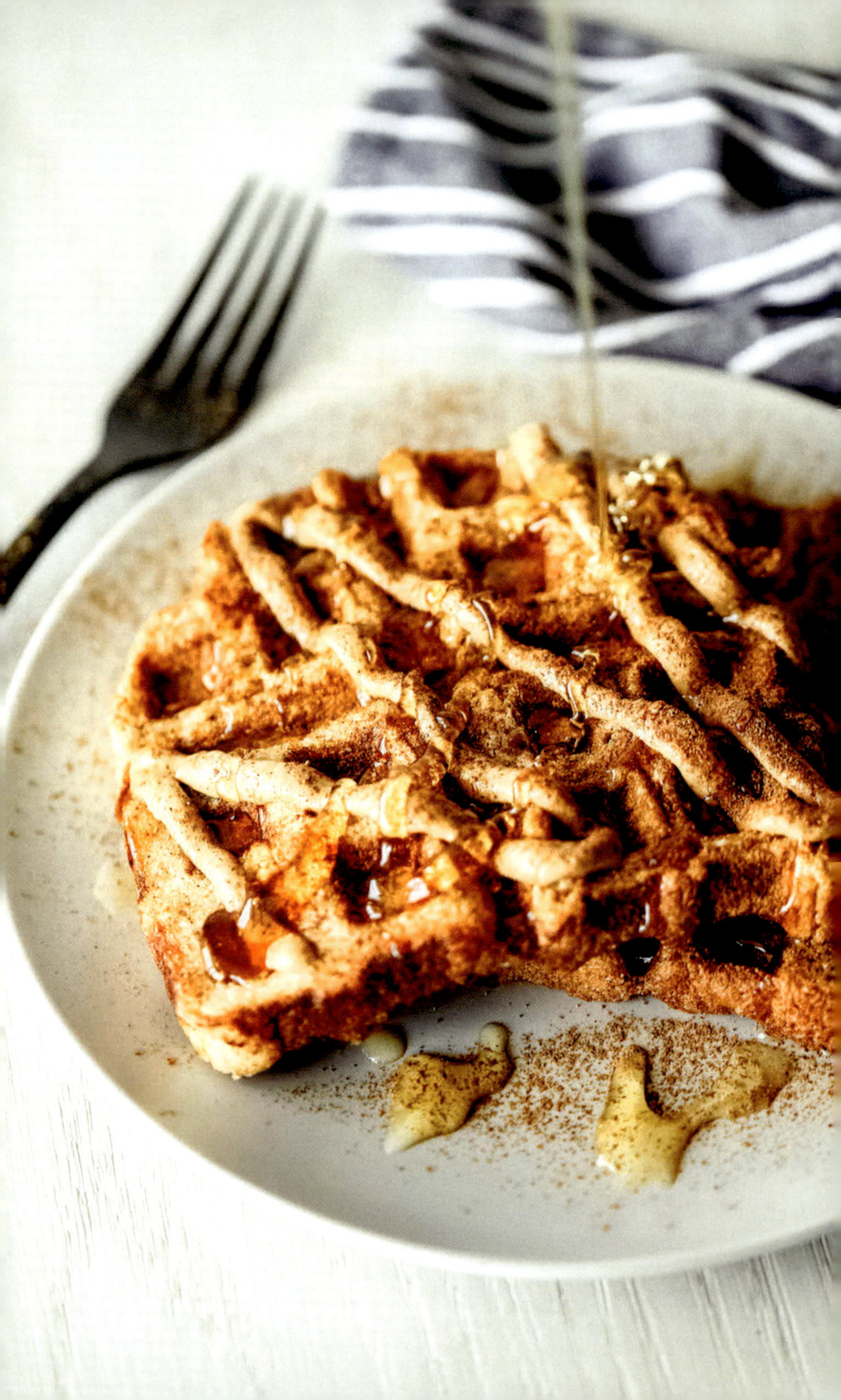

CINNAMON FRENCH TOAST CRUNCH

Makes 1 serving
340 calories/ 7F / 45C / 21P

---

4 Tbs. liquid egg whites
2 Tbs. Fairlife fat-free milk
1 Tbs. CSE Simply Vanilla Protein Powder
Dash vanilla
Dash cinnamon
2 slices Harper's Bran Bread
1 Tbs. OffBeat Cinnamon Bun Butter
½ Tbs. raw honey

1. Heat waffle iron.

2. Add the egg whites, milk, protein powder, vanilla and cinnamon to a shallow dish. Whisk all ingredients together until well combined.

3. Dip each slice of bread into egg mixture, coating each side evenly. Place one at a time onto greased waffle iron.

4. Top with Cinnamon Bun Butter and honey.

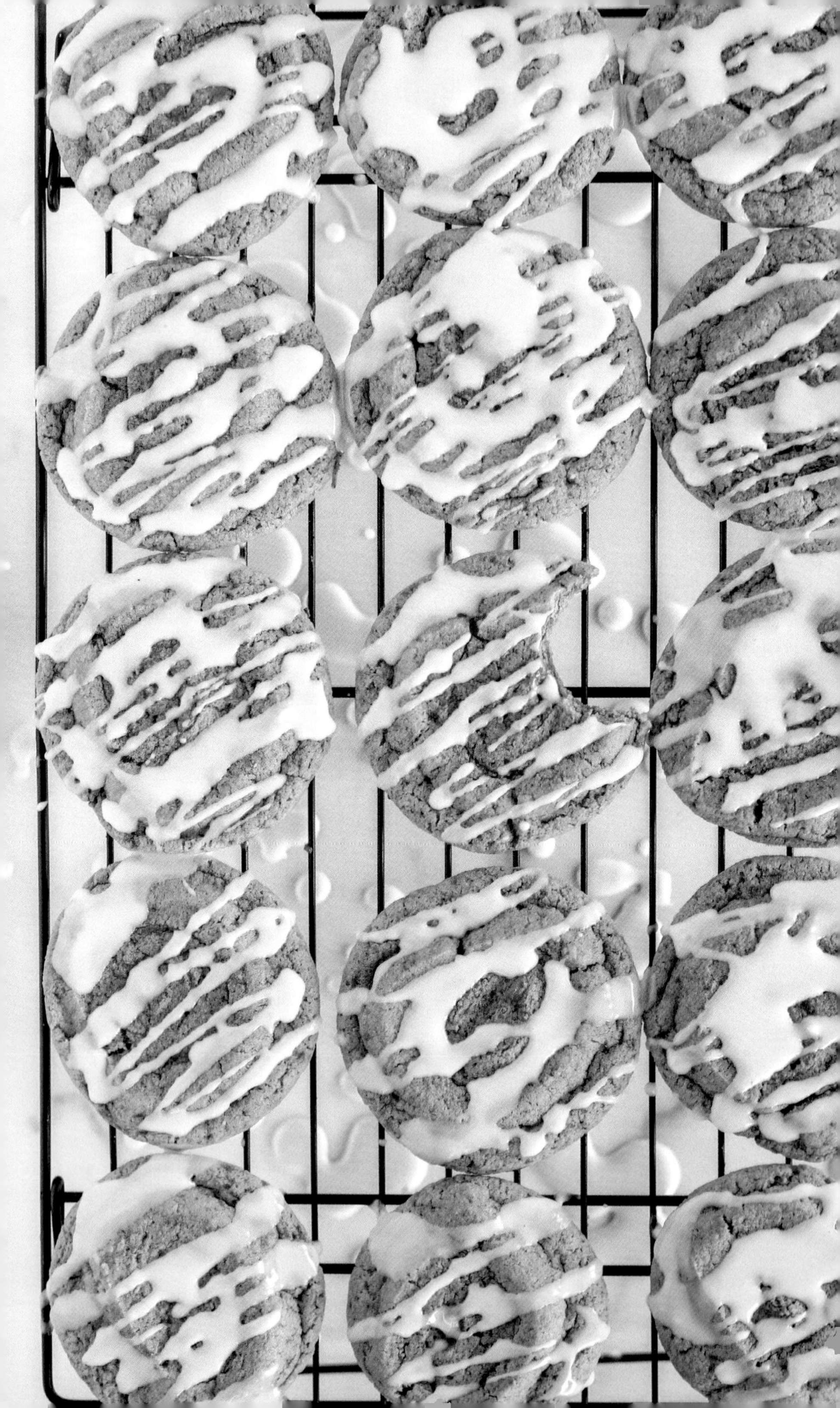

CINNAMON ROLL COOKIES
Makes 16 cookies
195 calories/ 8F / 28C / 4P / per cookie

½ cup grass-fed butter
¼ cup organic cane sugar
½ cup coconut sugar
1 large egg
½ tsp. vanilla extract
1 ½ cups (180g) whole wheat pastry flour
1 serving CSE Cinnamon Roll Protein Powder
½ tsp. baking soda
¼ tsp. sea salt
Filling:
¼ cup (56g) Cinnamon Bun Butter
Icing:
½ cup organic powdered sugar
1 Tbs. liquid egg whites

1. Preheat oven to 350 degrees.

2. Add the softened butter, cane sugar and coconut sugar to a mixing bowl. Mix together until smooth. Add the egg and vanilla; beat together until smooth.

3. In a separate bowl, add the flour, protein powder, baking soda and sea salt. Stir until incorporated. Add the dry ingredients to the wet ingredients and mix until just combined.

4. Lay a large piece of parchment paper out on the counter. Sprinkle a little flour over the top. Place the large ball of dough on the parchment paper. Using a floured rolling pin, roll the dough out into a large rectangle. Spread the Cinnamon Bun Butter evenly over the dough. Carefully roll the dough up lengthwise like a cinnamon roll. Once completely rolled up, gently slice into 16 equal-sized cookies. Place each cookie on a baking sheet lined with parchment paper and bake for 8-9 minutes. Let cool for a few minutes and then transfer to a cooling rack.

5. Make the icing by adding the powdered sugar and egg whites to a small bowl. Whisk together until well combined and smooth. Drizzle over the cooled cookies.

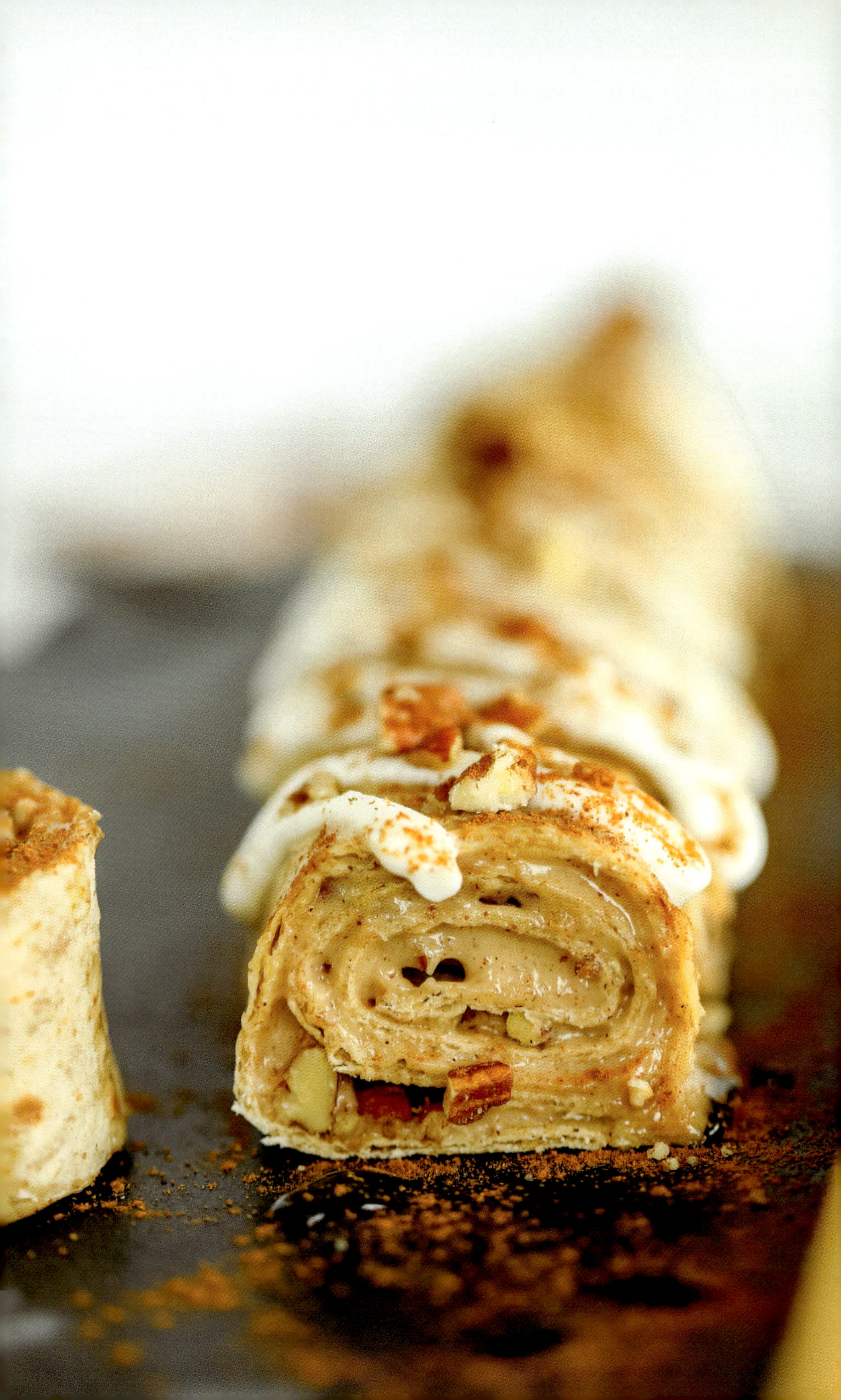

CINNAMON ROLL'D SUSHI
Makes 1 serving
350 calories/ 13F / 37C / 26.5P

¼ cup nonfat, plain Greek yogurt, divided
1 Tbs. OffBeat Cinnamon Bun Butter
⅔ serving (21g) CSE Cinnamon Roll Protein Powder
1 slice Joseph's Lavash Bread
Toppings:
1 Tbs. raw honey
Vanilla stevia drops, optional
1 Tbs. (7g) chopped pecans

1. Add three tablespoons Greek yogurt, Cinnamon Bun Butter, and protein powder to a small bowl. Mix until smooth.

2. Lay the bread out flat on a plate. Add the yogurt mixture to the center and spread out evenly to cover the bread.

3. Roll the bread up tight lengthwise and cut into 1-inch slices to create your "sushi" rolls.

4. Add the honey, remaining tablespoon of Greek yogurt and stevia (if desired) to a small bowl. Mix until smooth. Drizzle honey over the top of the sushi roll and garnish with chopped pecans. Enjoy!

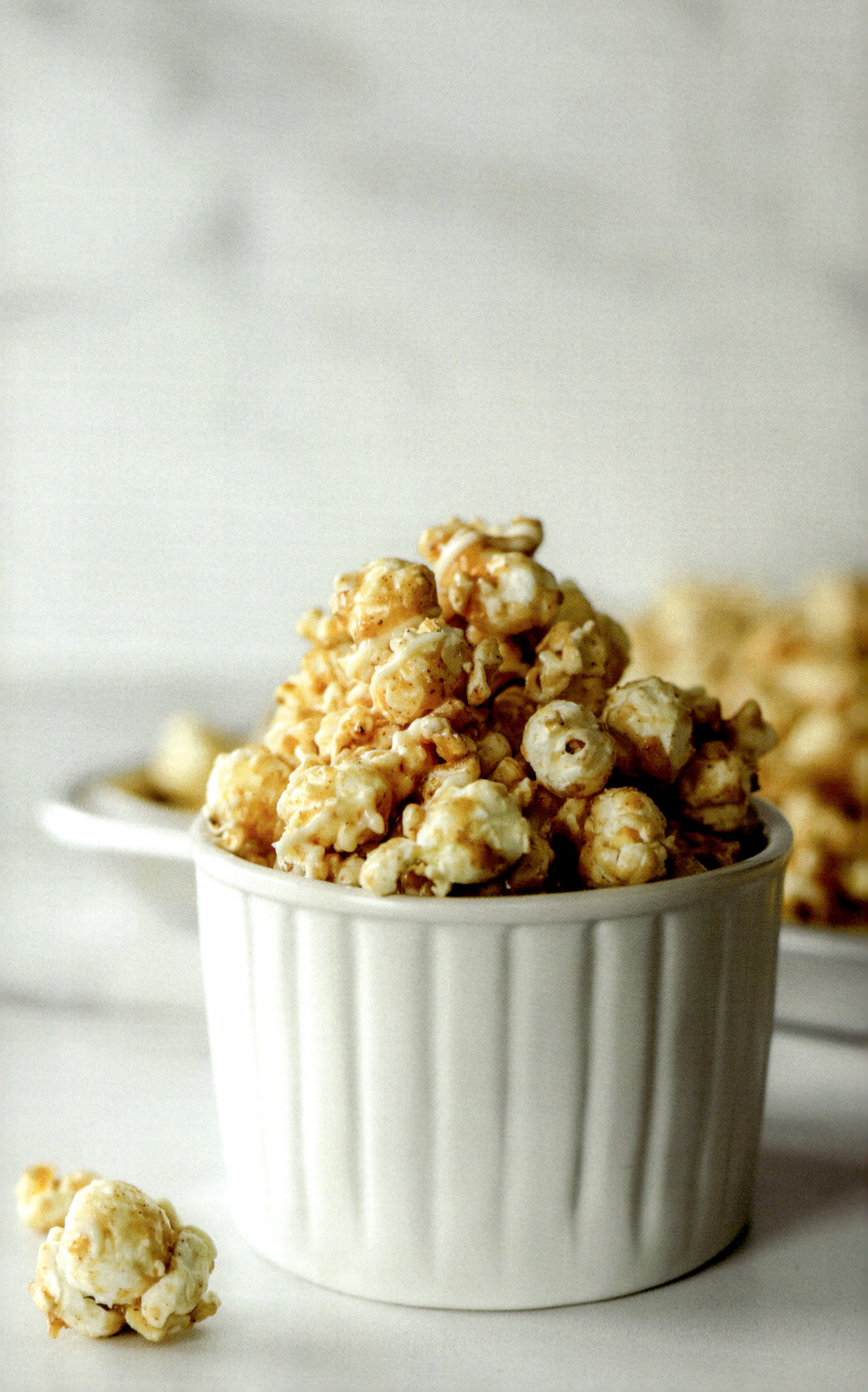

SNICKERDOODLE POPCORN
Makes 12 servings
185 calories / 5.5F / 30C / 4P / per serving

---

12 cups (½ cup kernels) air-popped popcorn
2 Tbs. white chocolate chips
¾ cup raw honey
⅓ cup OffBeat Cinnamon Bun Butter
1 serving CSE Simply Vanilla Protein Powder
Toppings:
Pinch sea salt
¼ cup melted white chocolate chips

1. Pop the popcorn into a large bowl. Set aside.

2. Add the white chocolate chips, honey and Cinnamon Bun Butter to a saucepan over low-medium heat. Melt down together until smooth and pourable. Remove from the heat and whisk in the protein powder until smooth.

3. Pour the mixture over the popcorn and stir until the popcorn is well coated.

4. Dump out onto a baking sheet lined with parchment paper and sprinkle with sea salt.

5. Melt the chocolate chips in the microwave for 30 seconds at a time until melted and smooth, stirring in between. Usually takes 60-90 seconds total. Drizzle the white chocolate over the popcorn and allow to cool. Enjoy!

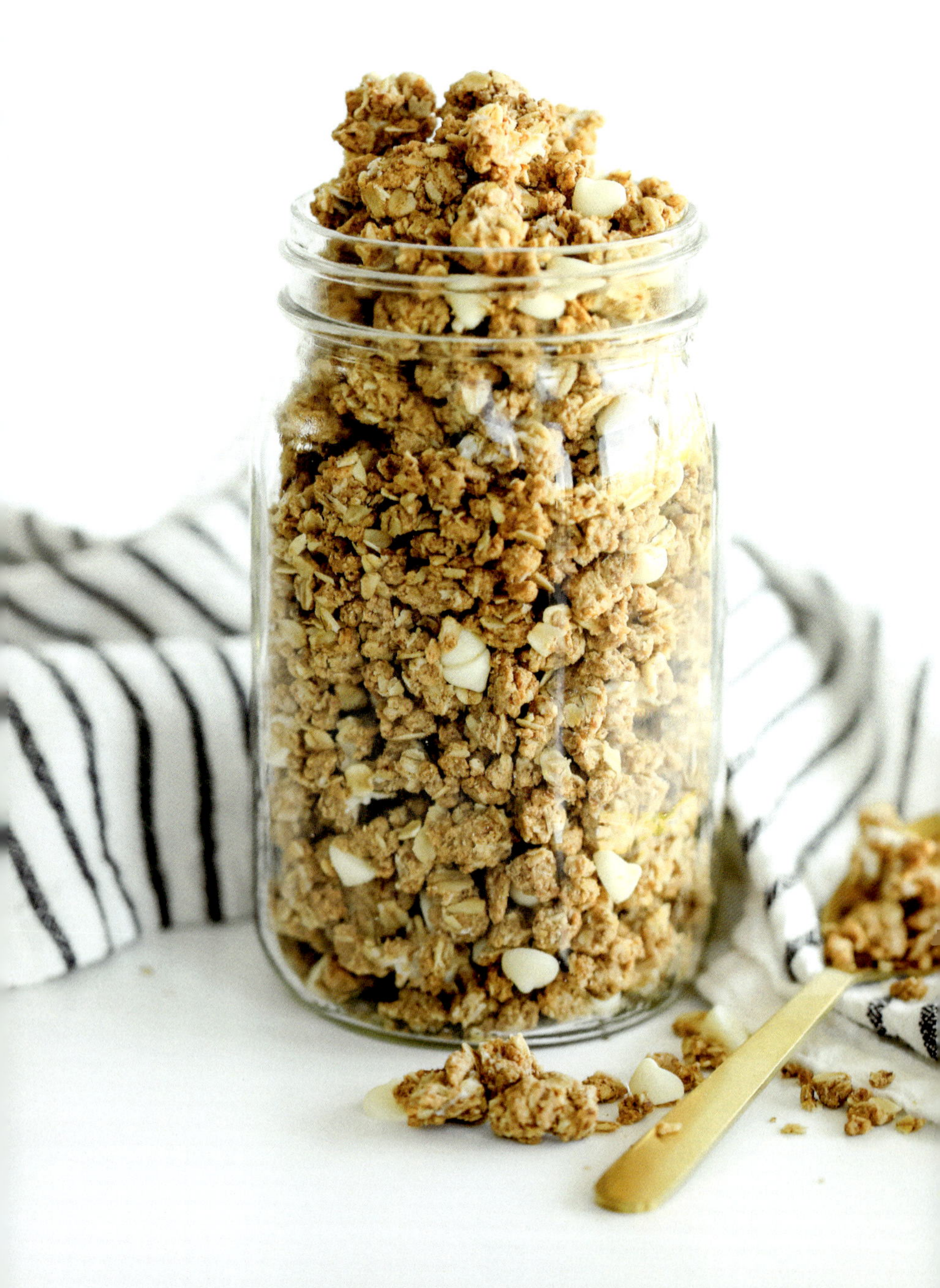

SNICKERDOODLE GRANOLA
Makes 24 servings
150 calories / 7.5F / 15C / 5P / per serving

12 oz. OffBeat Cinnamon Bun Butter
½ cup raw honey
2 servings CSE Simply Vanilla Protein Powder
¼ cup flaxseed meal
2 ½ cups old-fashioned rolled oats
½ tsp. sea salt
Topping:
¼ cup white or dark chocolate chips

1. Heat the oven to 350 degrees.

2. Add the Cinnamon Bun Butter, honey, protein powder, flaxseed meal, rolled oats and salt to a mixing bowl. Stir together until well combined.

3. Dump out onto a baking sheet lined with parchment paper and spread into a single layer. Bake for 5 minutes; flip and bake another 5 minutes. Remove from oven and let cool.

4. Sprinkle with chocolate chips once cooled. Store in an airtight container in the fridge. Enjoy with milk, almond milk, ice cream, or on yogurt.

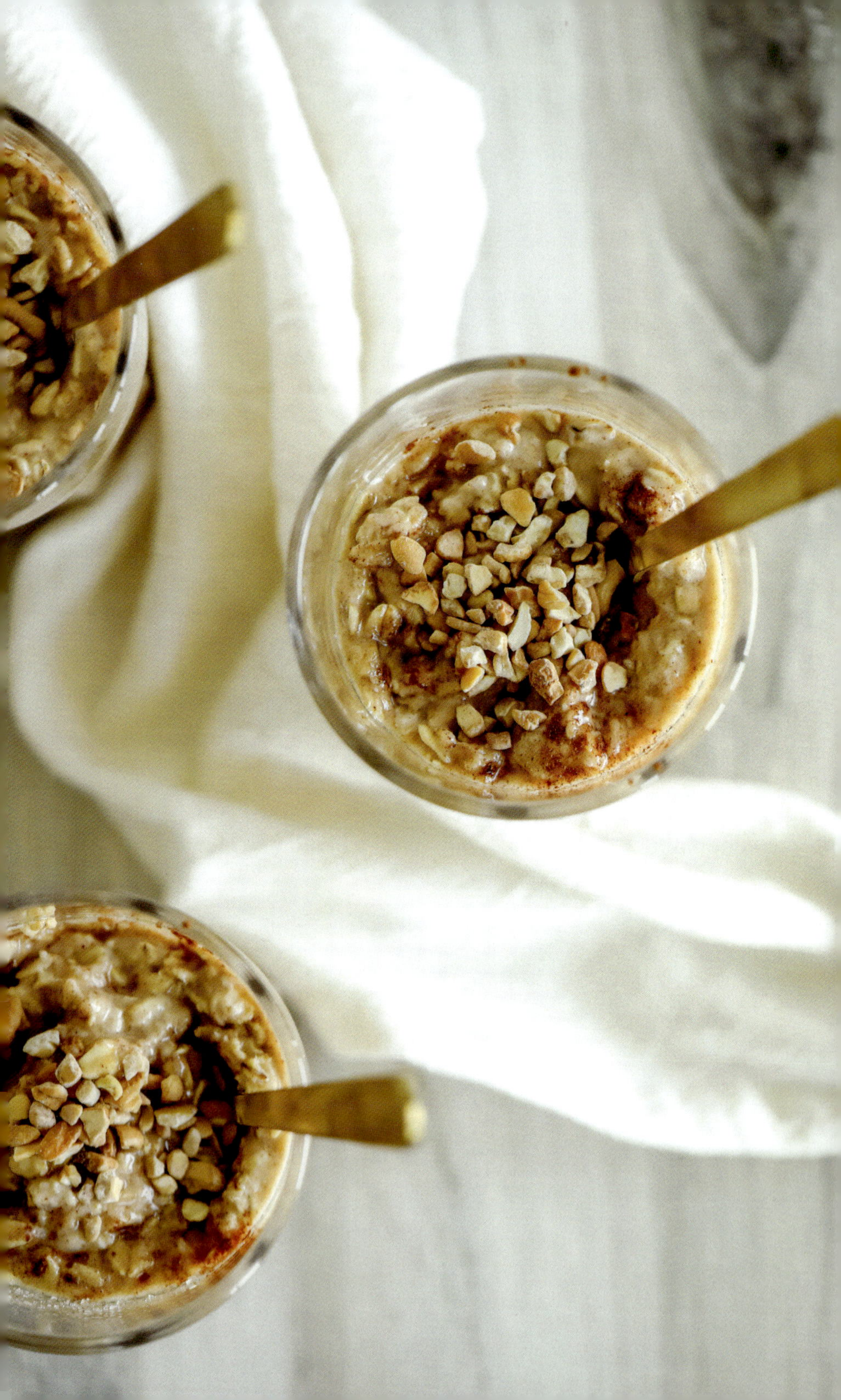

SNICKERDOODLE OVERNIGHT OATS

Makes 1 serving
365 calories / 13F / 37C / 25P

½ cup old-fashioned rolled oats
½ serving (16g) CSE Snickerdoodle Protein Powder
1 cup unsweetened vanilla almond milk
¼ cup plain, nonfat Greek yogurt
1 Tbs. (14g) OffBeat Cinnamon Bun Butter
Toppings:
½ Tbs. chopped pecans
½ tsp. turbinado sugar
Dash cinnamon

1. Add all the ingredients to a mason jar, cup or container. Mix until well combined.

2. Top with pecans, sugar and cinnamon. Cover and store in the fridge overnight.

3. Enjoy cold the next day. Store in the fridge up to 5 days. Enjoy!

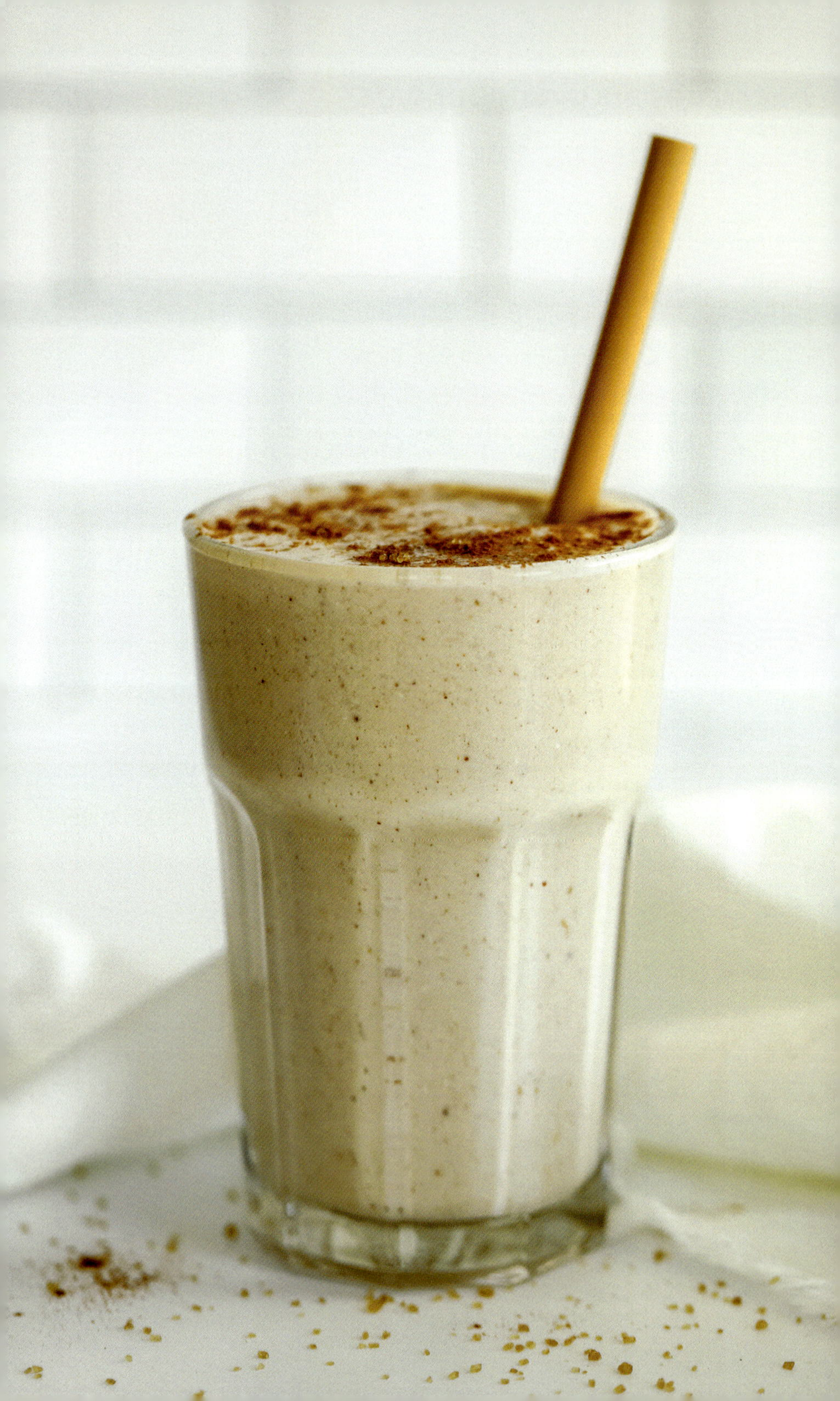

SNICKERDOODLE COOKIE SHAKE
Makes 1 serving
340 calories / 11F / 34C / 26P

---

1 cup unsweetened cashew milk
1 serving CSE Snickerdoodle Protein Powder
40g frozen banana slices
2 Tbs. old-fashioned rolled oats
18g OffBeat Cinnamon Bun Butter
6-8 (120g) ice cubes
Toppings:
Dash cinnamon
Pinch turbinado sugar

1. Add all of the shake ingredients to a high-powered blender. Blend on high until smooth. Pour into a cup.

2. Top with cinnamon and sugar. Enjoy!

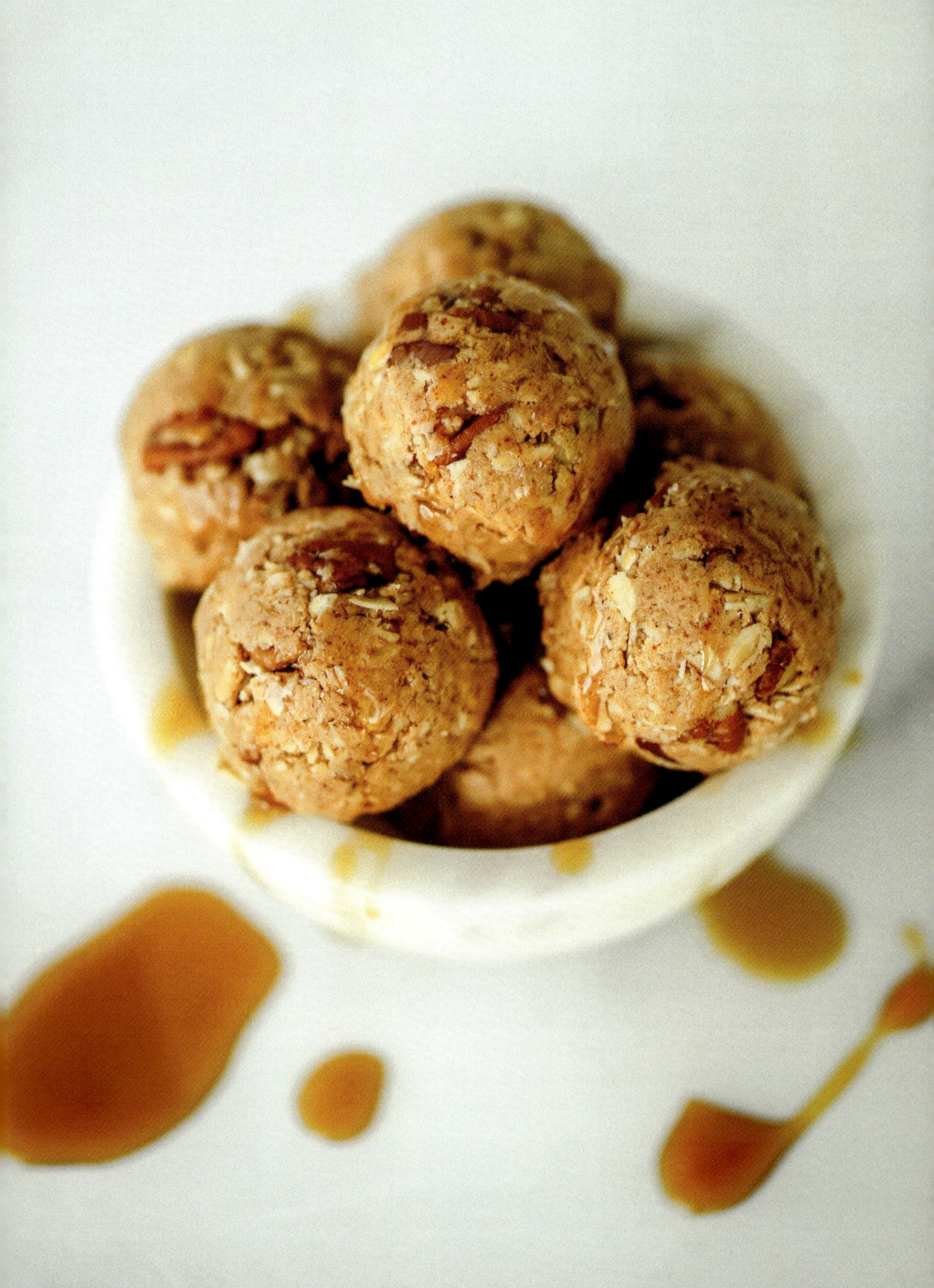

STICKY PECAN BITES
Makes 24 servings
100 calories / 5F / 11C / 3P / per bite

---

1 cup OffBeat Cinnamon Bun Butter
½ cup raw honey or pure maple syrup
1 serving CSE Cinnamon Roll Protein Powder
1 ½ cups old-fashioned rolled oats
Dash sea salt
2 Tbs. pecans
Topping:
1 Tbs. pure maple syrup

1. Add all the ingredients to a large bowl and mix until well combined.

2. Using a small cookie scoop, scoop into balls and place in a container. Drizzle one tablespoon of maple syrup over the top of all the bites. Cover and store in the fridge or freezer.

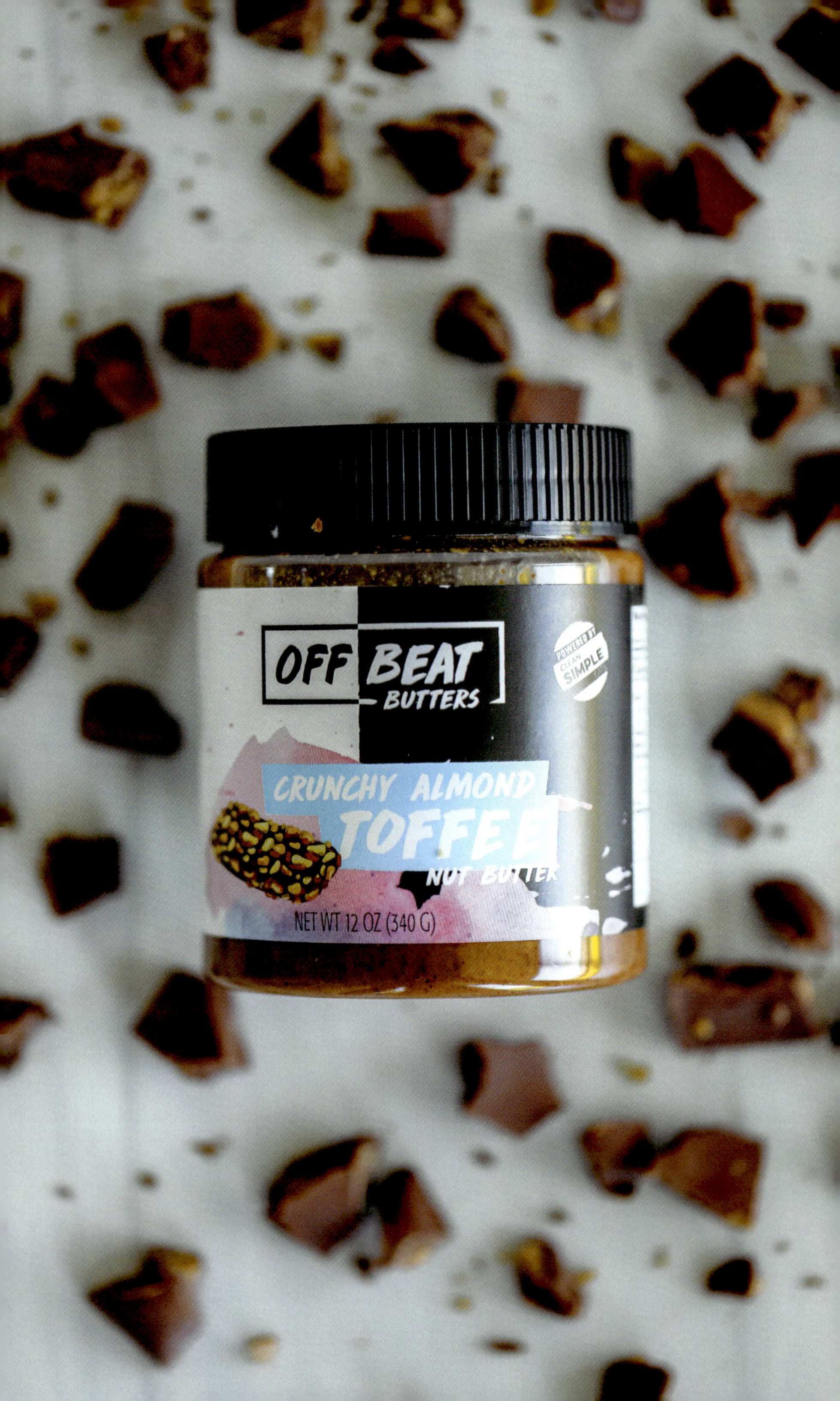
OFF BEAT BUTTERS
POWERED BY CLEAN SIMPLE
CRUNCHY ALMOND TOFFEE
NUT BUTTER
NET WT 12 OZ (340 G)

I'M NOT ADDICTED TO CHOCOLATE. CHOCOLATE IS ADDICTED TO ME.

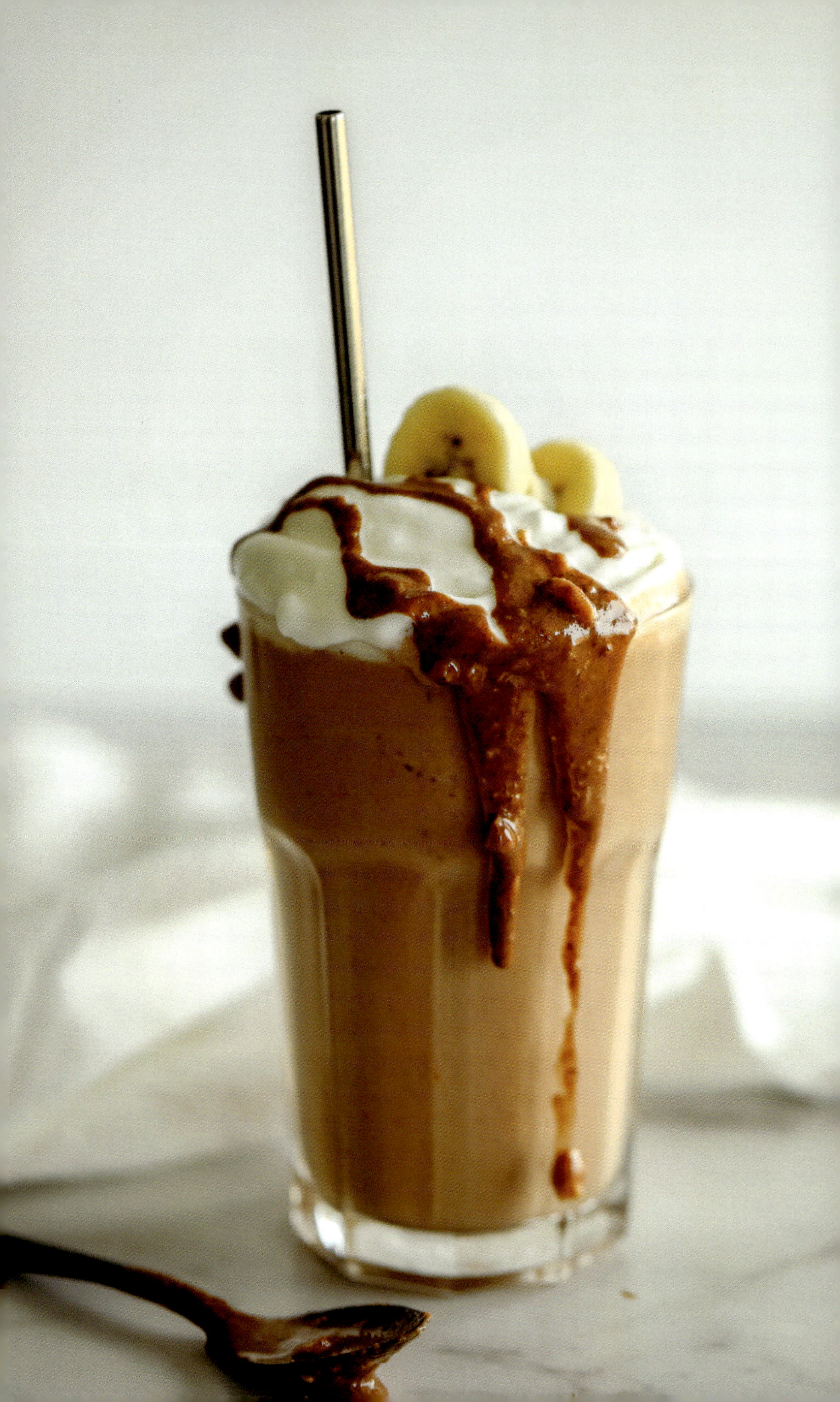

CHOCOLATE CARAMEL BANANA SHAKE
Makes 1 serving
350 calories / 13.5F / 33C / 27P

---

1 cup unsweetened almond milk
1 serving CSE Caramel Toffee Protein Powder
1 Tbs. (14g) OffBeat Crunchy Almond Toffee
   or Salted Caramel Butter
80g frozen banana slices
1 Tbs. low-fat cottage cheese
1 Tbs. cocoa powder
6-8 (120g) ice cubes
Topping:
2 Tbs. spray whipped cream

1. Add all of the ingredients to a high-powered blender. Blend on high until smooth.

2. Pour into a cup and top with whipped cream. Enjoy!

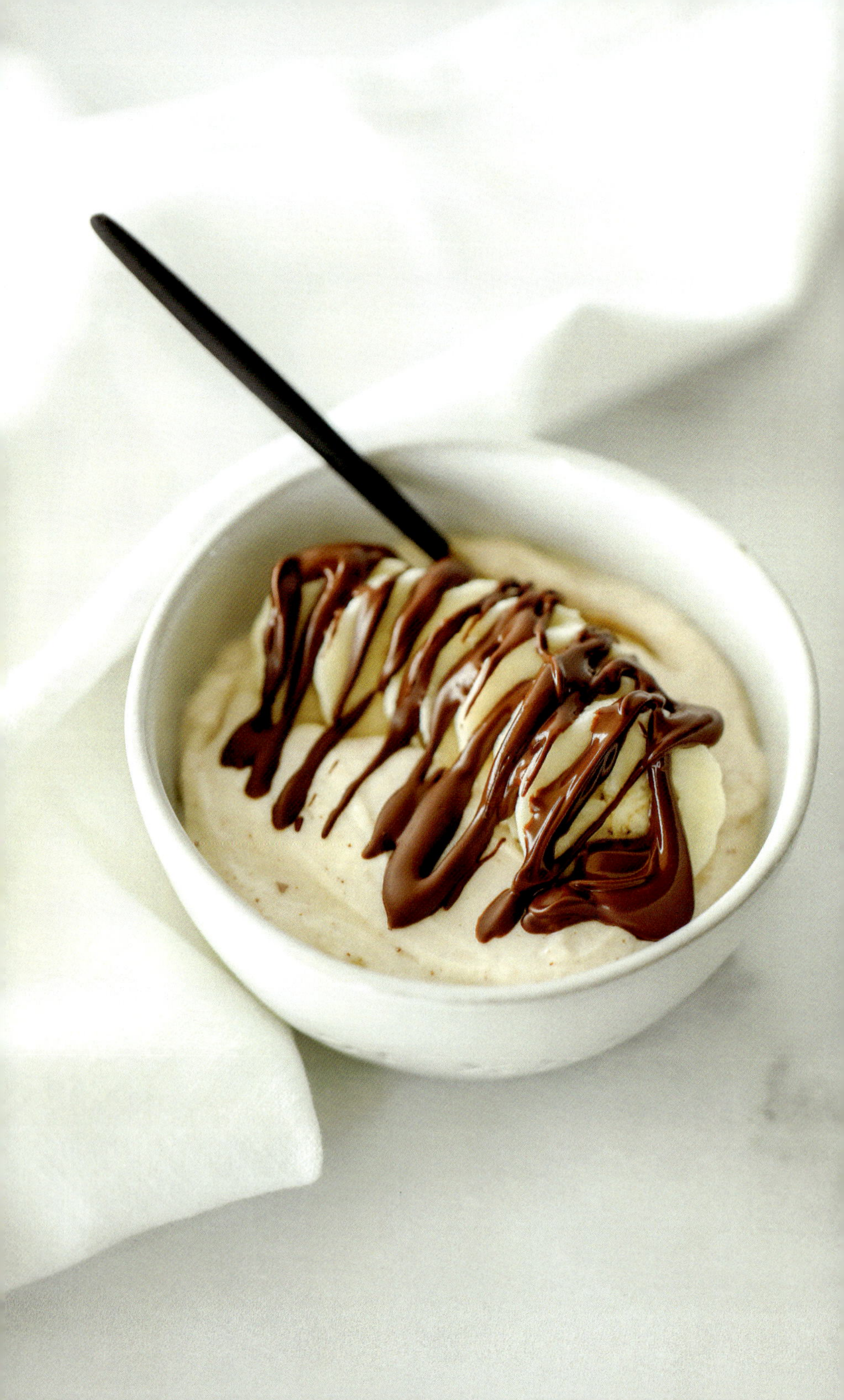

CHOCOLATE CARAMEL PROTEIN PARFAIT

Makes 1 serving
225 calories / 7.5F / 22.5C / 20.5P

½ cup nonfat, plain Greek yogurt
1 Tbs. unsweetened almond milk
10g CSE Caramel Toffee Protein Powder
½ Tbs. (7g) OffBeat Crunchy Almond Toffee Butter
45g bananas or 90g apples
2 tsp. mini chocolate chips

1. Add the Greek yogurt, almond milk, protein powder and Crunchy Almond Toffee Butter to a bowl. Stir until smooth.

2. Slice up a banana or apple. Top with sliced bananas or apples and mini chocolate chips. Enjoy!

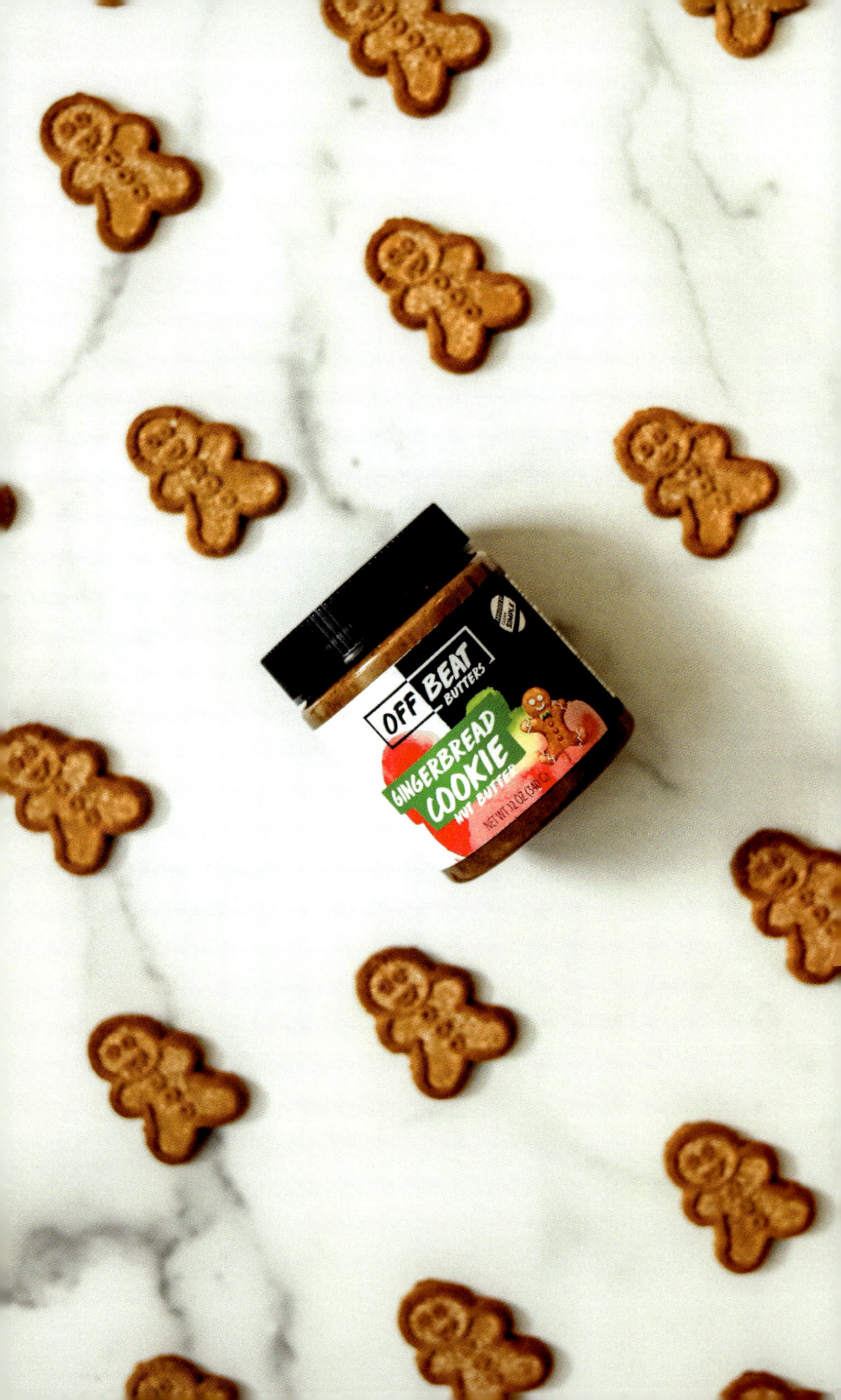
OFF BEAT BUTTERS
GINGERBREAD COOKIE
NUT BUTTER
NET WT 12 OZ (340 g)

SAVE A GINGERBREAD MAN; EAT THE BUTTER

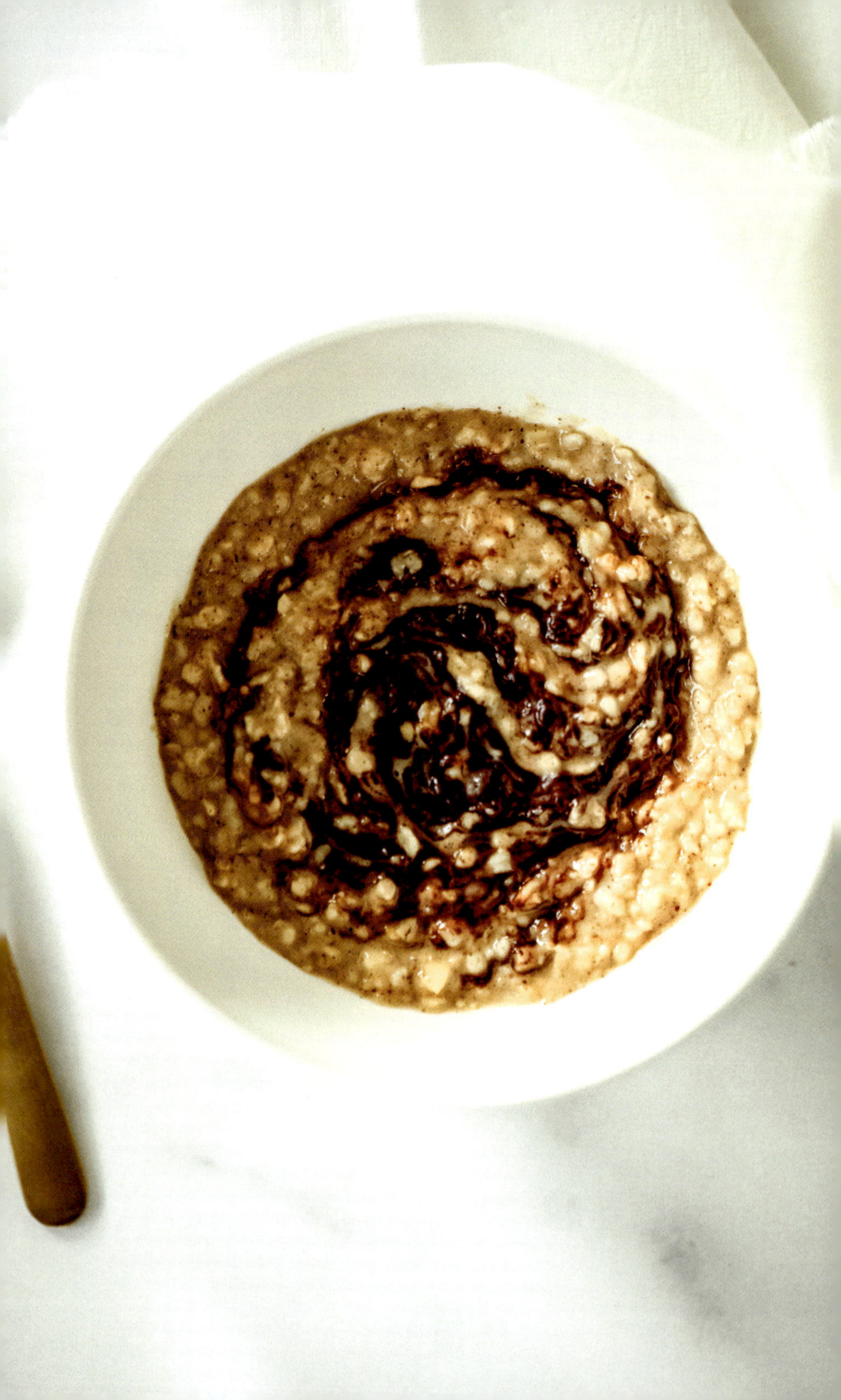

CARAMEL GINGY CHOCOLATE CHIP OATMEAL
Makes 1 serving
350 calories / 12F / 35C / 26.5P

⅓ cup old-fashioned rolled oats
½ cup water
3 Tbs. (46g) liquid egg whites
1 Tbs. (14g) OffBeat Gingerbread Cookie Butter
¾ serving (24g) CSE Caramel Toffee Protein Powder
Topping:
10g dark chocolate chips

1. Add the oats, water, and egg whites to a microwave-safe bowl. Whisk until the egg whites are well combined. Microwave for 1-2 minutes.

2. Stir in the Gingerbread Cookie Butter. Let cool for a couple minutes, then stir in the protein powder.

3. Top with chocolate chips. Enjoy!

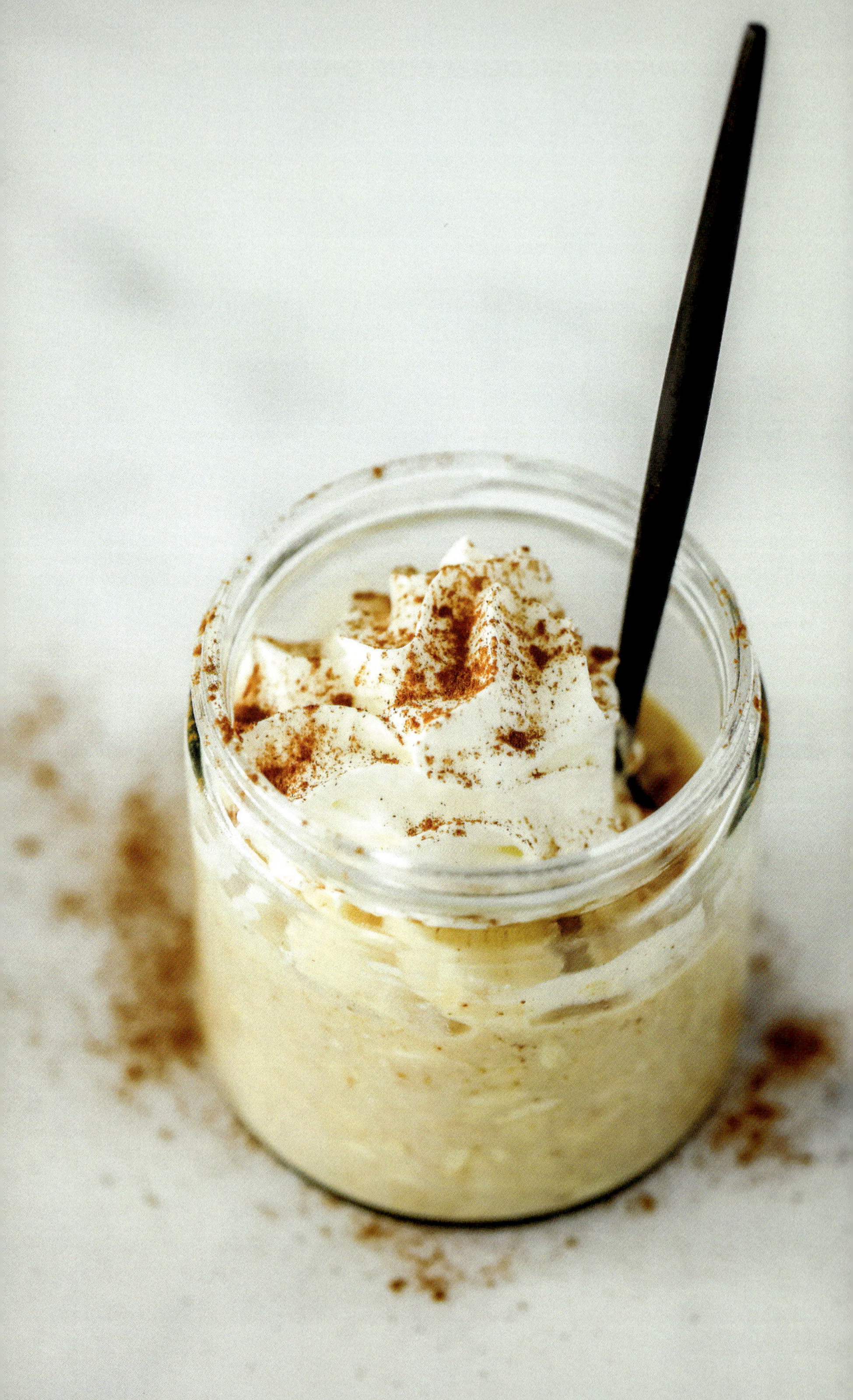

CHRISTMAS SPICED OVERNIGHT OATS
Makes 1 serving
355 calories / 11F / 44C / 22P

⅓ cup old-fashioned rolled oats
⅔ cup almond milk eggnog
¾ (24g) serving CSE Eggnog Protein Powder
1 Tbs. OffBeat Gingerbread Cookie Butter
20g banana slices
Toppings:
2 Tbs. spray whipped cream
Dash cinnamon

1. Add all of the ingredients to a bowl or a jar and mix well. Cover and refrigerate overnight.

2. Top with spray whipped cream and enjoy cold.

Stays in the fridge up to 5-7 days

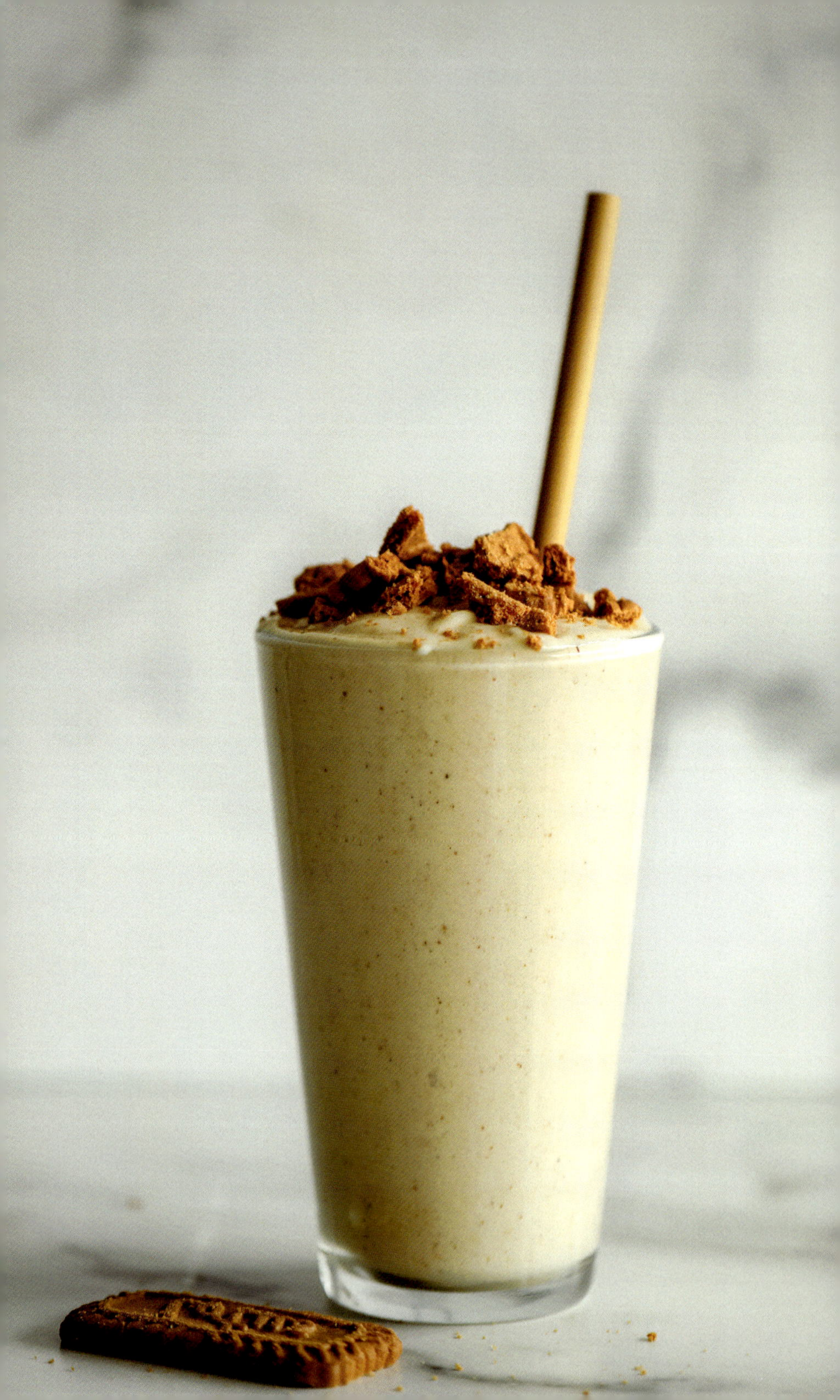

EGGNOG BISCOFF SHAKE

Makes 1 serving
390 calories / 14F / 37C / 30P

---

1 cup unsweetened almond milk
2 Tbs. Califia Farms Almondmilk Creamer Nog
1 serving CSE Eggnog Protein Powder
½ Tbs. OffBeat Gingerbread Cookie Butter
¼ cup low-fat cottage cheese
¼ tsp. xanthan gum
2 Biscoff cookies
150g ice cubes
Toppings:
2 Biscoff cookies

1. Add all ingredients to a high-powered blender. Blend on high until smooth.

2. Pour into a cup. Crumble the cookies on top and enjoy with a spoon.

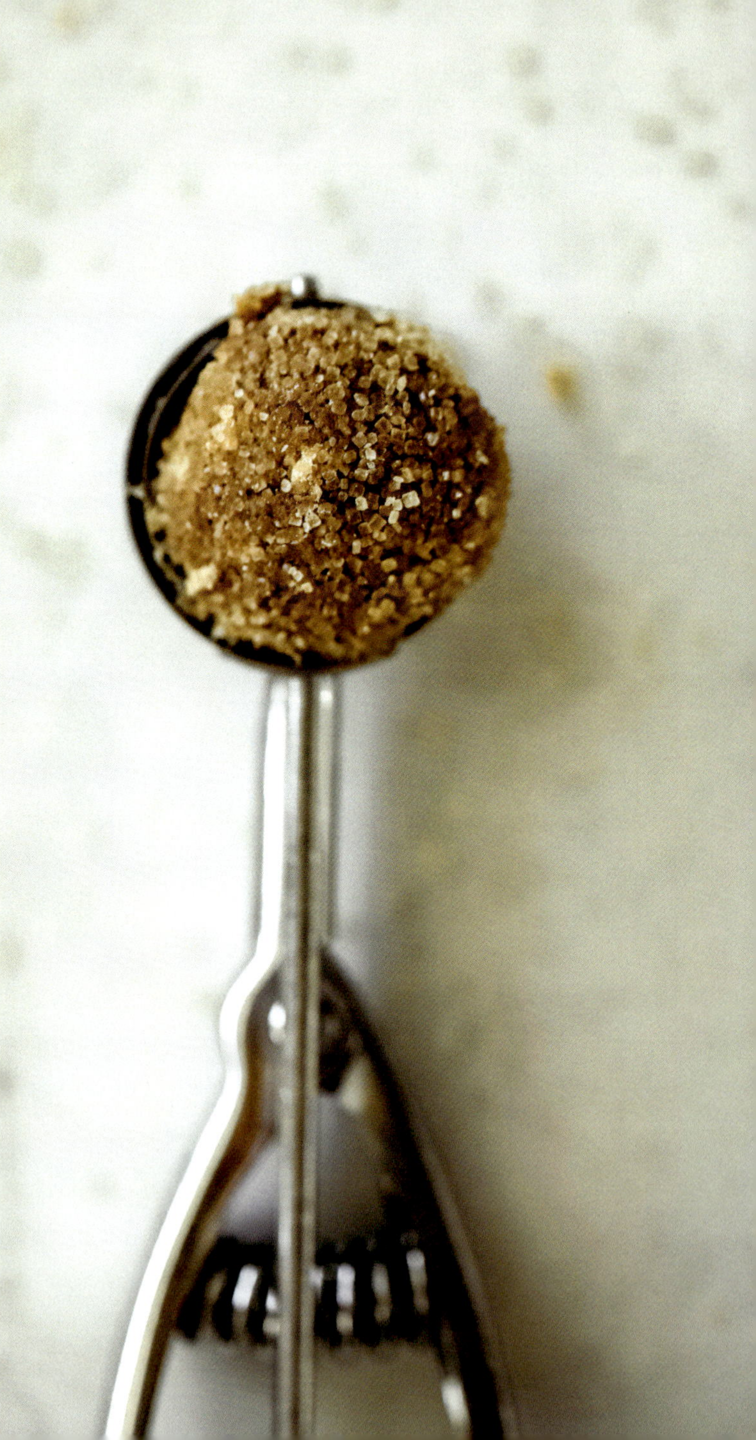

GINGERBREAD COOKIE BITES
Makes 26 servings
100 calories / 4F / 13C / 2.5P / per bite

---

1 cup OffBeat Gingerbread Cookie Butter
½ cup raw honey
1 serving CSE Simply Vanilla Protein Powder
Dash sea salt
1 ½ cups old-fashioned rolled oats
¼ cup turbinado sugar

1. Add the Gingerbread Cookie Butter, honey, protein, sea salt and oats together in a bowl. Mix until well combined.

2. Using a small cookie scoop, scoop into balls. Roll in sugar and store in the fridge or freezer. Enjoy!

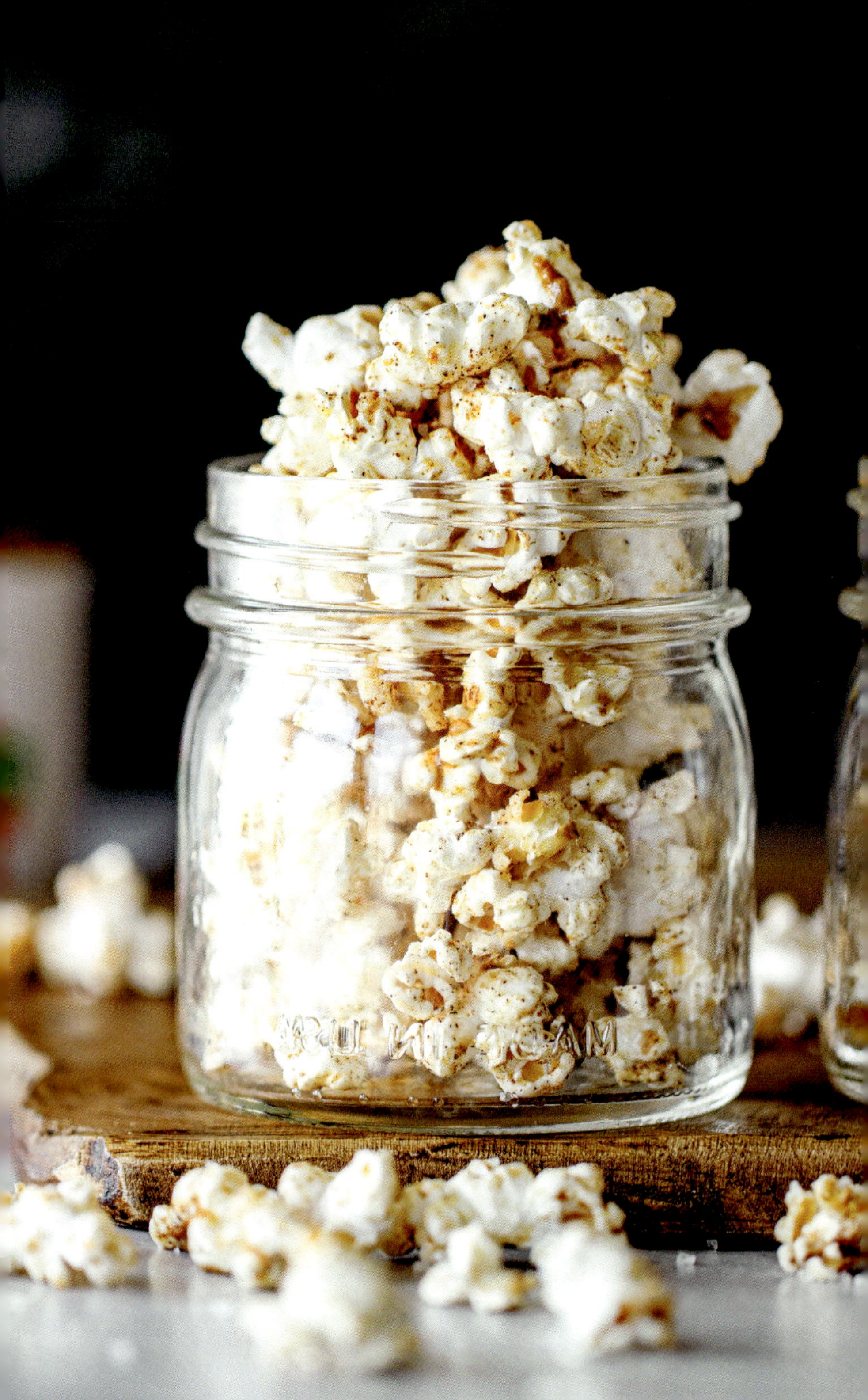

GINGERBREAD COOKIE POPCORN
Makes 4 servings
105 calories / 9F / 5C / 1.5P / per serving

½ cup popcorn kernels
2 Tbs. grass-fed butter
2 Tbs. OffBeat Gingerbread Cookie Butter
Dash cinnamon
Dash sea salt

1. Add the popcorn kernels to an air popper. Pop into a large bowl; set aside.

2. Add the butter to a small bowl and melt in the microwave for 10-20 seconds. Add the Gingerbread Cookie Butter to the melted butter and stir until combined.

3. Pour the butters over the top of the popcorn and toss to coat. Sprinkle with cinnamon & sea salt. Enjoy!

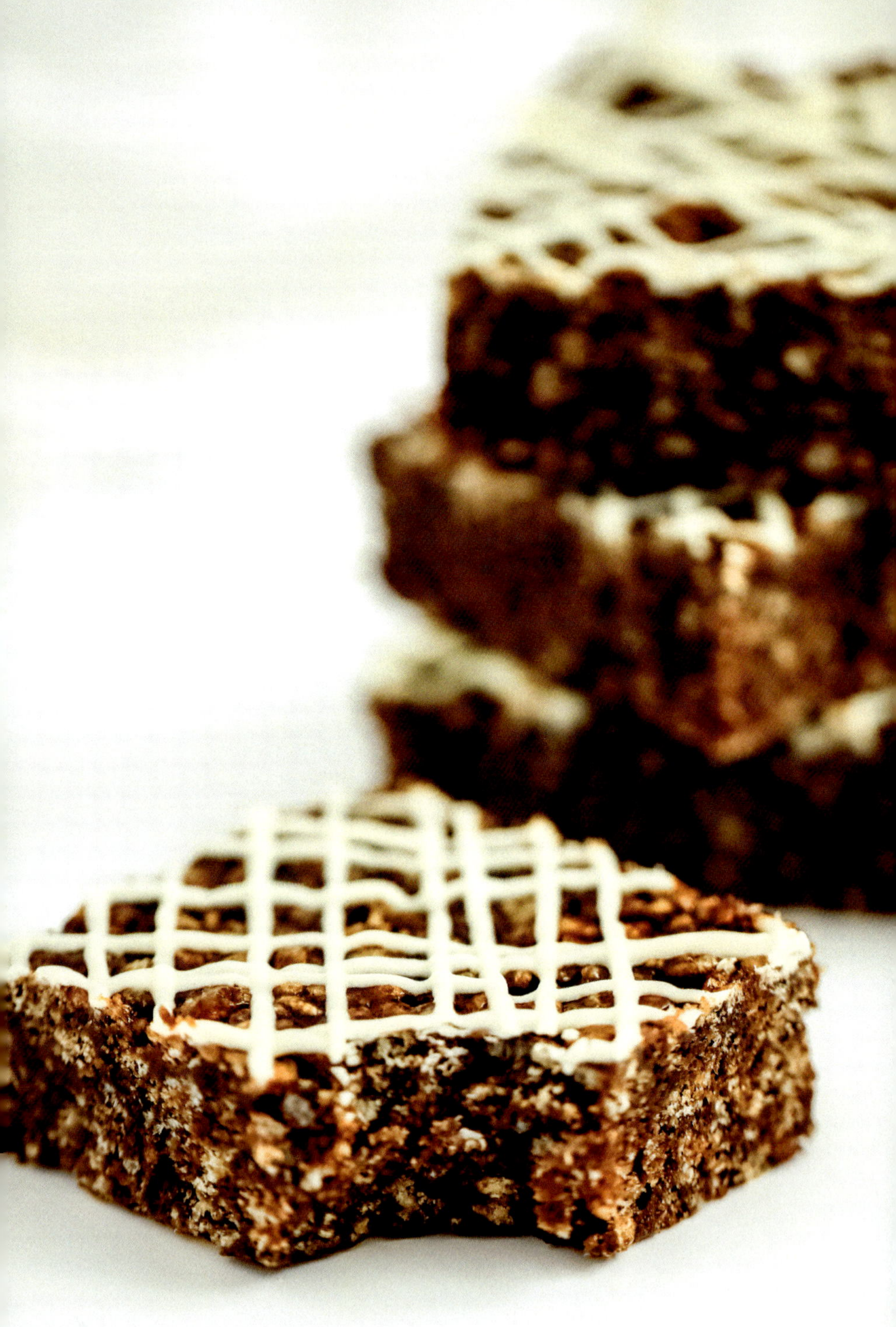

GINGERBREAD RICE KRISPIES *

Makes 9 servings
274 calories / 12F / 40C / 4P / per serving

---

4 cups Rice Krispies cereal
1 cup OffBeat Gingerbread Cookie
   or Cinnamon Bun Butter
½ cup honey
3 Tbs. molasses
1 tsp. vanilla
1 tsp. ginger
½ tsp. allspice
½ tsp. nutmeg
½ tsp. cloves
Melted white chocolate for drizzling, optional

1. Line and grease a 9×9 pan with parchment paper. In a large mixing bowl, add the Rice Krispies cereal.

2. In a small pot on the stove, add the Gingerbread Cookie Butter, honey and molasses and stir until well combined. While stirring, bring the mixture to a low simmer and then immediately take off the heat and stir in the vanilla, ginger, allspice, nutmeg, and cloves.

3. Pour the wet ingredients over the Rice Krispies cereal and stir together well, until all of the cereal is well coated with the mixture.

4. Pour the gingerbread Rice Krispies into a pan and spread them evenly across the pan, so the top is smooth and as flat as possible. Press into the pan. Drizzle with white chocolate, if desired. Enjoy!

**OffBeat Fam Recipe Submitted by Alex Daynes*

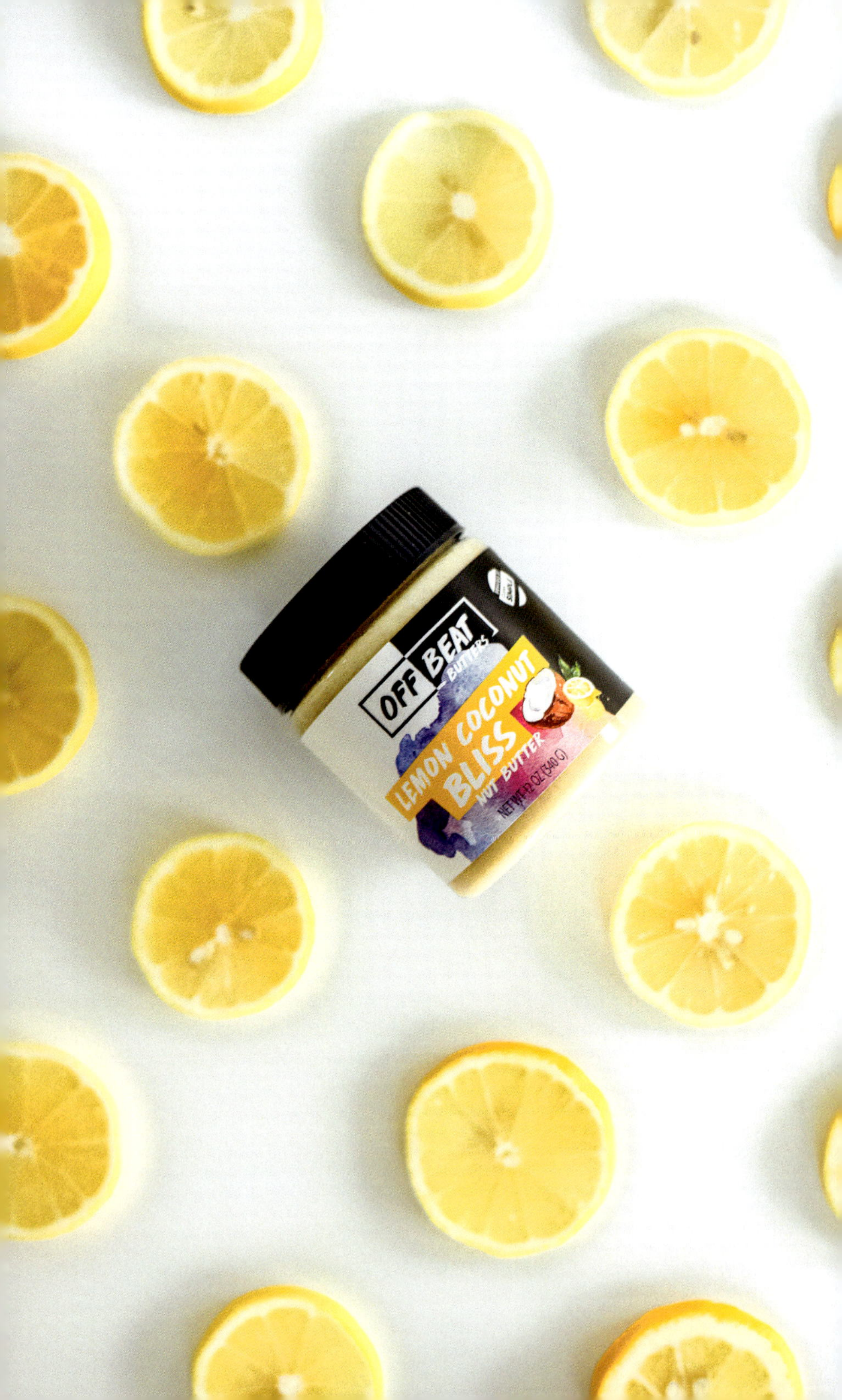

OFF BEAT
BUTTERS
LEMON COCONUT
BLISS
NUT BUTTER
NET WT 12 OZ (340 G)

WHEN LIFE GIVES YOU OFFBEAT BUTTER, EAT IT ALL AND HIDE THE EVIDENCE

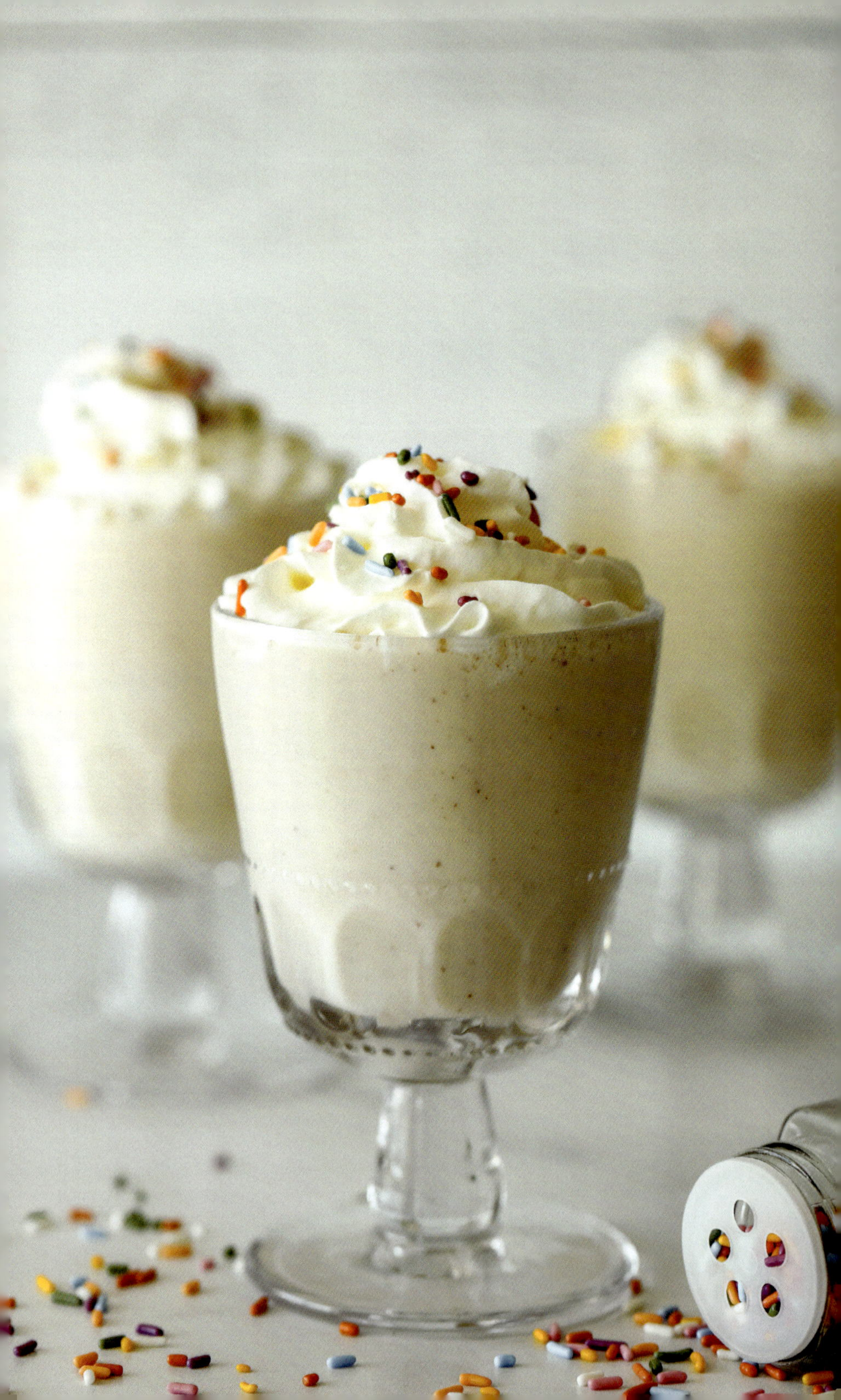

BIRTHDAY CAKE MILKSHAKE
Makes 1 serving
245 calories / 9F / 23C / 17.5P

¾ cup unsweetened almond milk
½ serving CSE Birthday Cake Protein Powder
   or Simply Vanilla Protein Powder
½ cup birthday cake or vanilla high-protein ice cream
½ Tbs. (7g) OffBeat Aloha, Salted Caramel,
   or Lemon Coconut Bliss Butter
8-10 (120g) ice cubes
Toppings:
2 Tbs. spray whipped cream
1 tsp. sprinkles

1. Add all of the ingredients to a high-powered blender. Blend on high until smooth.

2. Pour into a cup. Top with whipped cream and sprinkles. Enjoy!

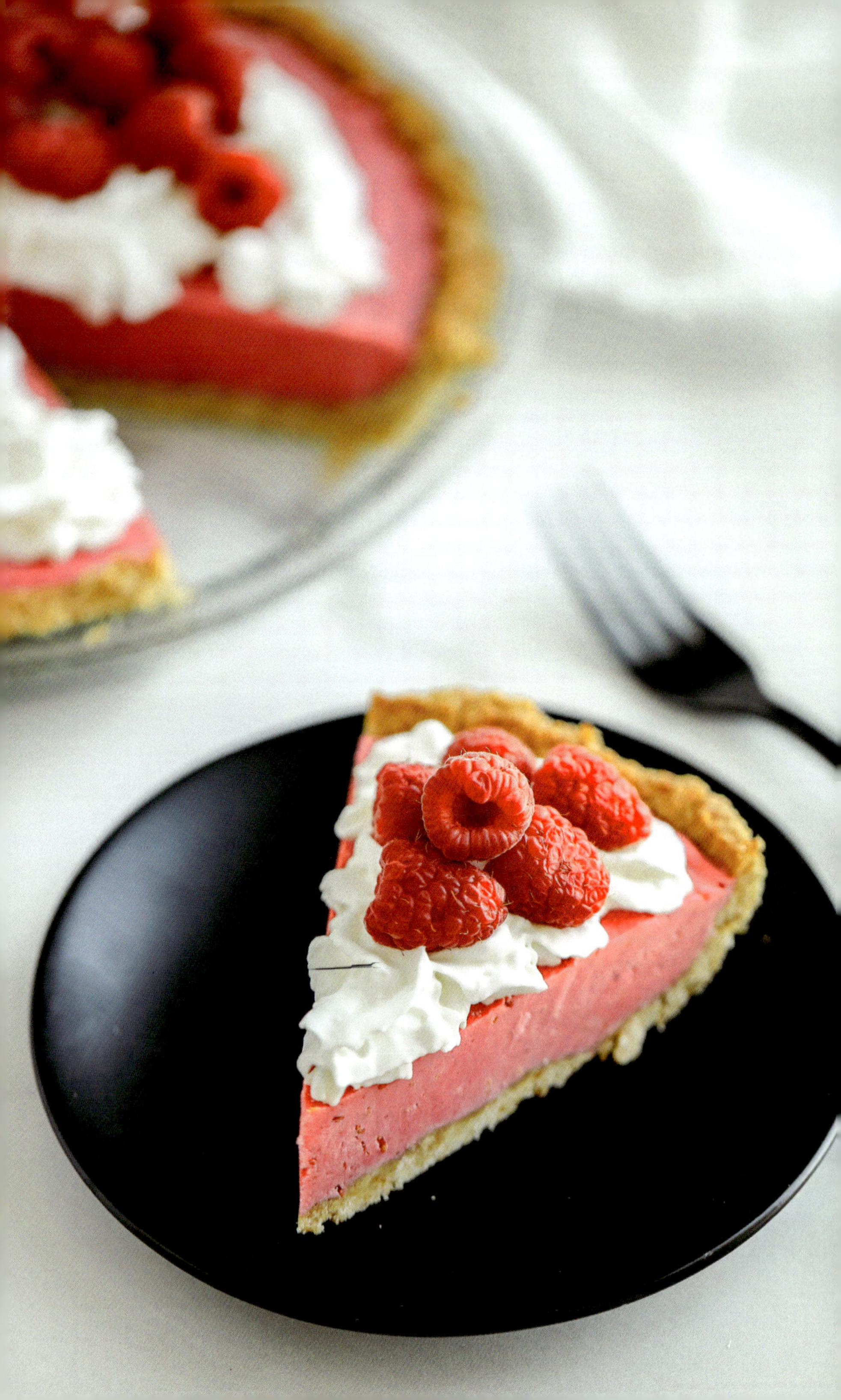

FROZEN RASPBERRY SORBET PIE
Makes 8 servings
300 calories / 15F / 21.5C / 4.5P / per serving

Pie Crust:
¼ cup OffBeat Lemon Coconut Bliss
  Butter or natural coconut butter
¼ cup melted grass-fed butter
¼ cup coconut sugar
½ serving (16g) CSE Simply
  Vanilla Protein Powder
2 Tbs. flaxseed meal
1 cup almond flour
½ tsp. vanilla extract
¼ tsp. sea salt

Pie Filling:
1 cup canned coconut cream
2 Tbs. pure maple syrup
2 cups fresh raspberries
¼ cup xylitol natural
  sweetener
½ Tbs. fresh lemon juice
Toppings per serving:
2 Tbs. spray whipped cream
6 fresh raspberries

1. Preheat the oven to 400 degrees.

2. Add the Lemon Coconut Bliss Butter, melted butter, coconut sugar, protein powder, flaxseed meal, almond flour, vanilla extract and sea salt to a large bowl. Mix until well combined.

3. Press the crust dough into the bottom and up the sides of a greased pie pan. Bake for 8-10 minutes. Remove from the oven and let cool completely.

4. Add the coconut cream, pure maple syrup, raspberries, xylitol and lemon juice to a blender. Blend until smooth.

5. Pour the mixture into the pie pan over the crust. Smooth out the top and freeze until firm.

6. Let thaw about 10-20 minutes before eating. Top each individual serving with whipped cream and fresh raspberries. Enjoy!

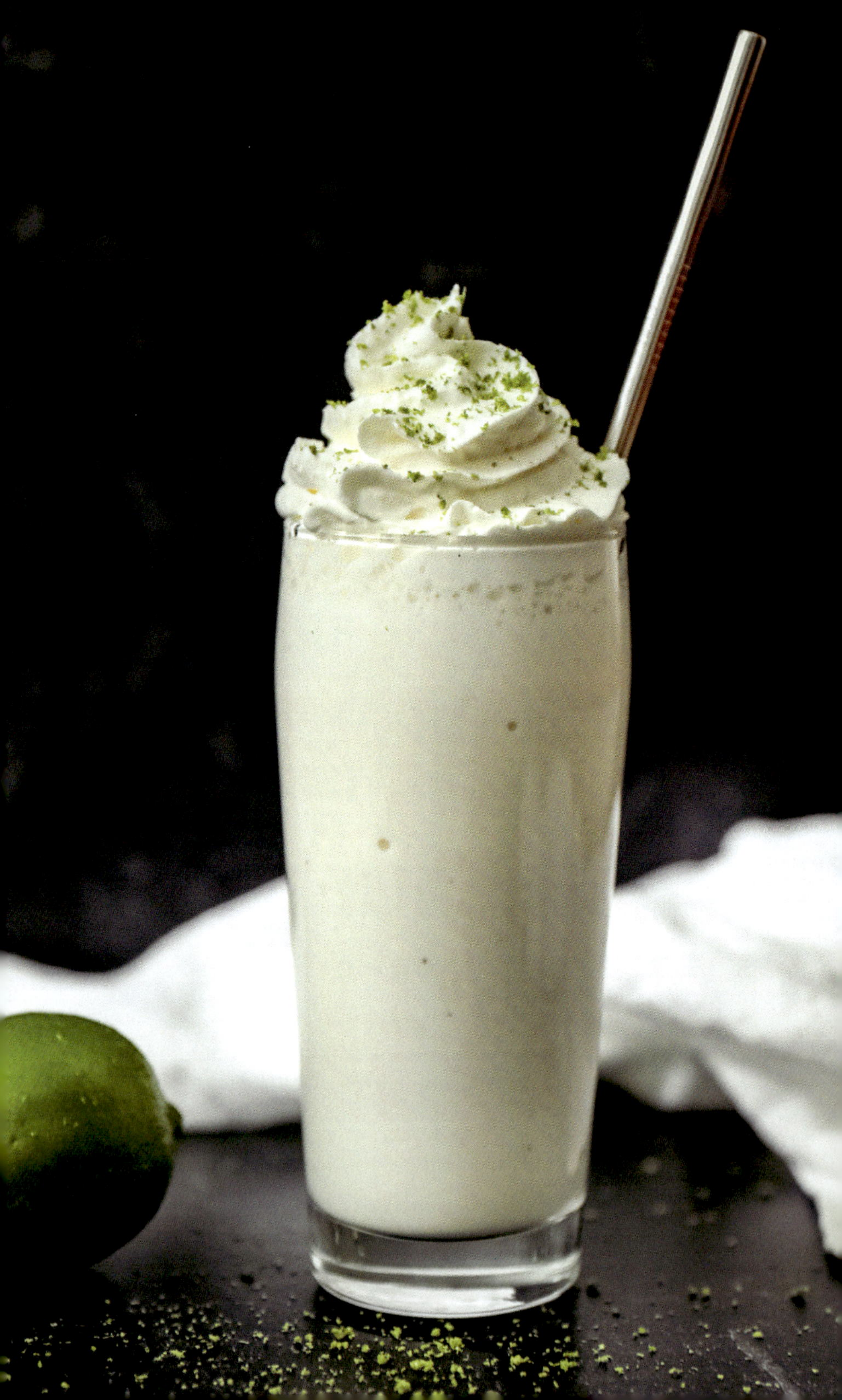

KEY LIME SHAKE*
Makes 1 serving
390 calories / 11F / 42C / 29P

½ cup fat-free milk
½ cup Key Lime Halo Top Ice Cream
30g frozen bananas
2 Tbs. CSE Bananas Foster
   or Simply Vanilla Protein Powder
1 Tbs. OffBeat Lemon Coconut Bliss Butter
6-8 ice cubes
Topping:
2 Tbs. spray whipped cream

1. Add all of the ingredients to a blender and blend until smooth.
Top with spray whipped cream.

OffBeat Fam Recipe Submitted by Becky Haugen

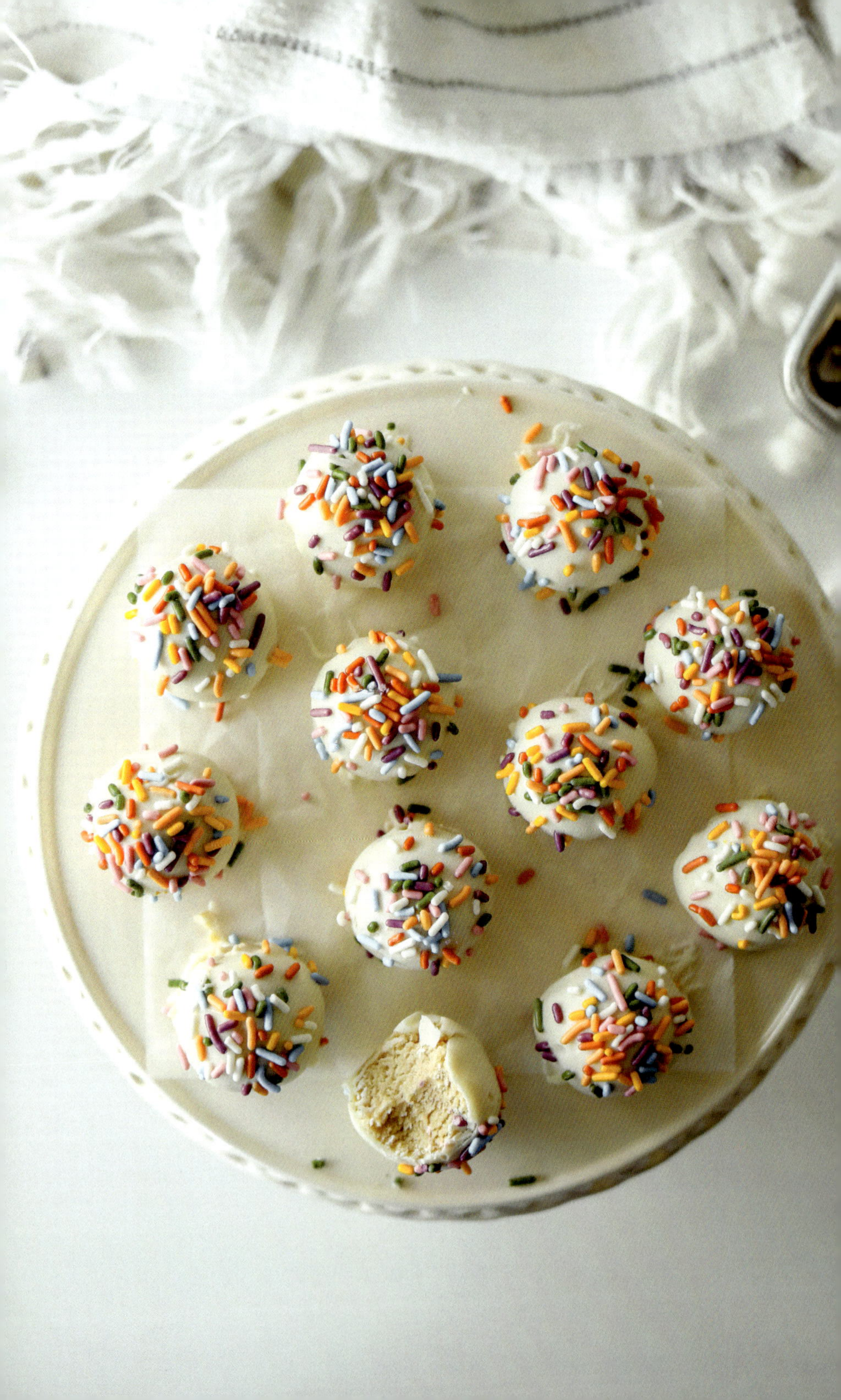

LEMON CAKE POPS

Makes 26 servings
150 calories / 9.5F / 12C / 4P / per cake pop

---

12 oz. OffBeat Lemon Coconut Bliss Butter
½ cup raw honey
2 servings CSE Cake Batter Protein Powder
1 cup almond flour
Pinch sea salt
Dash vanilla extract
Toppings:
50g white chocolate chips
1 Tbs. rainbow sprinkles

1. Add the Lemon Coconut Bliss Butter, honey, protein powder, almond flour, sea salt and vanilla extract to a bowl. Mix until well combined. Place in the fridge to harden for 30 minutes.

2. Remove from the fridge. Using a small cookie scoop, scoop into balls and place on a baking sheet lined with parchment paper. Return to the fridge while preparing the topping.

3. Add the white chocolate chips to a microwave-safe bowl. Heat for 30 seconds at a time until completely melted. Drizzle the melted chocolate over one ball at a time and immediately add the sprinkles, so they will stick to the chocolate before it hardens. Store in the fridge. Enjoy!

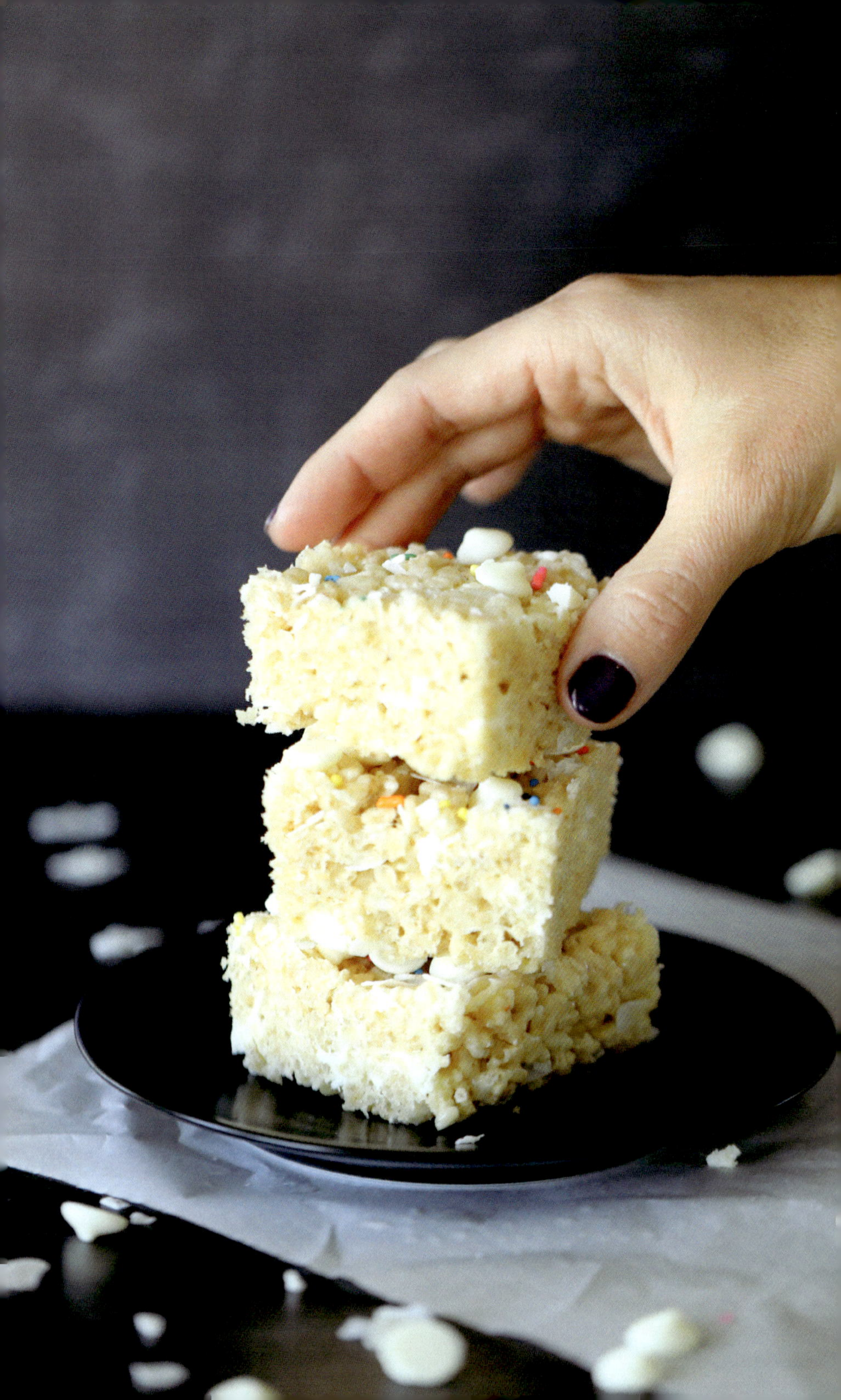

LEMON COCONUT RICE KRISPIE TREATS
Makes 12 servings
140 calories / 5F / 21C / 1.5P / per serving

½ cup OffBeat Lemon Coconut Bliss Butter
2-3 cups mini marshmallows
6 cups Rice Krispies cereal
¼ cup white chocolate chips
¼ cup unsweetened flaked coconut

1. In a large saucepan, melt the Lemon Coconut Bliss Butter over low heat. Add the marshmallows and stir until completely melted. Remove from heat.

2. Add Rice Krispies cereal to the saucepan. Stir until well coated. Fold in white chocolate chips and flaked coconut.

3. Spray a 9x13 baking pan with cooking spray. Pour mixture into the pan and press evenly. Let cool, then cut into squares.

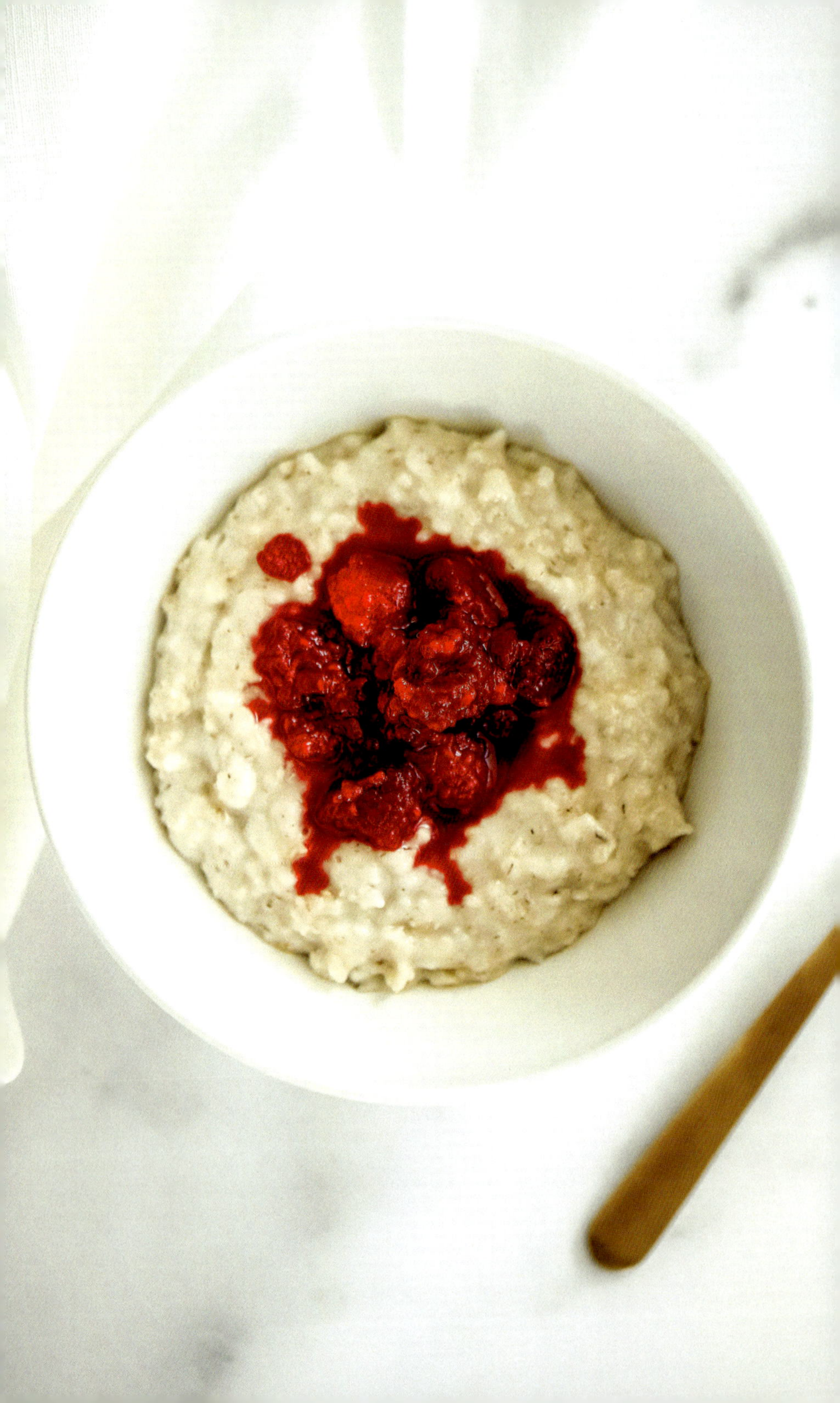

LEMON RASPBERRY BLISS OATMEAL
Makes 1 serving
330 calories / 9F / 38C / 26P

⅓ cup old-fashioned rolled oats
½ cup water
3 Tbs. (46g) liquid egg whites
50g frozen raspberries
1 Tbs. (14g) OffBeat Lemon Coconut Bliss Butter
¾ serving CSE Simply Vanilla Protein Powder

1. Add the oats, water, egg whites, and raspberries to a micro-wave-safe bowl. Whisk until the egg whites are well combined. Microwave for 1-2 minutes.

2. Stir in the Lemon Coconut Bliss Butter. Let cool for a couple minutes, then stir in the protein powder.

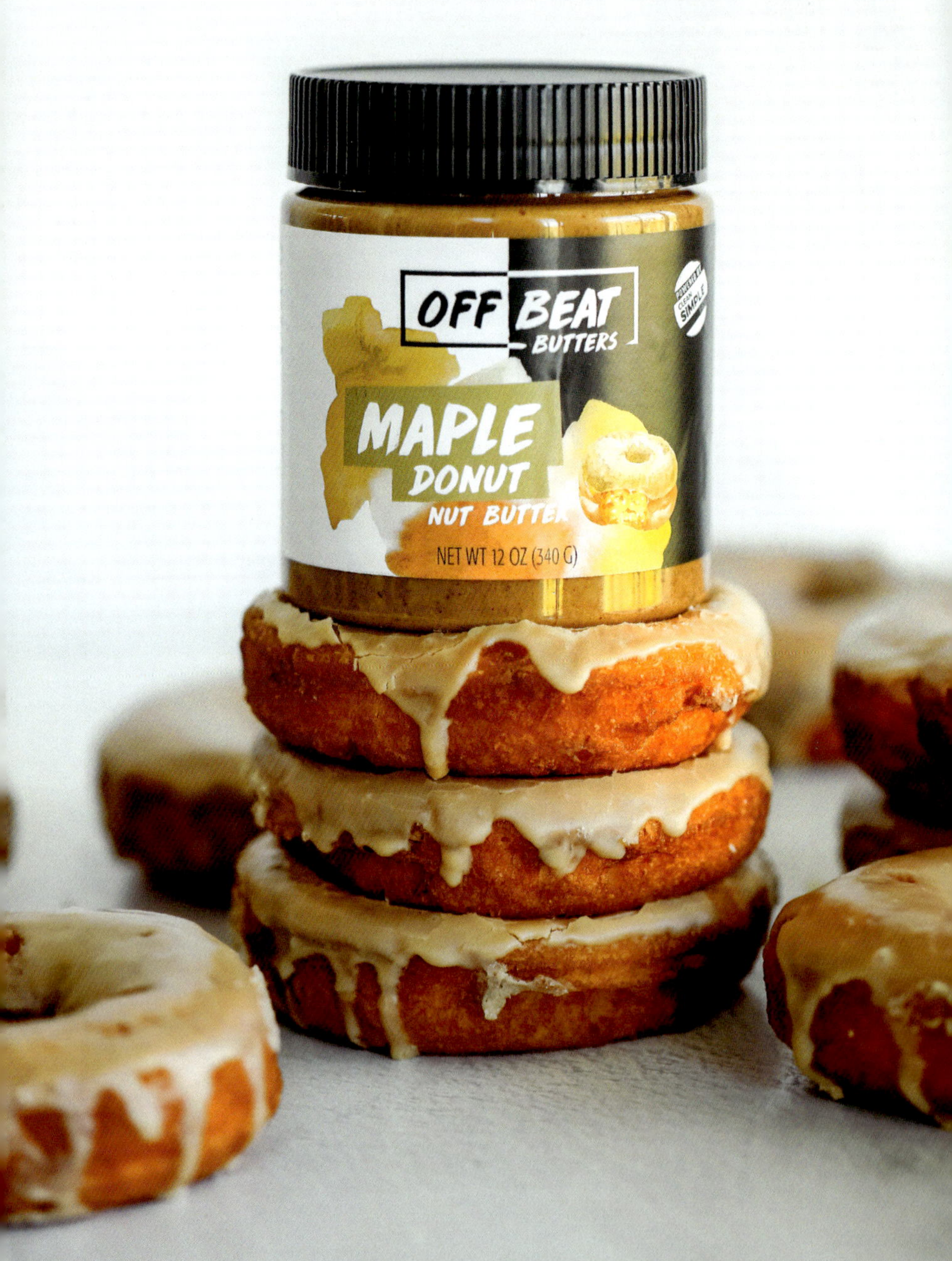

OFF BEAT
BUTTERS
POWERED BY CLEAN SIMPLE
MAPLE
DONUT
NUT BUTTER
NET WT 12 OZ (340 G)

YOU CAN'T BUY HAPPINESS, BUT YOU CAN BUY DONUTS AND THAT'S KIND OF THE SAME THING

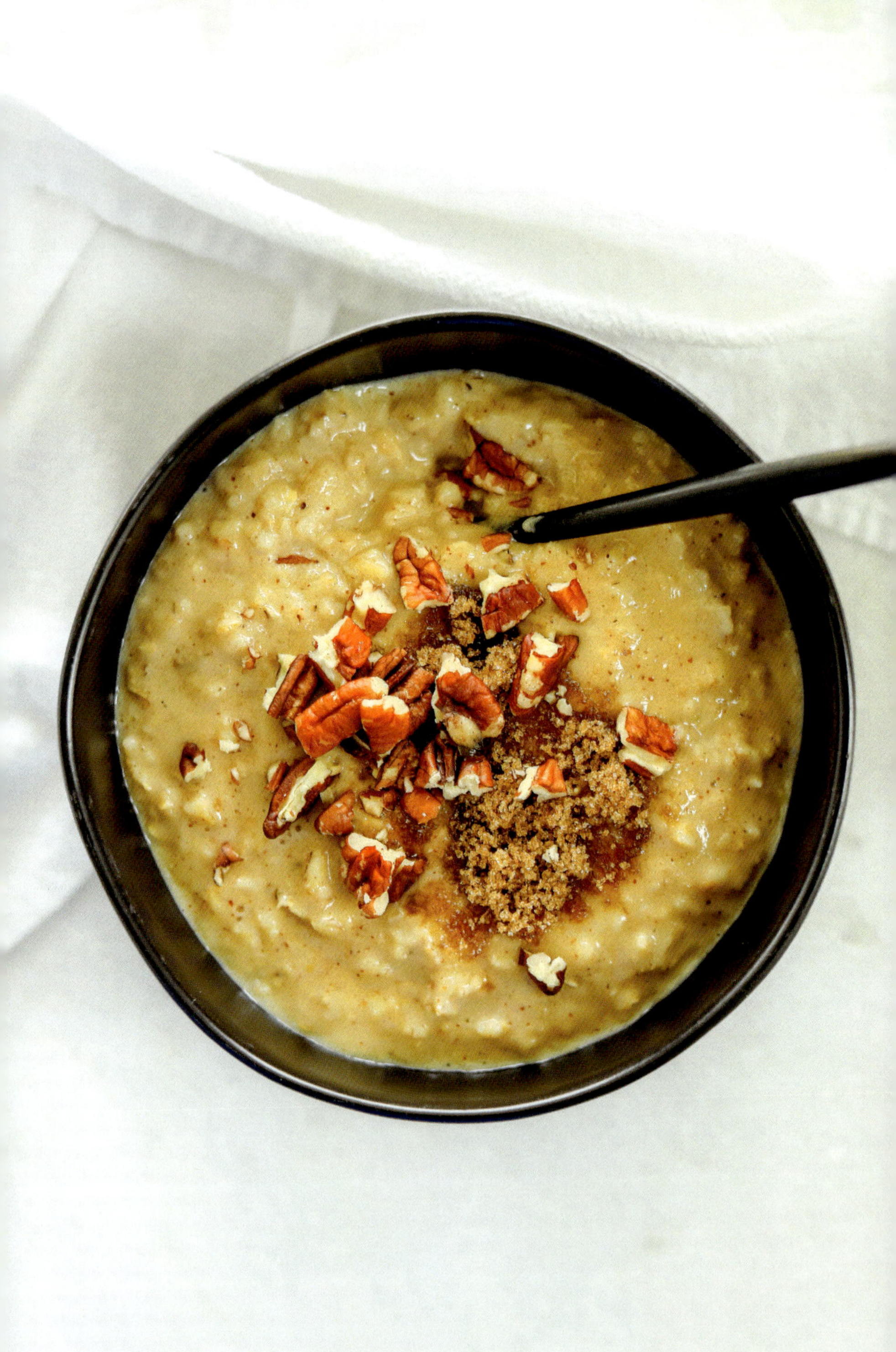

MAPLE BROWN SUGAR OATMEAL

Makes 1 serving
340 calories / 12F / 31C / 26.5P

⅓ cup old-fashioned rolled oats
½ cup water
30g liquid egg whites
14g OffBeat Maple Donut Butter
25g nonfat, plain Greek yogurt
Vanilla stevia drops, optional for sweetness
¾ serving (24g) CSE Maple Donut Protein Powder
Toppings:
1 Tbs. chopped pecans
1 tsp. coconut or brown sugar

1. Add the oats, water, and egg whites to a microwave-safe bowl. Whisk until the egg whites are well combined. Microwave for 1-2 minutes.

2. Stir in the Maple Donut Butter, yogurt and stevia until well combined. Let cool for a couple minutes, then stir in the protein powder.

3. Top with chopped pecans and sugar. Enjoy!

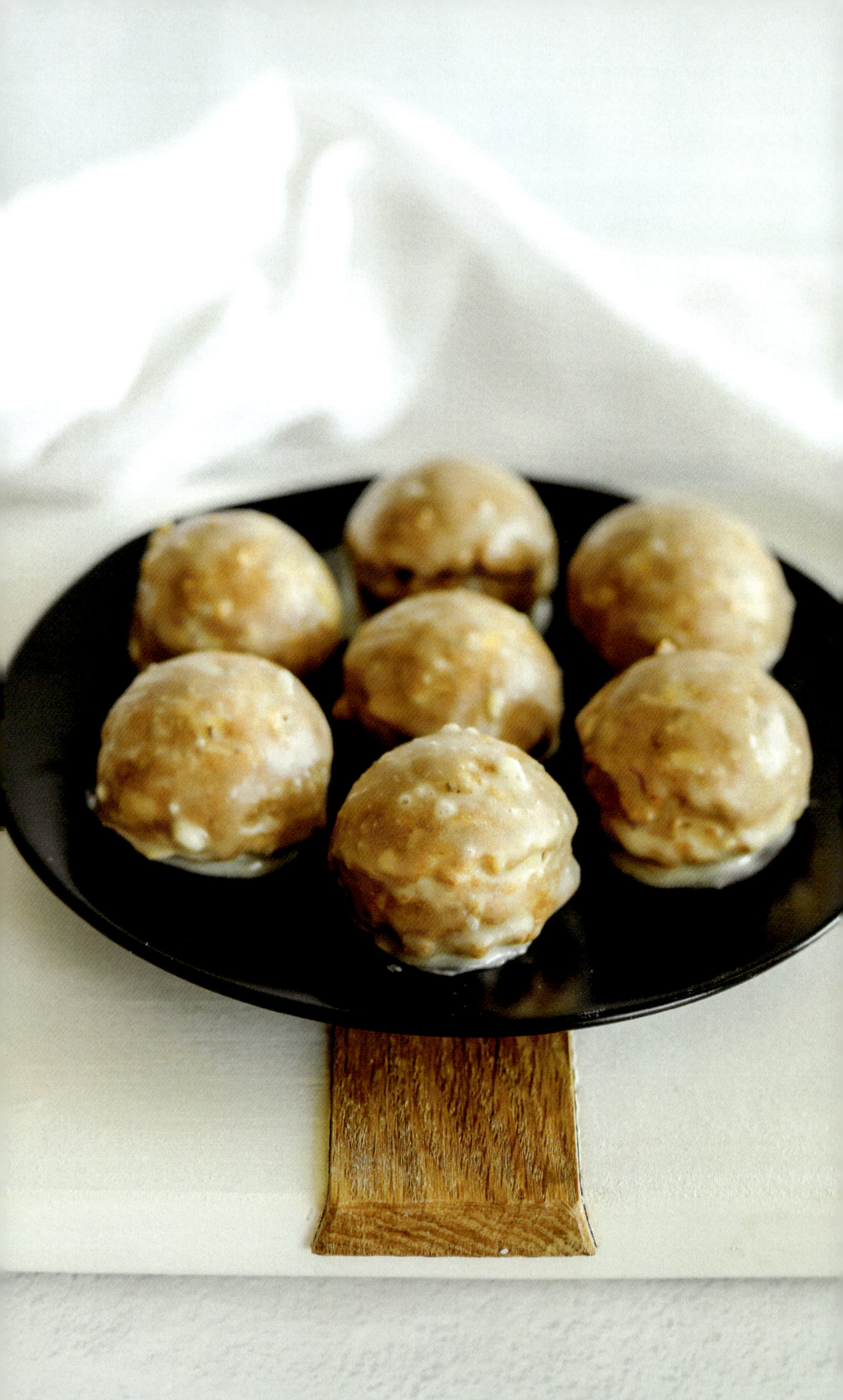

MAPLE DONUT HOLE POWER BITES
Makes 24 servings
110 calories / 5F / 14.5C / 3P / per bite

1 cup OffBeat Maple Donut Butter
½ cup raw honey
1 serving CSE Maple Donut Protein Powder
1 ½ cups old-fashioned rolled oats
Dash sea salt
Dash vanilla extract
Frosting:
½ cup powdered sugar
1 Tbs. liquid egg whites

1. Add the Maple Donut Butter, honey, protein powder, oats, sea salt and vanilla to a mixing bowl. Mix until well combined. Set aside.

2. In a small bowl, whisk together the powdered sugar and egg whites. Set aside.

3. Using a cookie scoop, scoop the power bite mixture into balls and place on a baking sheet lined with parchment paper. Drizzle the frosting over the top of each one and store in the fridge until the frosting hardens. Move all the bites to a container, cover and store in the fridge or freezer.

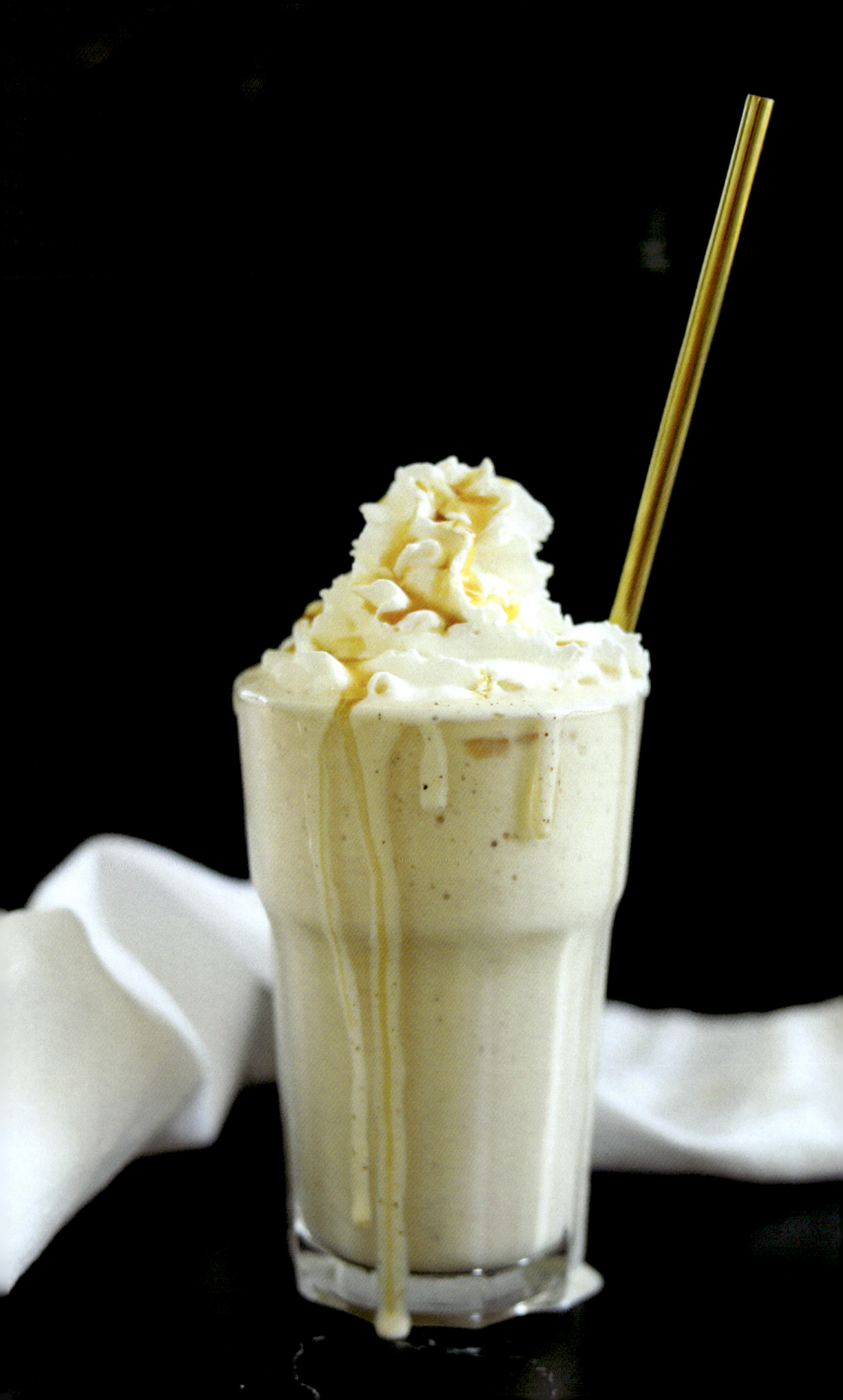

MAPLE DONUT MILKSHAKE
Makes 1 serving
340 calories / 10F / 35C / 27P

---

1 cup fat-free milk
1 serving CSE Maple Donut Protein Powder
20g OffBeat Maple Donut Butter
40g frozen banana slices
1 tsp. pure maple syrup
Dash sea salt
6-8 (120g) ice cubes

1. Add all of the ingredients to a blender. Blend on high until smooth. Pour into a cup and enjoy!

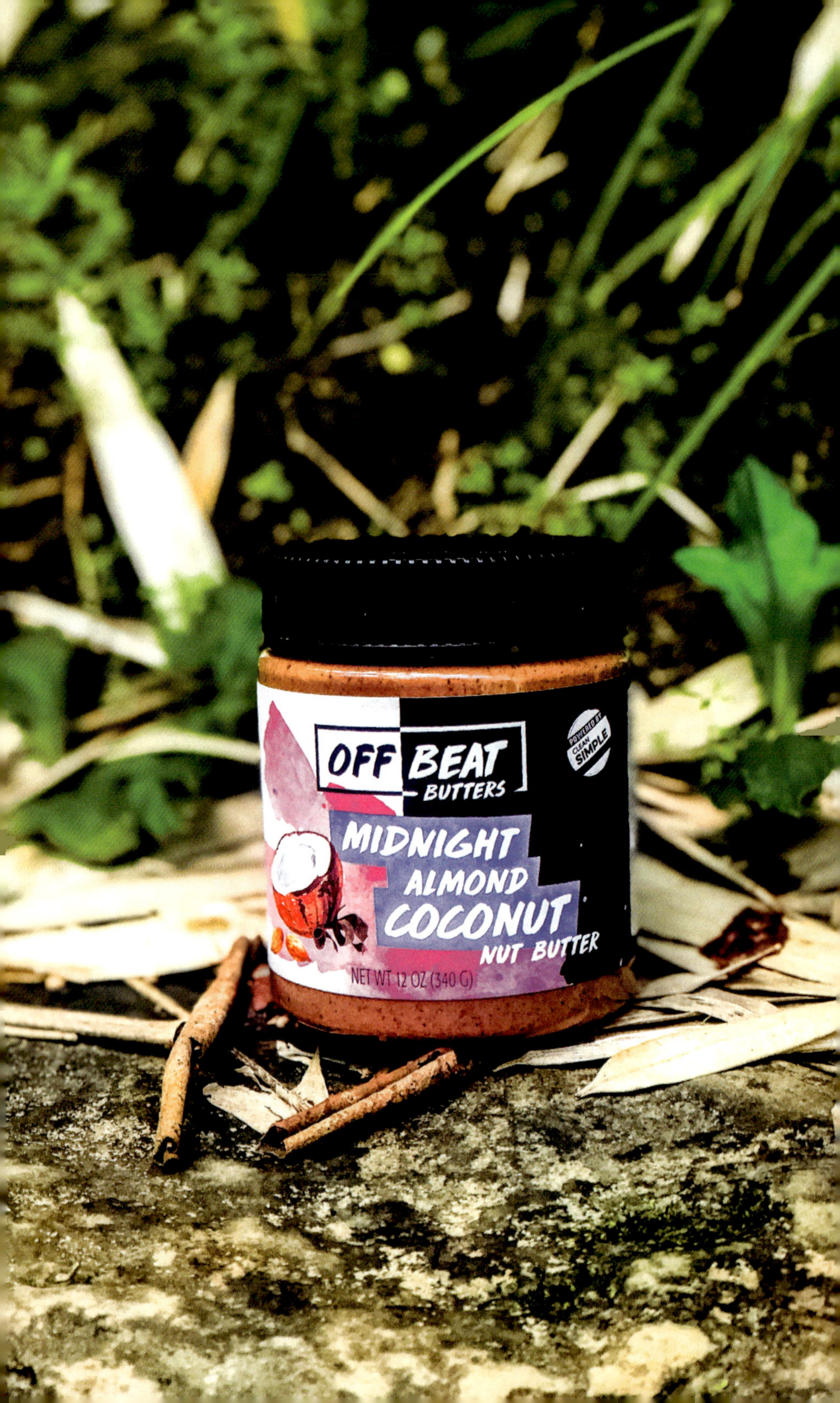
OFF BEAT
BUTTERS
POWERED BY
CLEAN SIMPLE
MIDNIGHT
ALMOND
COCONUT
NUT BUTTER
NET WT 12 OZ (340 G)

COME TO THE DARK SIDE... WE HAVE CHOCOLATE

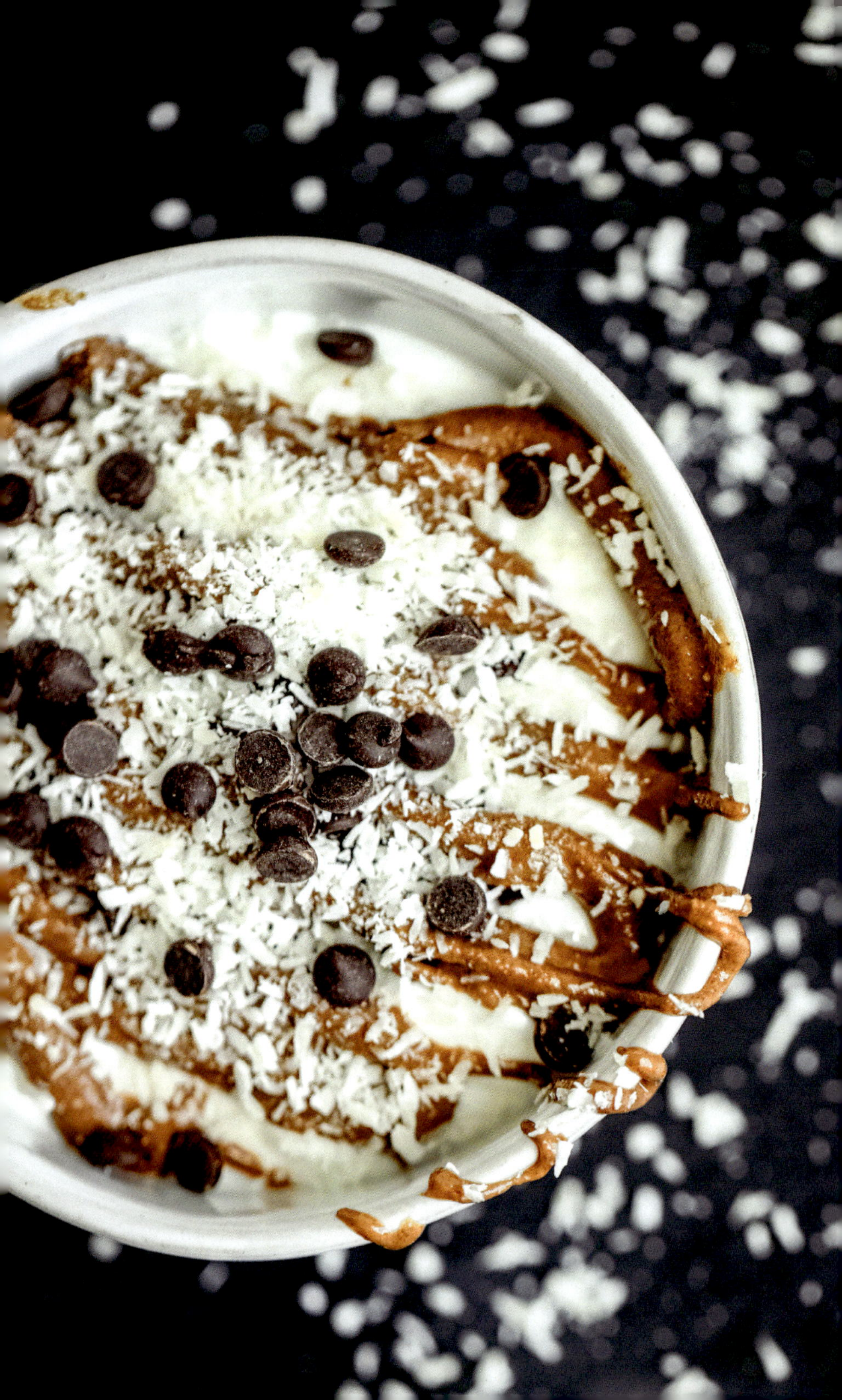

ALMOND JOY PARFAIT
Makes 1 serving
270 calories / 13F / 15C / 21P

¾ cup nonfat, plain Greek yogurt
Vanilla stevia drops, to taste
¼ tsp. coconut extract
Toppings:
1 Tbs. OffBeat Midnight Almond Coconut Butter
10g dark chocolate chips
5g shredded coconut

1. Add the Greek yogurt, stevia and coconut extract to a bowl. Stir until well combined.

2. Drizzle the Midnight Almond Coconut Butter over the yogurt, sprinkle with dark chocolate chips and shredded coconut. Enjoy!

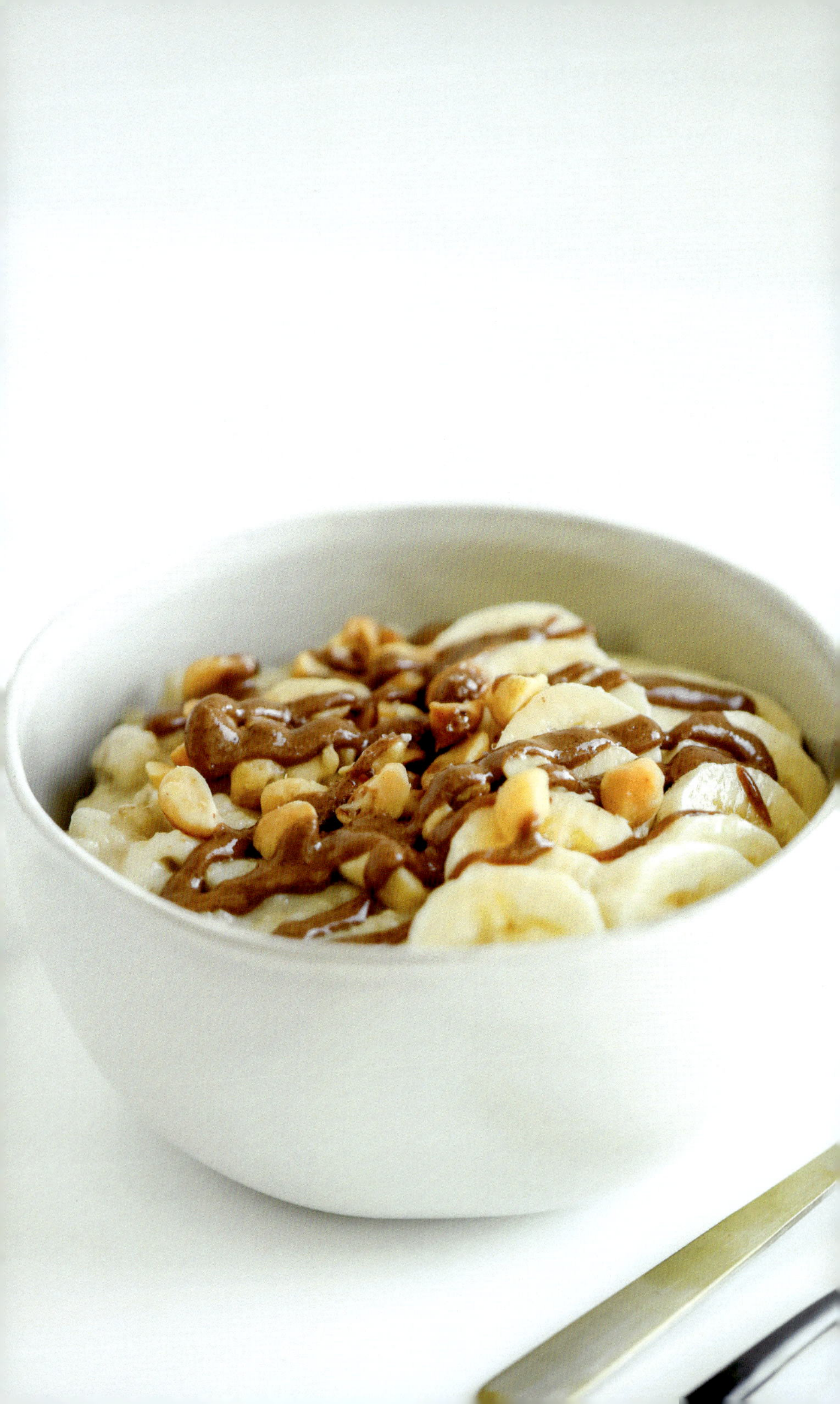

CHOCOLATE COCONUT MACADAMIA OATMEAL
Makes 1 serving
340 calories / 11.5F / 34C / 25.5P

⅓ cup old-fashioned rolled oats
½ cup water
3 Tbs. (46g) liquid egg whites
¾ serving (25g) CSE Coconut Cream Protein Powder
8g OffBeat Midnight Almond Coconut Butter
  or dark chocolate chips
Toppings:
40g sliced bananas
8g chopped macadamia nuts
Dash sea salt

1. Add the oats, water, and egg whites to a microwave-safe bowl. Whisk until the egg whites are well combined. Microwave for 1-2 minutes.

2. Stir in the Midnight Almond Coconut Butter. Let cool for a couple minutes, then stir in the protein powder.

3. Top with sliced bananas, macadamia nuts, and sea salt. Enjoy!

*To make the oatmeal extra chocolatey, add a dash of cocoa powder when you add the protein powder and stir until well combined.

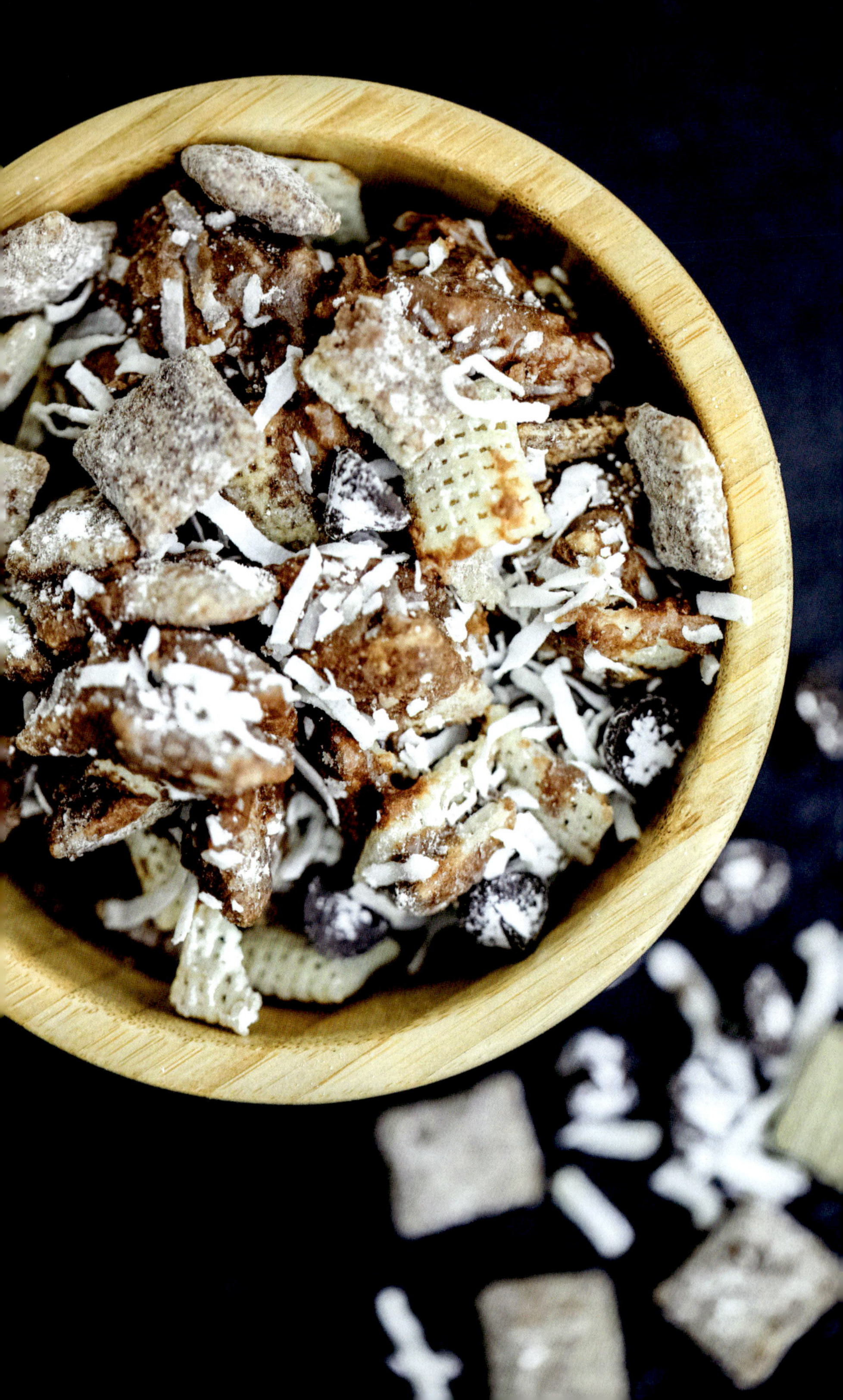

MIDNIGHT ALMOND COCONUT BUDDIES

Makes 16 servings
190 calories / 6.5F / 31C / 4P / per serving (½ cup or 45g)

¾ cup raw honey
½ cup OffBeat Midnight Almond Coconut Butter
1 serving CSE Brownie Batter Protein Powder
2 Tbs. cocoa powder
2 Tbs. powdered sugar
6 cups Chocolate Rice Chex cereal
¼ cup unsweetened shredded coconut
30g dark chocolate chips

1. In a small saucepan, melt together the honey and Midnight Almond Coconut Butter until smooth.

2. Place Chocolate Chex cereal into a large bowl. Pour hot mixture of honey and nut butter over the top and gently stir until cereal is well coated.

3. Pour the contents from the bowl into a large zip top bag. Add the protein powder, cocoa powder and powdered sugar to the bag. Seal the bag and shake well.

4. Add the shredded coconut and chocolate chips to the bag and shake again. Pour mixture out onto wax or parchment paper to cool. Store leftovers (if there are any!) in the fridge.

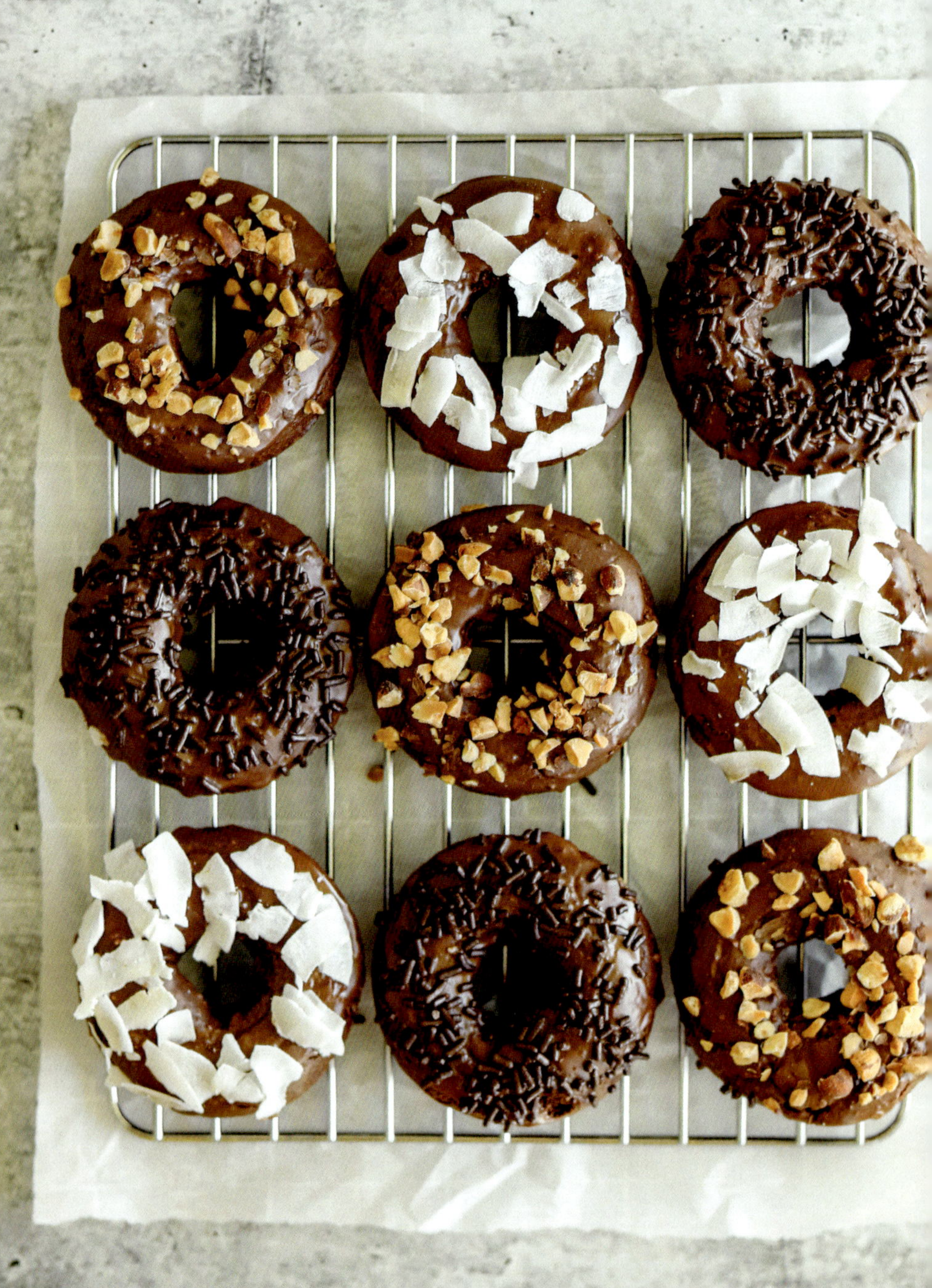

MIDNIGHT ALMOND COCONUT DONUTS *
Makes 15 donuts
200 calories / 8F / 27C / 4P / per donut

1 ½ cups white whole wheat flour
1 tsp. baking powder
¼ tsp. baking soda
¼ tsp. salt
½ cup cocoa powder
½ cup raw honey
¼ cup melted coconut oil
¼ cup pure maple syrup
3 Tbs. almond milk
2 eggs
½ tsp. vanilla extract

100 grams OffBeat Midnight Almond Coconut Butter

Glaze:
½ cup powdered sugar
1 Tbs. cocoa powder
2 Tbs. almond milk

Optional Toppings:
Additional OffBeat drizzle
Coconut flakes
Chopped almonds

1. Preheat the oven to 350 degrees.

2. In a mixing bowl, add the flour, baking powder, baking soda, salt, and cocoa powder. Whisk the dry ingredients together and set aside.

3. In another bowl or stand mixer, add the honey, coconut oil, maple syrup, and almond milk and beat together for a few minutes. Add in the eggs, vanilla, and the Midnight Almond Coconut Butter and mix well.

4. Add the dry ingredients to the wet ingredients and beat on low until combined.

5. Spray donut pan with cooking spray. Pour the donut batter into a piping or Ziploc bag and cut off one of the corners. Pipe the batter into the donut molds.

6. Bake for 6-8 minutes. Allow the donuts to cool in the pan for a few minutes before transferring to a wire rack to cool completely.

7. Whisk together the powdered sugar, cocoa powder, and almond milk until a smooth glaze has formed.

8. Dip each donut into the chocolate glaze then place it back on the wire rack to allow it to set.

9. Top with optional toppings (not included in macros) and enjoy!

OffBeat Fam Recipe Submitted by Alex Daynes

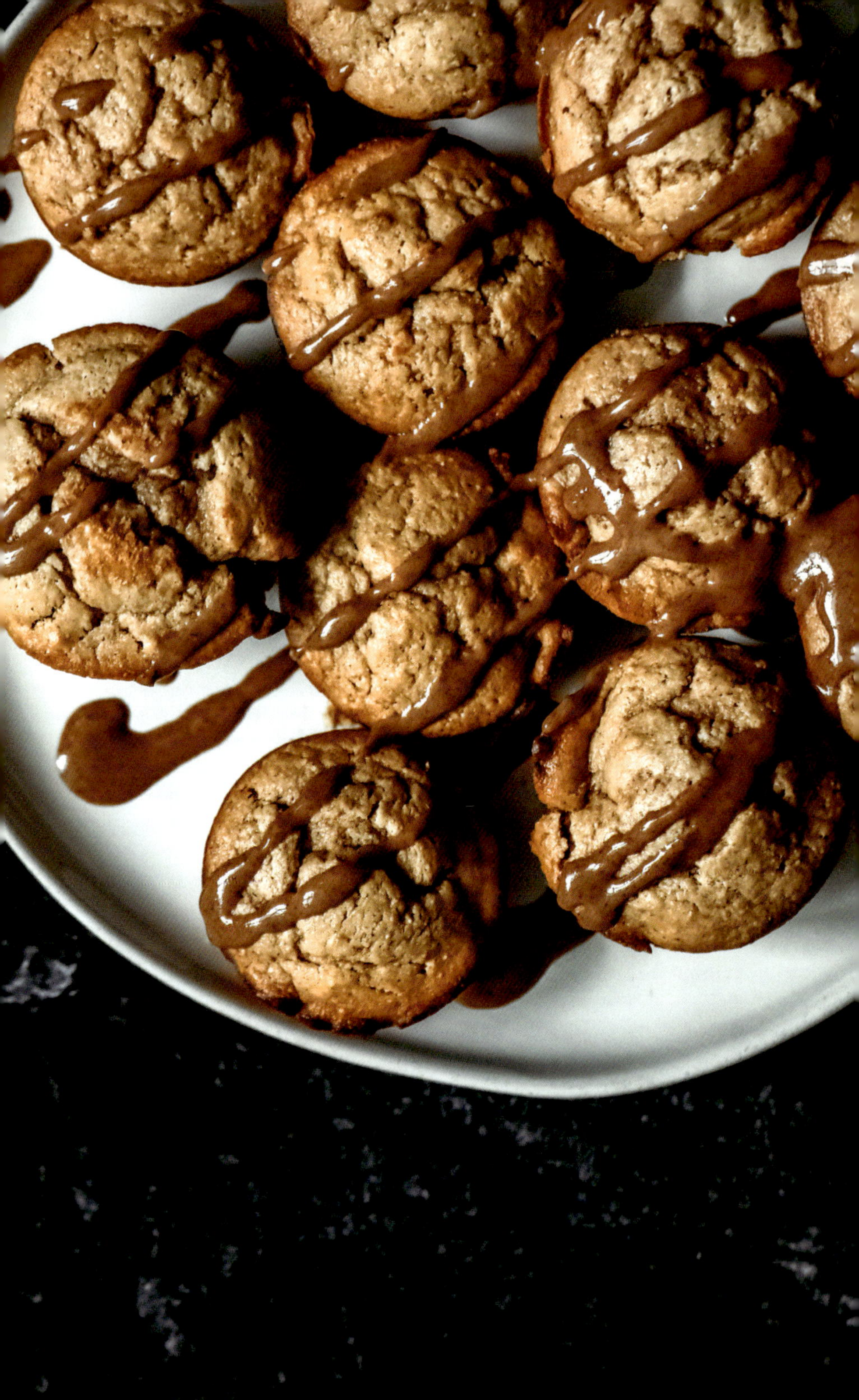

MIDNIGHT ALMOND COCONUT MUFFINS
Makes 14 muffins
150 calories / 4F / 23C / 7P / per muffin

---

2 (240g) ripe bananas
½ cup raw honey
6 Tbs. OffBeat Midnight Almond Coconut Butter, divided
½ cup unsweetened applesauce
1 large egg
1 tsp. vanilla extract
1 ½ cups CSE Vanilla Pancake & Waffle Mix
1 serving CSE Simply Vanilla Protein Powder
2 Tbs. flaxseed meal
1 tsp. baking soda
¼ tsp. sea salt

1. Preheat the oven to 350 degrees.

2. Mash the bananas in a large mixing bowl. Beat in the honey and three tablespoons of Midnight Almond Coconut Butter. Add in the applesauce, egg and vanilla; mix well and set aside.

3. In a separate bowl, combine the CSE Pancake & Waffle Mix, protein powder, flaxseed meal, baking soda and sea salt. Add the wet ingredients to the dry ingredients and whisk together until just combined.

4. Line a muffin tin with liners. Scoop about ¼ cup of the batter into each muffin cup. Bake for 15-16 minutes. Transfer from the pan to the cooling rack. Drizzle with remaining nut butter.

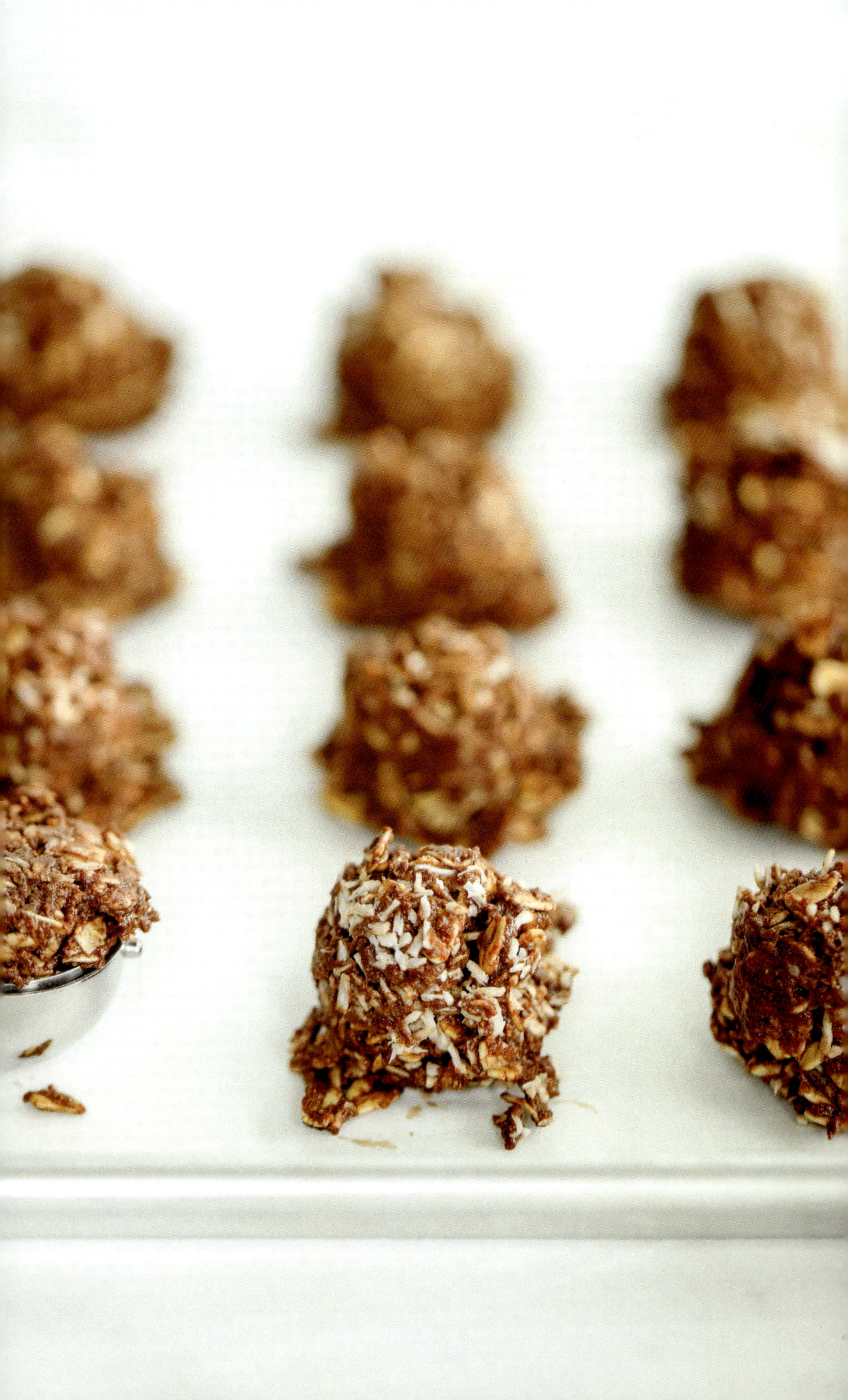

NO-BAKE MIDNIGHT COCONUT COOKIES
Makes 12 cookies
150 calories / 10F / 14C / 4P / per cookie

¼ cup coconut oil
¼ cup coconut sugar
1 Tbs. raw honey
2 Tbs. unsweetened almond milk
2 Tbs. cocoa powder
⅓ cup OffBeat Midnight Almond Coconut Butter
¼ cup unsweetened shredded coconut
1 cup old-fashioned rolled oats
1 serving CSE Coconut Cream Protein Powder

1. Add the coconut oil, coconut sugar, honey, almond milk and cocoa powder to a pot. Melt the ingredients over medium-high heat. Whisk constantly until mixture starts to bubble. Turn heat off.

2. Stir in the Midnight Almond Coconut Butter, unsweetened shredded coconut and rolled oats. Add the protein powder last. Mix until well combined.

3. Using a small cookie scoop, scoop rounded cookies onto a baking sheet lined with parchment paper. Let cool and enjoy!

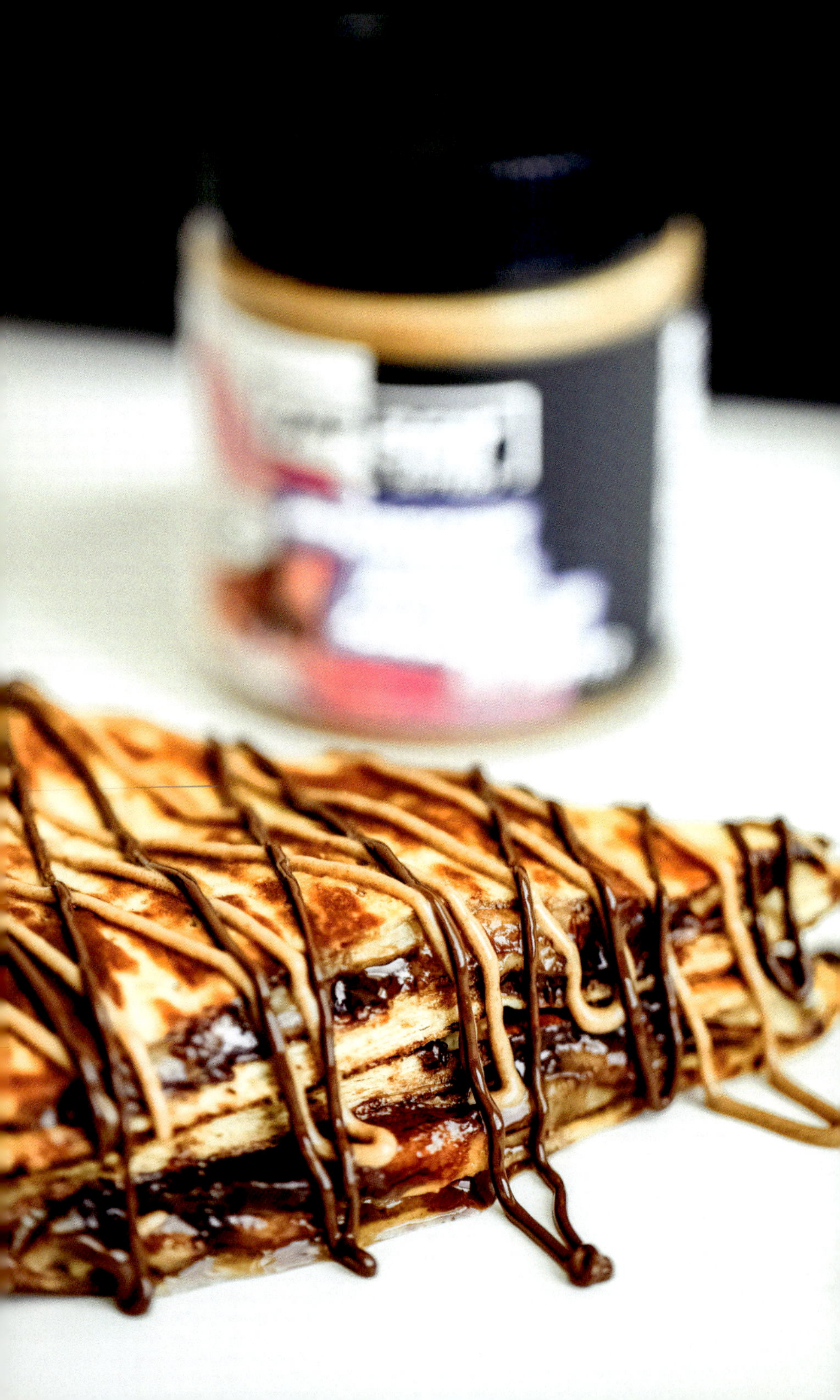

OOEY-GOOEY CHOCOLATE BANANA QUESADILLAS
Makes 1 serving
310 calories / 12F / 40C / 12P

1 Flatout Wrap or Joseph's Flatbread Wrap
1 Tbs. OffBeat Midnight Almond Coconut Butter
50g banana slices
1 tsp. (7g) raw honey
5g mini chocolate chips

1. Lay the wrap out on a plate.

2. Spread the Midnight Almond Coconut Butter in the center of the wrap. Top with banana slices, honey, and chocolate chips.

3. Fold all the edges in over the top, so all the ingredients are enclosed.

4. Heat a pan to medium heat and spray with cooking spray. Place the quesadilla fold side down in the pan. Cover with a lid and cook for 2-3 minutes per side or until crispy on the outside and heated through.

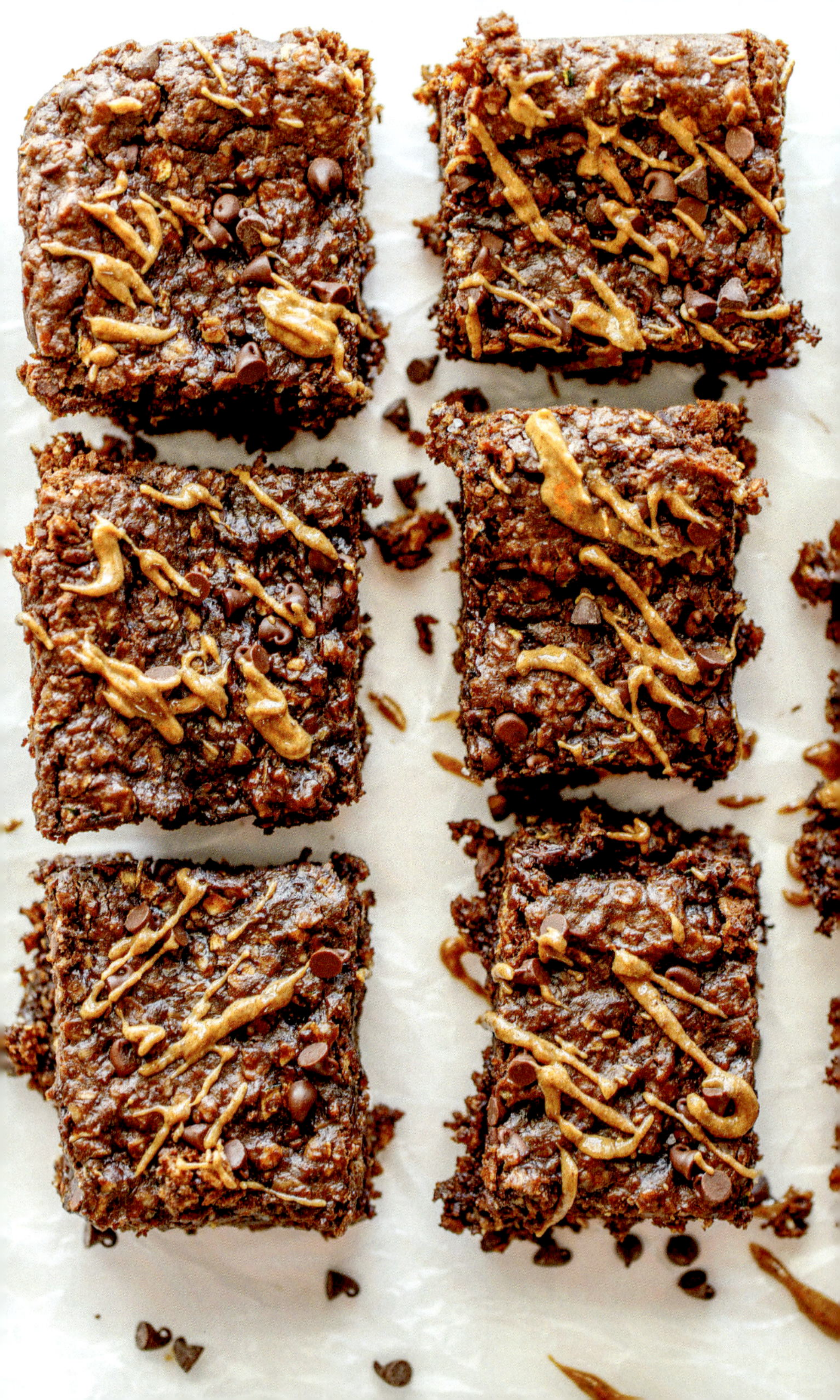

ZUCCHINI MONSTER BARS*
Makes 12 servings
350 calories / 21F / 34C / 9P / per serving

---

12 oz. OffBeat Midnight Almond Coconut Butter
¼ cup raw honey
1 large egg
1 tsp. vanilla
1 cup shredded zucchini squash
1½ cups old-fashioned rolled oats
¼ cup flaxseed meal
¼ cup cacao powder
½ tsp. baking soda
1 cup mini chocolate chips

1. Preheat the oven to 350 degrees.

2. Add Midnight Almond Coconut Butter, honey, egg, vanilla and zucchini to a large bowl. Mix until well combined. Stir in the remaining ingredients.

3. Spray an 8x8 baking pan with cooking spray. Spread mixture into the pan and bake for 12-15 minutes.

*Will still look a little gooey in the middle. Enjoy!

OffBeat Fam Recipe Submitted by Amy Newton

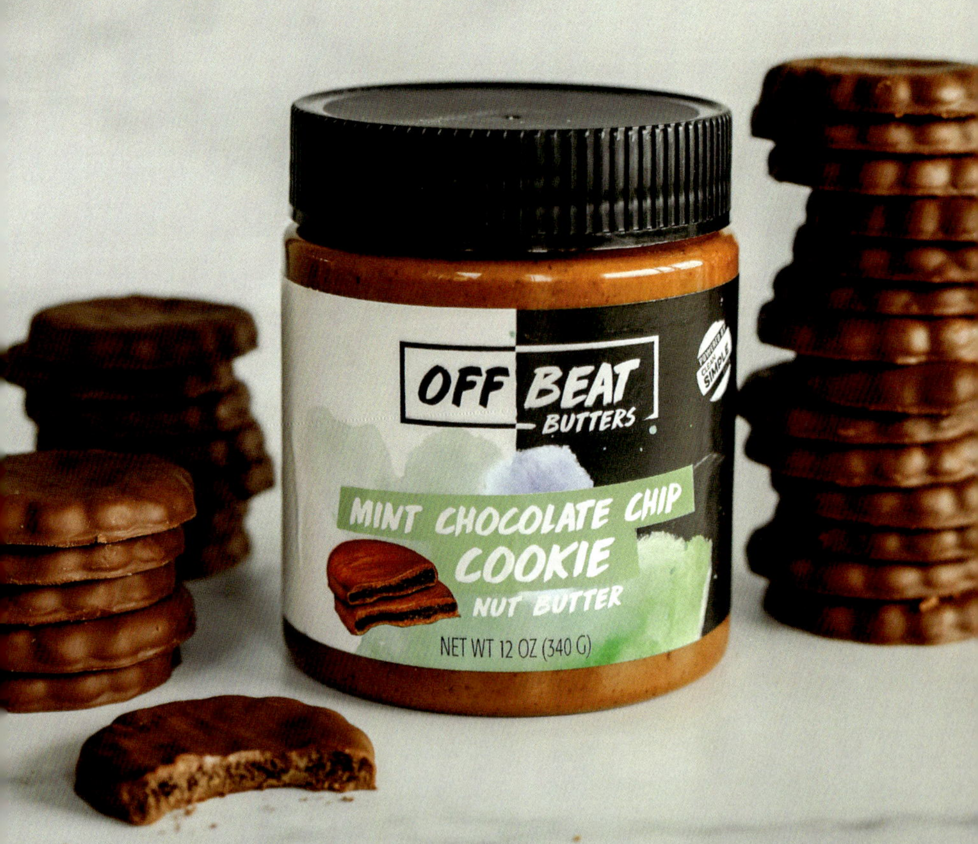

OFF BEAT
BUTTERS
MINT CHOCOLATE CHIP
COOKIE
NUT BUTTER
NET WT 12 OZ (340 G)

MINT CHOCOLATE IS MORE THAN A FLAVOR, IT'S A WHOLE VIBE

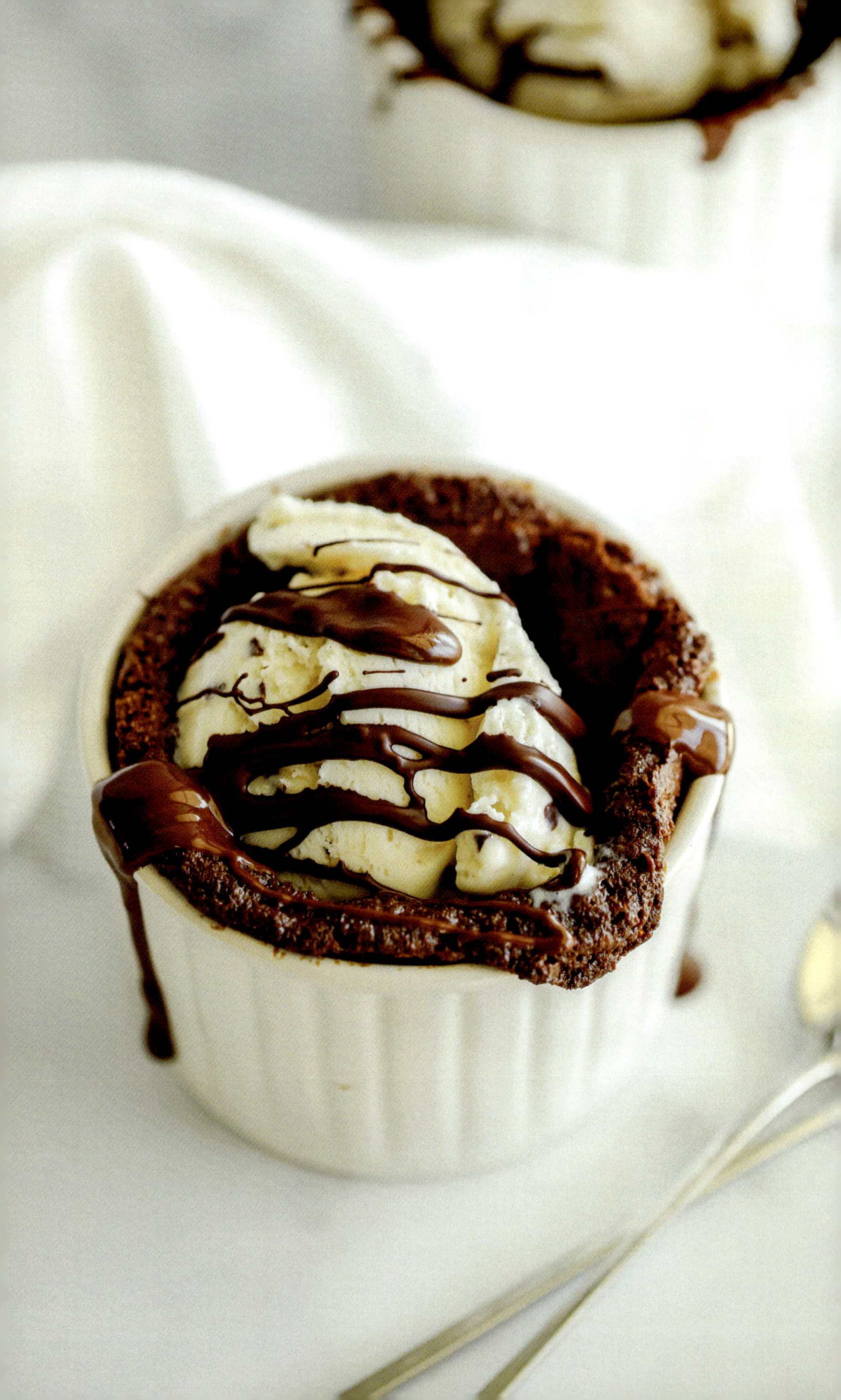

MINT BROWNIE AIR FRYER PAZOOKIE
Makes 8 servings
285 calories / 17.5F / 30C / 6P / per serving

---

1 cup OffBeat Mint Chocolate Chip Cookie Butter
1 cup brown sugar or coconut sugar
1 egg
1 tsp. baking soda
¼ cup semi-sweet chocolate chips
Optional Toppings:
1 serving mint chip high protein ice cream
1 banana
1 serving OffBeat Mint Chocolate Chip Cookie Butter

1. Line the basket of the air fryer with tin foil. Turn the air fryer to 350 degrees and let it run for ten minutes while you make the dough.

2. Add the Mint Chocolate Chip Cookie Butter, brown sugar, egg and baking soda together in a large bowl. Mix with a wooden spoon until well combined. Fold in the chocolate chips.

3. Spray the foil with cooking spray and press the dough into the foil in the bottom of the air fryer basket. Bake for 5-7 minutes or until you've reached your desired doneness.

4. Remove the basket from the air fryer and set on a hot pad. Add toppings, grab a fork and enjoy straight from the basket.

*Toppings are not included in macros.

*Oven instructions: Preheat the oven to 350 degrees. Spray eight mini (8-10 oz.) baking dishes. Add ⅓ of the mixture into each one. Bake for 10-12 minutes or until you've reached your desired doneness. They should still be a little gooey.

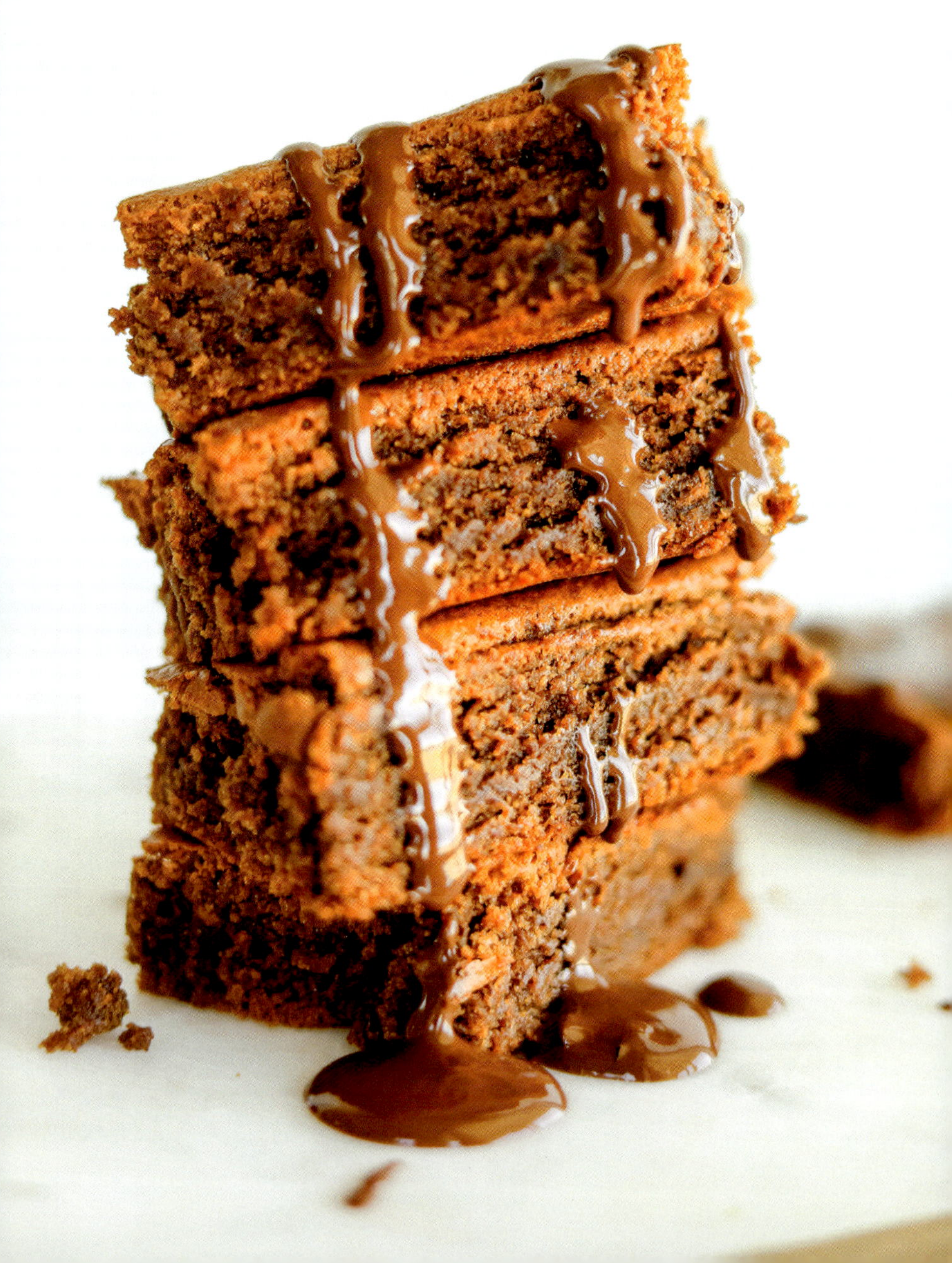

MINT CHOCOLATE CHIP COOKIE BROWNIE*

Makes 16 servings
210 calories / 14F / 19C / 5P / per brownie

12 oz. OffBeat Mint Chocolate Chip Cookie Butter
½ cup coconut sugar
¼ cup maple syrup
2 eggs
1 Tbs. coconut oil
¼ tsp. baking soda
⅛ tsp. salt
Glaze:
1 Tbs. OffBeat Mint Chocolate Chip Cookie Butter
1 Tbs. chocolate chips

1. Preheat the oven to 350 degrees. Line a 9x9 inch baking pan with parchment paper.

2. Combine Mint Chocolate Chip Cookie Butter, coconut sugar, maple syrup, and eggs and mix until well combined.

3. Mix in the coconut oil.

4. Add the baking soda and salt.

5. Pour batter into the pan and bake for 20-25 minutes. Let cool completely.

6. For the glaze, melt the nut butter and chocolate chips in the microwave. Drizzle on top of brownies. Enjoy!

OffBeat Fam Recipe Submitted by Tori Landavazo

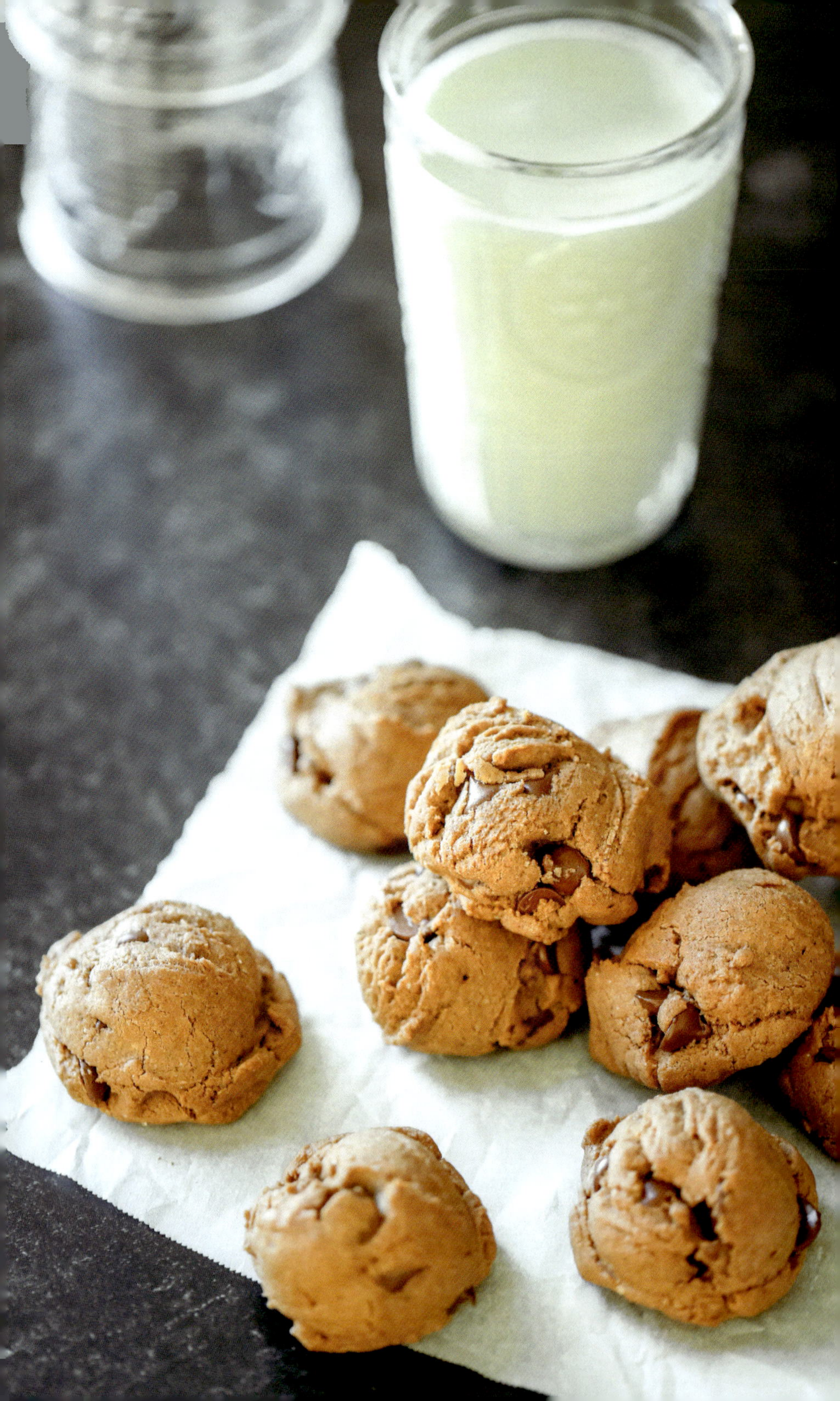

MINT CHOCOLATE CHIP COOKIES
Makes 16 cookies
150 calories / 9F / 14C / 4P / per cookie

½ cup grass-fed butter
¼ cup OffBeat Mint Chocolate Chip Cookie Butter
1 serving CSE Mint Chocolate Cookie Protein Powder
⅓ cup organic cane sugar
1 large egg
1 tsp. vanilla extract
1 cup organic unbleached all-purpose flour
2 Tbs. cocoa powder
¼ tsp. sea salt
¼ tsp. baking soda
2 oz. dark chocolate chips

1. Preheat the oven to 350 degrees.

2. Add the butter, Mint Chocolate Chip Cookie Butter, protein powder and the sugar to a mixing bowl. Beat together until smooth. Add the egg and vanilla. Mix until combined.

3. In a separate bowl, add the flour, cocoa powder, sea salt and baking soda and stir until combined. Add the wet ingredients to the dry ingredients and mix until just combined. Fold in the chocolate chips.

4. Using a cookie scoop, scoop the cookie dough onto a baking sheet lined with parchment paper. Bake for 8-10 minutes. Remove from the oven and allow to cool for a few minutes. Transfer to a cooling rack. Store leftover cookies in the fridge.

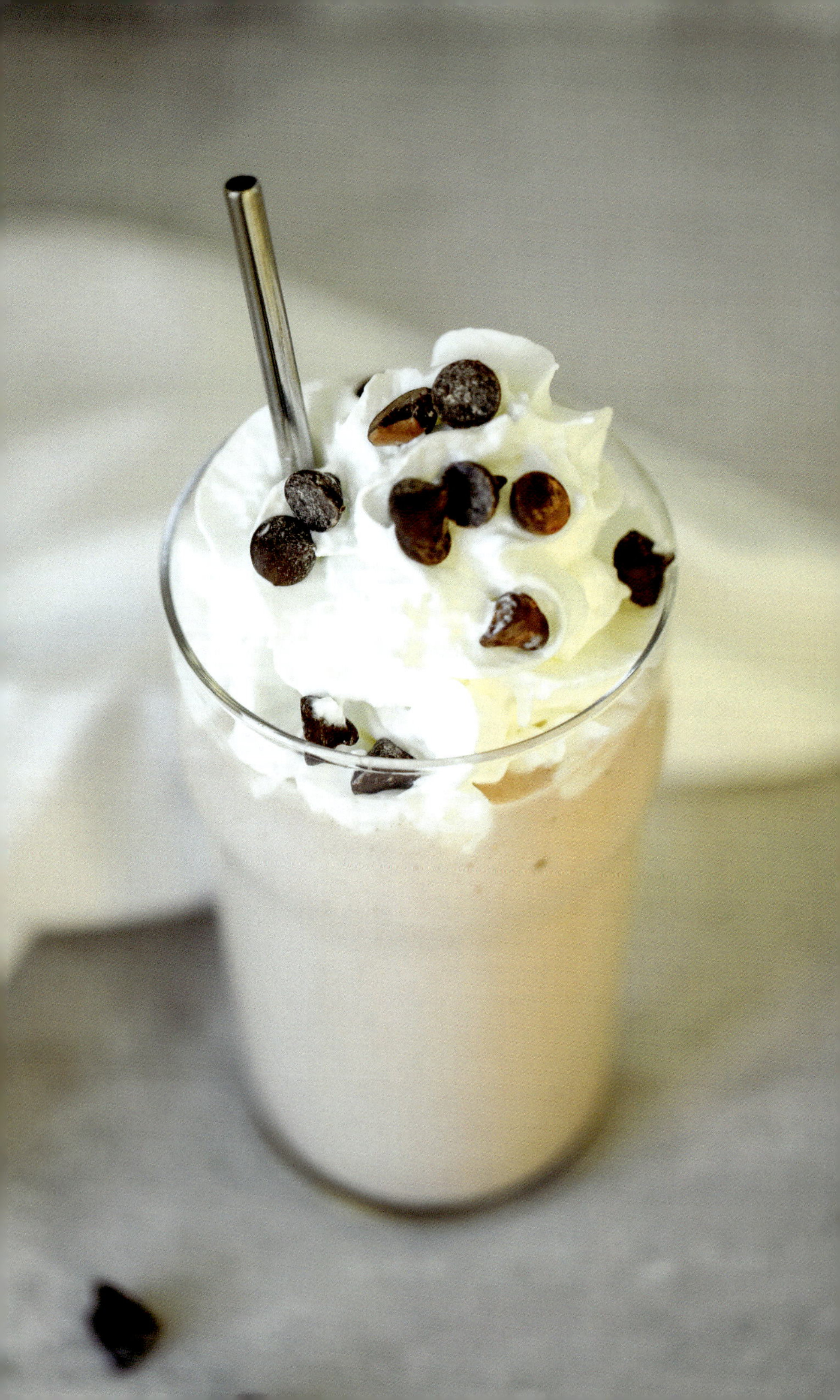

MINT CHOCOLATE COOKIE SHAKE

Makes 1 serving
240 calories / 9F / 16C / 23P

---

1 cup unsweetened almond milk
¾ serving (24g) CSE Mint Chocolate Cookie Protein Powder
½ Tbs. OffBeat Mint Chocolate Chip Cookie Butter
1 Tbs. old-fashioned rolled oats
6-8 (120g) ice cubes
Toppings:
2 Tbs. spray whipped cream
5g dark chocolate chips

1. Add all of the ingredients to a high-powered blender and blend until smooth.

2. Pour into a cup. Top with whipped cream and dark chocolate chips. Enjoy with a spoon!

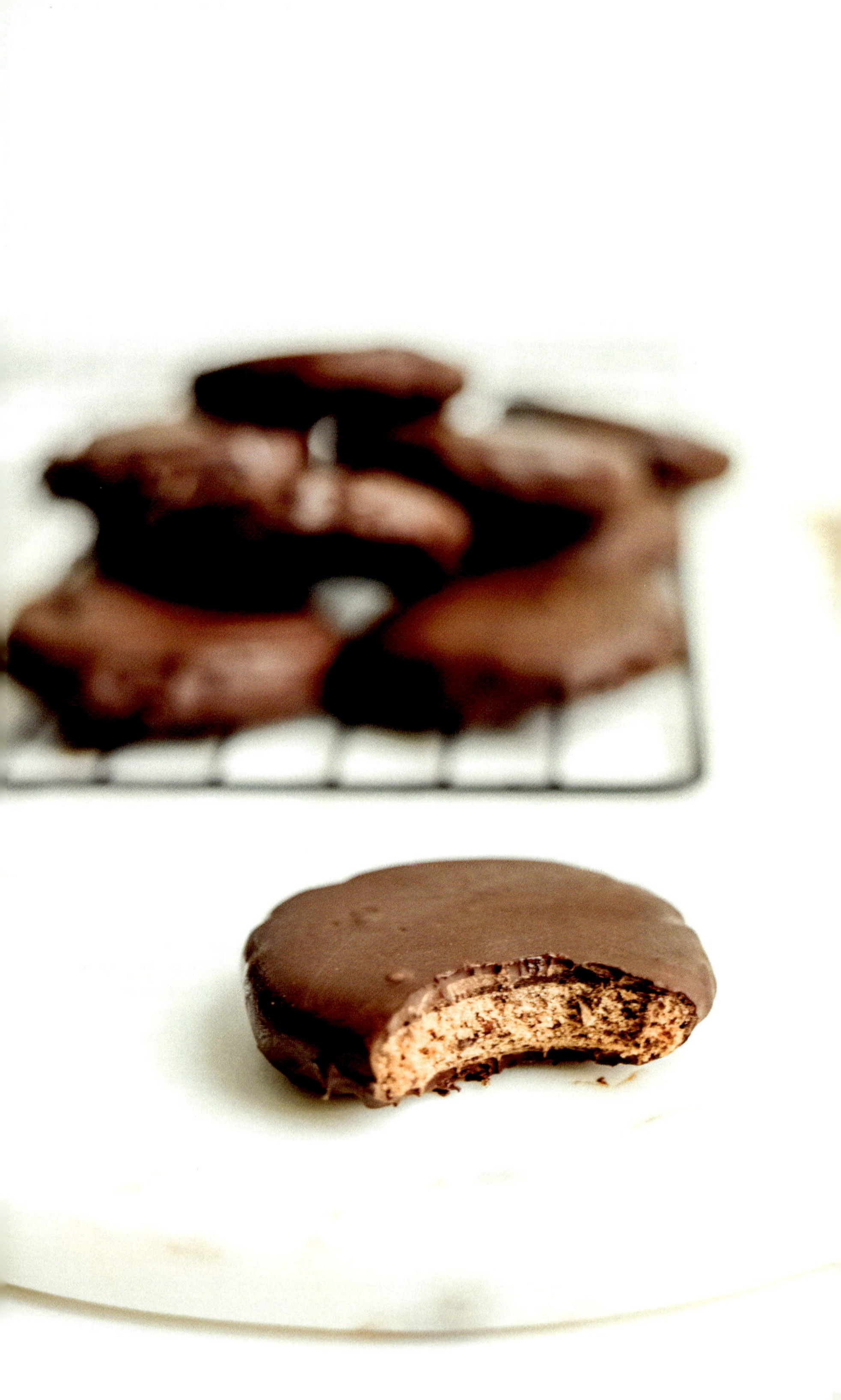

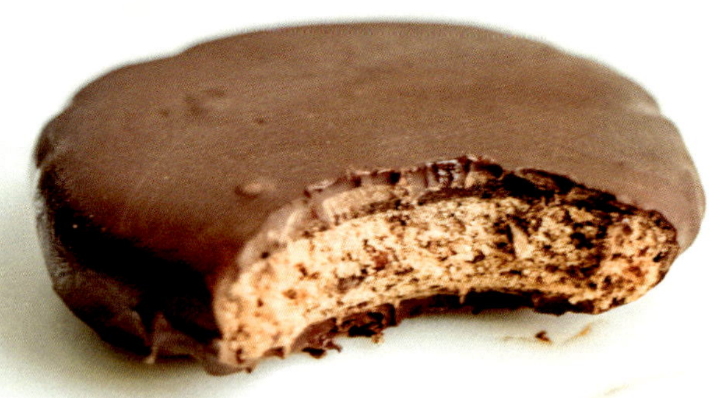

MINT CHOCOLATE COOKIES

Makes 36 cookies
120 calories / 7.5F / 13C / 3.5P / per cookie

12 oz. OffBeat Mint Chocolate Chip Cookie Butter
½ cup raw honey
2 servings CSE Brownie Batter Protein Powder
1 cup CSE Vanilla Pancake & Waffle Mix
½ tsp. vanilla extract
Dash sea salt
2 cups dark chocolate chips
1 Tbs. coconut oil

1. Add the Mint Chocolate Chip Cookie Butter, honey, protein powder, CSE Pancake & Waffle Mix, vanilla and salt together in a bowl. Mix until well combined. Using a small cookie scoop, scoop them onto a baking sheet lined with parchment paper (makes 36 cookies). Using the bottom of a glass jar or cup, smash the balls flat and then round out the edges with your hands to form into a cookie. Place the cookies in the freezer for 30 minutes or until hardened.

2. Place the dark chocolate and coconut oil into a small saucepan over low heat to melt (or melt in a bowl in the microwave). Stir continuously until completely melted, then turn the heat off. Drop each cookie into the chocolate one at a time and scoop them out with a fork, letting the excess chocolate drip off into the pan. Place the chocolate dipped cookies back onto the parchment paper and then place them in the freezer to harden.

3. Once frozen, transfer to a storage container or bag. When ready to eat, let cookies sit out 5-10 minutes to thaw before taking a bite. Enjoy!

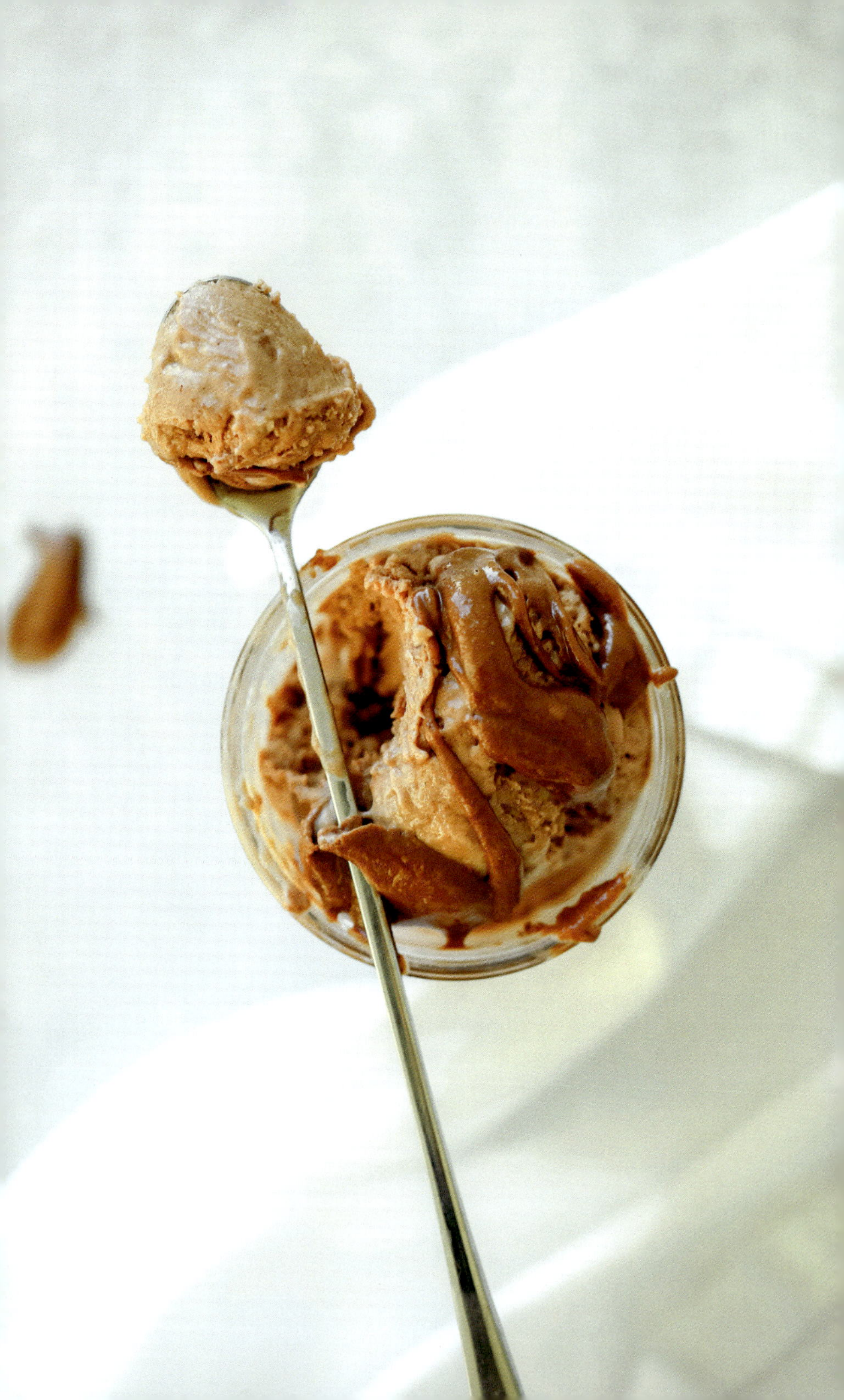

MINT CHOCOLATE ICE CREAM

Makes 4 servings
230 calories / 7.5F / 30C / 13P / per serving

400g frozen banana slices
2 servings CSE Mint Chocolate Cookie Protein Powder
¼ cup OffBeat Mint Chocolate Chip Cookie Butter
¼ cup unsweetened almond milk
Optional Toppings:
Melted chocolate
OffBeat Mint Chocolate Chip Cookie Butter

1. Add all of the ingredients to a high-powered blender. Blend until thick and smooth, scraping down the sides in between.

2. Scrape out into a loaf pan lined with parchment paper. Freeze for 2-3 hours. Use an ice cream scoop to scoop the ice cream into a bowl. Divide into four equal servings. Top the ice cream with melted chocolate or extra Mint Chocolate Chip Cookie Butter. Enjoy!

*Toppings are not included in macros.

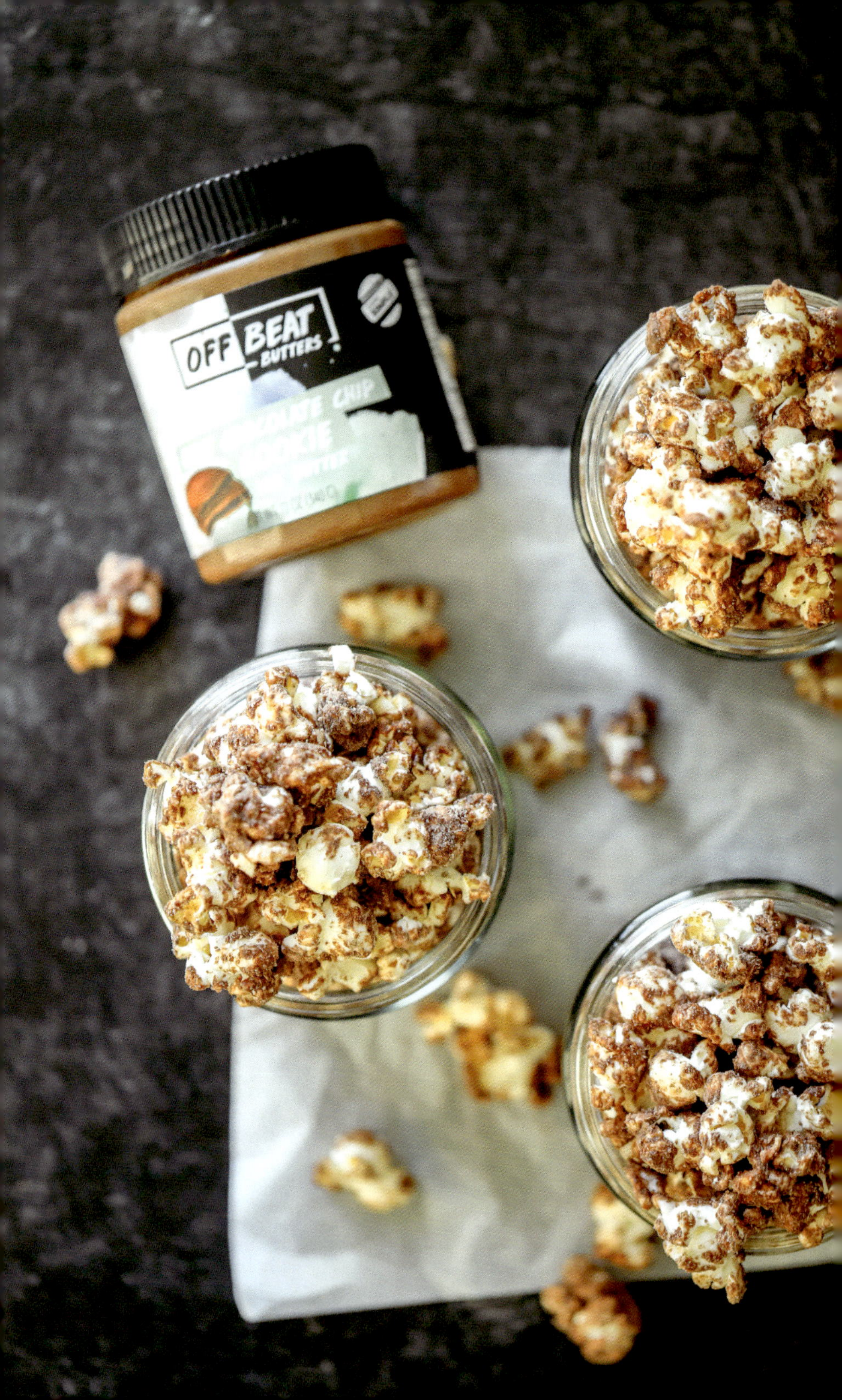
OFF BEAT
BUTTERS
CHIP
COOKIE

MINT CHOCOLATE POPCORN
Makes 8 servings
170 calories / 10F / 15.5C / 5P / per serving

80g popcorn kernels
½ cup dark chocolate chips
¼ cup OffBeat Mint Chocolate Chip Cookie Butter
2 Tbs. grass-fed butter
1 tsp. vanilla extract
1 serving CSE Mint Chocolate Cookie Protein Powder

1. Use an air popper to pop the kernels in a large bowl and set aside.

2. Add the chocolate chips, Mint Chocolate Chip Cookie Butter, and butter to a small saucepan. Melt over low heat until smooth. Remove from heat and whisk in the vanilla extract.

3. Pour the melted chocolate mixture over the popcorn and mix gently until the popcorn is well coated. Immediately add the protein powder and toss until the popcorn is well coated.

4. Divide into eight servings (approximately 1.25oz per serving) and enjoy!

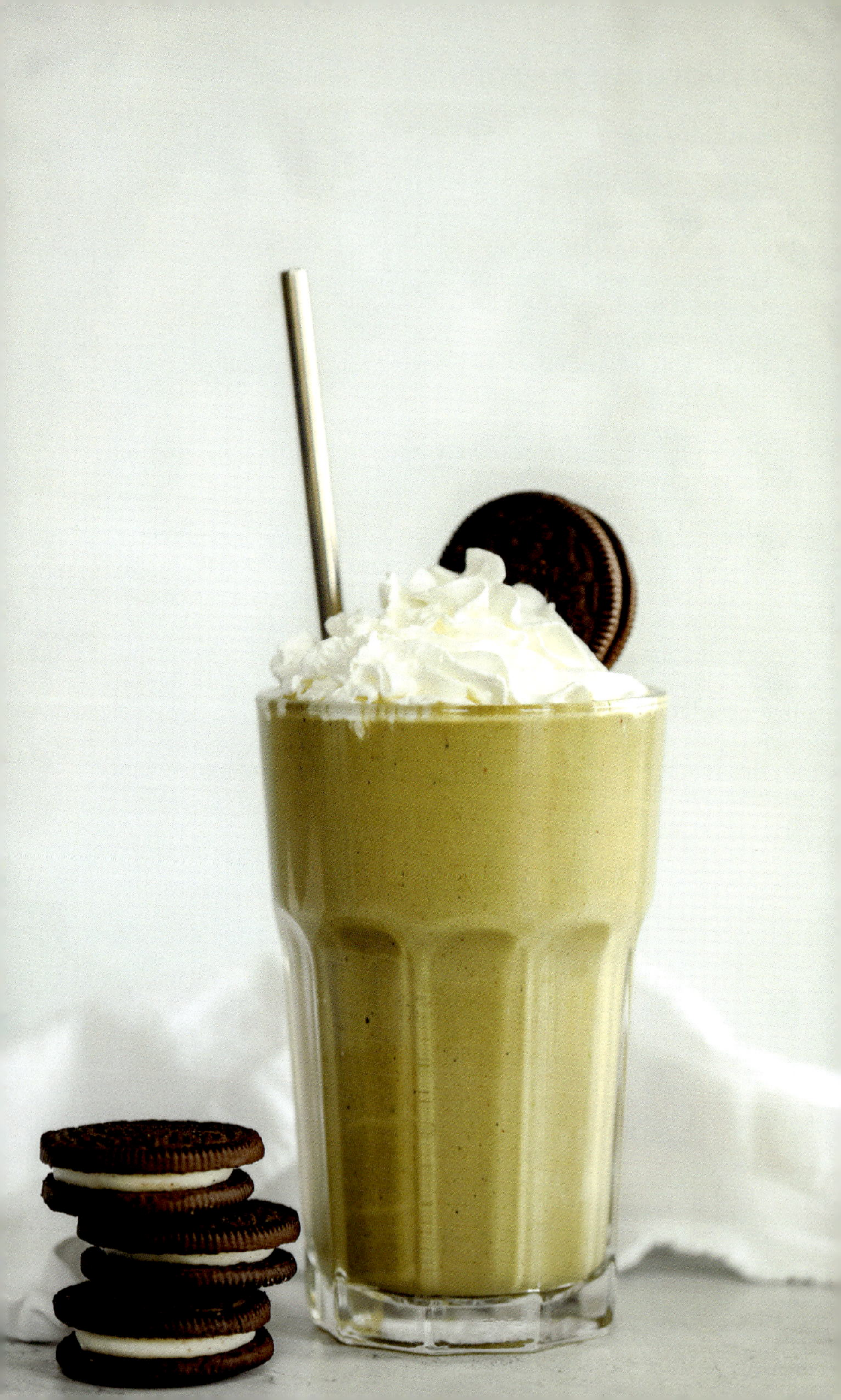

MINT COOKIES & CREAM SHAKE

Makes 1 serving
360 calories / 13.5F / 29C / 27P

---

1 cup unsweetened almond milk
¾ (24g) serving CSE Mint Chocolate Cookie Protein Powder
½ (7g) Tbs. OffBeat Mint Chocolate Chip Cookie Butter
¼ cup low-fat cottage cheese
1 Newman's Own creme filled chocolate cookies
1 cup spinach
¼ tsp. xanthan gum
8-10 (150g) ice cubes

Toppings:
2 Tbs. spray whipped cream
1 Newman's Own creme filled chocolate cookies, crumbled

1. Add all of the ingredients to a high-powered blender. Blend until smooth and thick.

2. Pour into a cup and top with spray whipped cream and cookie crumbles. Enjoy with a spoon!

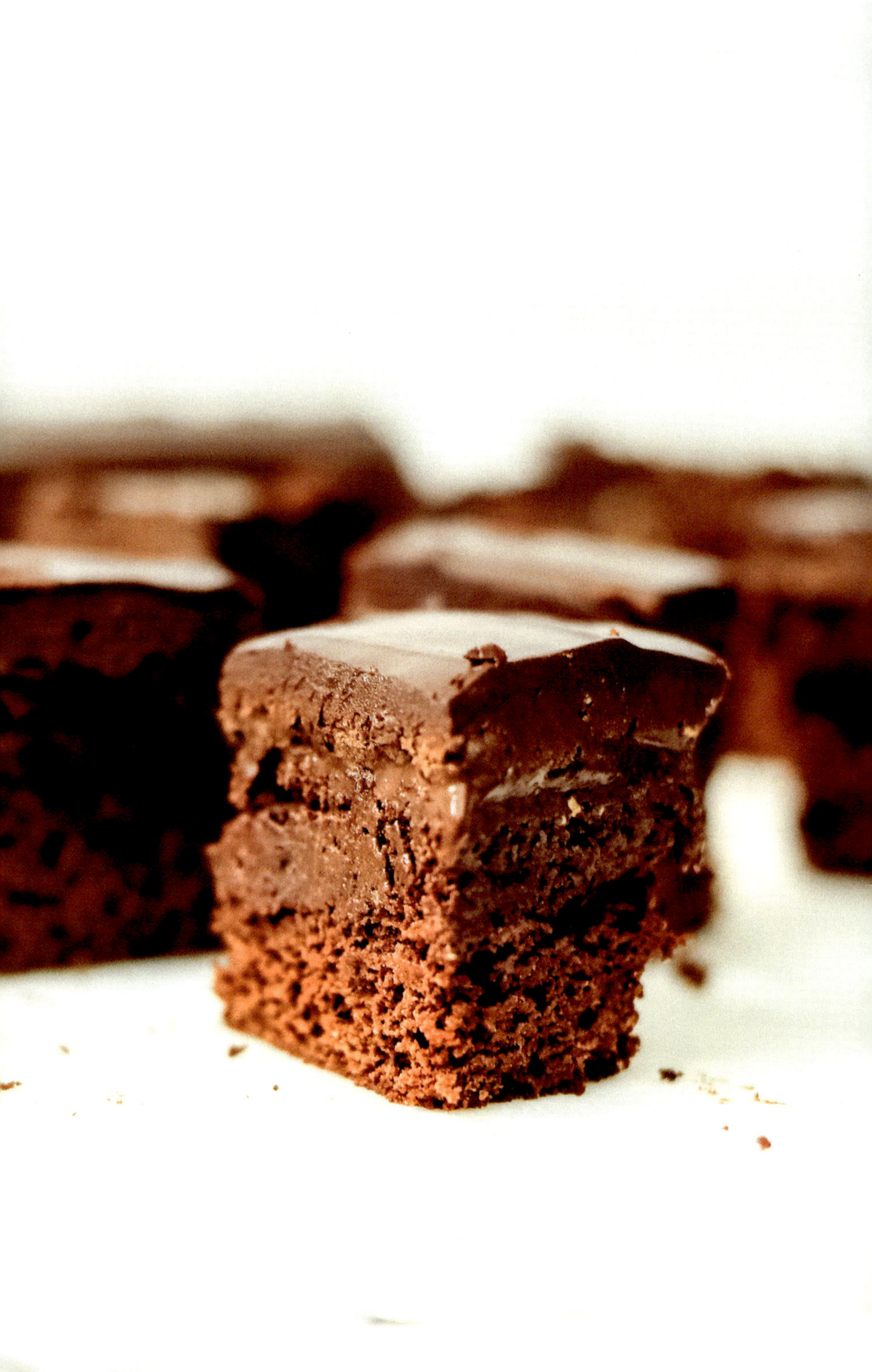

THIN MINT CHOCOLATE BROWNIE
Makes 36 brownies
100 calories / 4.5C / 12F / 2.5P / per brownie

¾ cup oat flour
½ cup cocoa powder
1 serving CSE Brownie Batter
   or Mint Chocolate Cookie Protein Powder
½ tsp. baking powder
⅛ tsp. sea salt
2 Tbs. grass-fed butter
½ cup raw honey
1 large egg
2 egg whites
½ cup unsweetened applesauce
1 Tbs. vanilla extract
Toppings:
1 cup OffBeat Mint Chocolate Chip Cookie Butter
2 Tbs. grass-fed butter
½ cup dark chocolate chips

1. Preheat oven to 350 degrees.

2. Stir the dry ingredients together in a small bowl; set aside.
3. In a separate bowl, beat the butter and honey together. Add
the eggs, egg whites, applesauce and vanilla; mix well. Add the
wet ingredients to the dry ingredients and mix until just combined.

4. Pour into a greased 8x8 glass baking dish. Bake for 20-25
minutes, then let cool.

5. Once the brownies are cool, pour Mint Chocolate Chip Cookie
Butter over the top and spread out evenly. Place in the freezer
until the chocolate has set.

6. Place the butter and chocolate chips in a bowl. Microwave 30
seconds at a time until melted and smooth, stirring in between.
Pour over the brownies and spread out smooth. Return to the
fridge or freezer for about 1 hour or until the chocolate has set.
Allow brownies to sit out at room temperature for about 5-10 minutes before slicing. Slice into 36 brownie bites and enjoy!

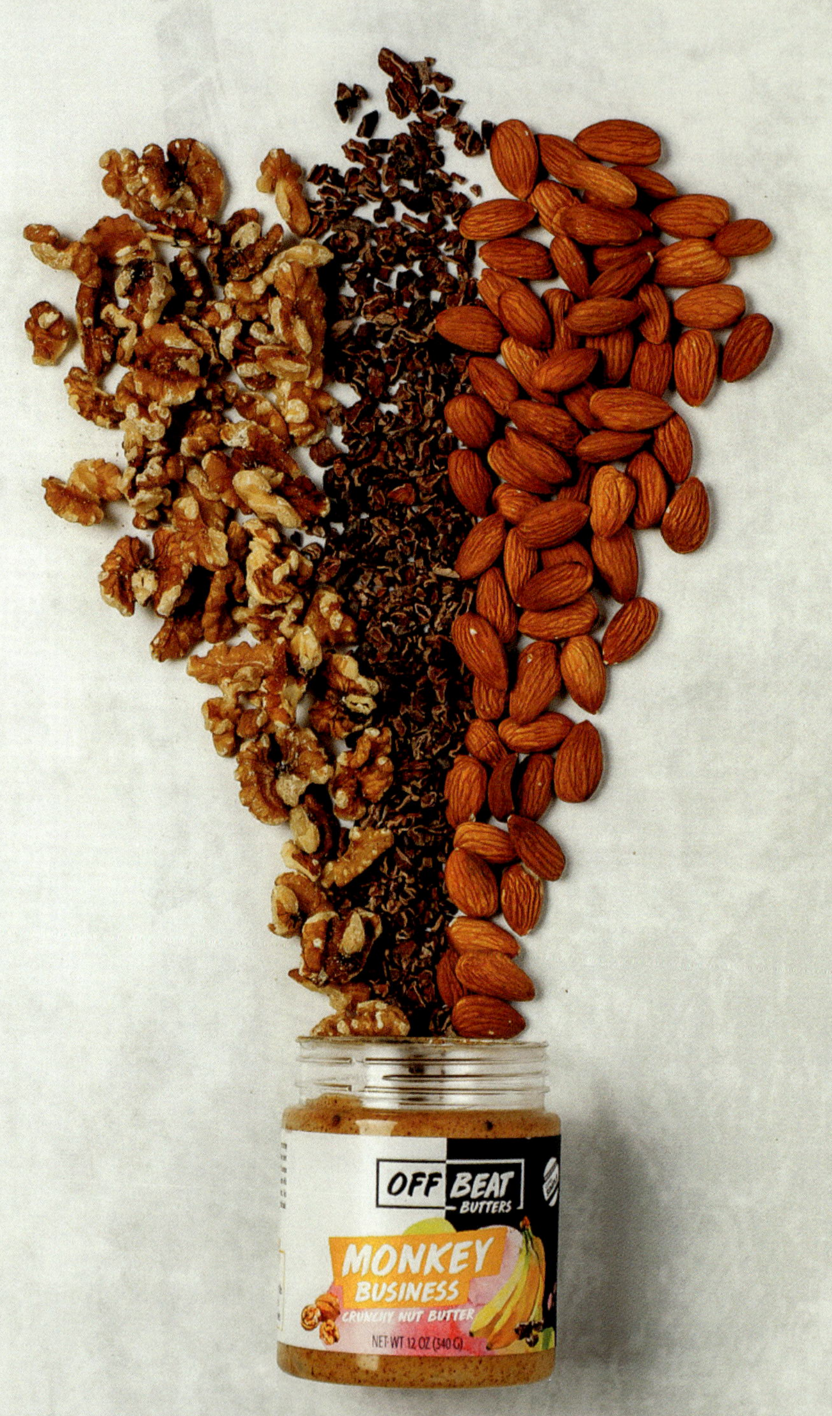

OFF BEAT
BUTTERS
MONKEY
BUSINESS
CRUNCHY NUT BUTTER
NET WT 12 OZ (340 G)

BANANAS MAKE EVERYTHING MORE A-PEELING

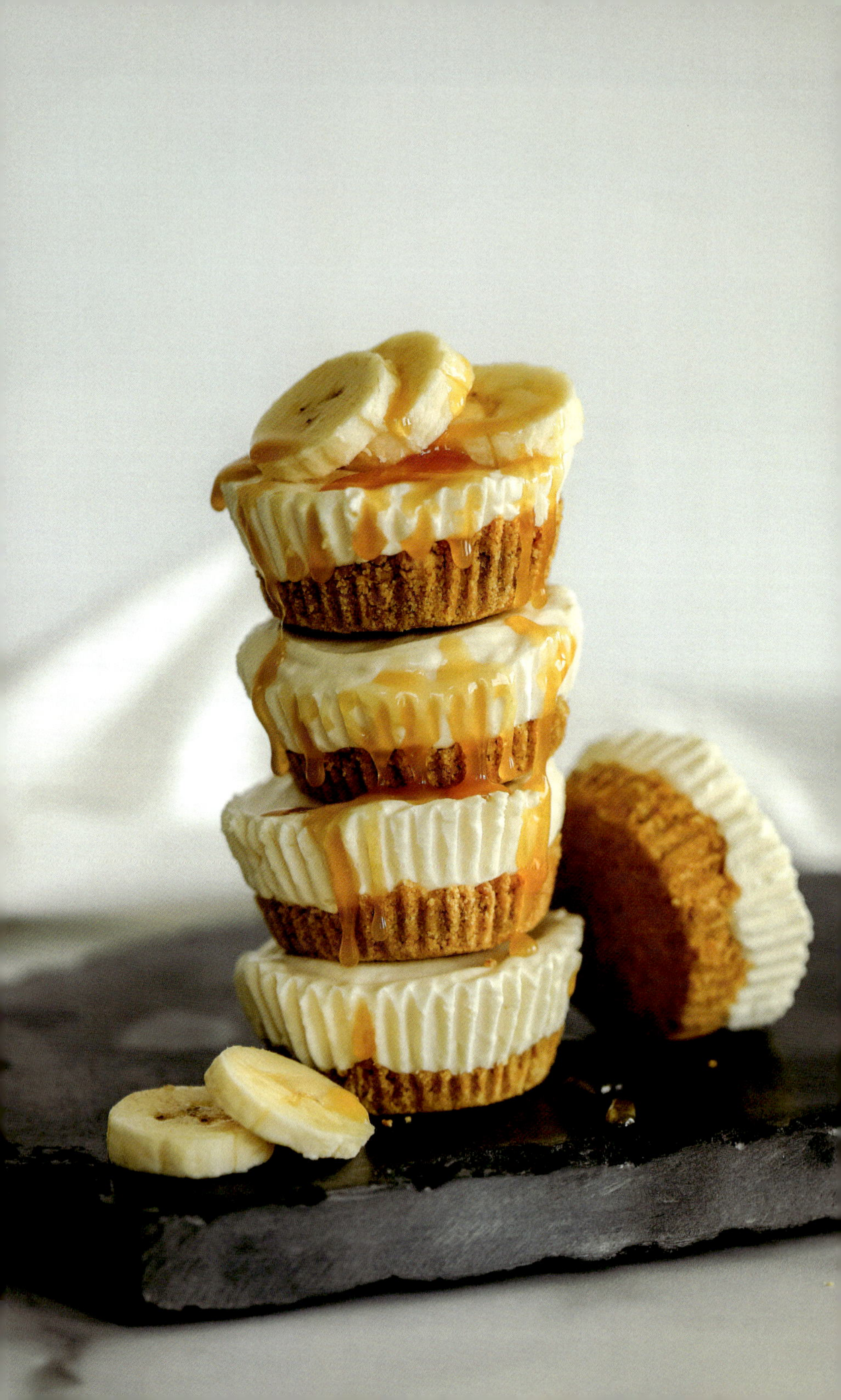

BANANA CHEESECAKE CUPS

Makes 12 servings
165 calories / 10F / 11.5C / 7P / per cup

Crust:
1 cup graham cracker crumbs
2 Tbs. grass-fed butter
1 Tbs. OffBeat Monkey Business Butter
Cheesecake:
8 oz. organic cream cheese, room temperature
2 servings (72g) CSE Bananas Foster Protein Powder
1 ½ cups Truwhip Skinny
⅔ cup plain, nonfat Greek yogurt

1. Place 12 cupcake liners in a muffin tin. Set aside.

2. Add the graham cracker crumbs to a bowl. Melt the butter. Add the melted butter and Monkey Business Butter to the bowl with the graham crackers. Stir until well combined. Weigh the mixture and divide evenly into the 12 cupcake liners. Press into the bottom and freeze.

3. Add the softened cream cheese to a mixing bowl and beat until smooth. Slowly mix in the protein powder until well combined. Add the Truwhip and Greek yogurt; beat until smooth. Weigh the mixture and divide evenly into the cupcake liners. Using a small, rubber spatula or spoon, smooth out the top of each one.

4. Cover with foil and freeze for 2+ hours. When ready to eat, remove the cupcake liner and let thaw outside of the freezer for about 5-10 minutes. Enjoy!

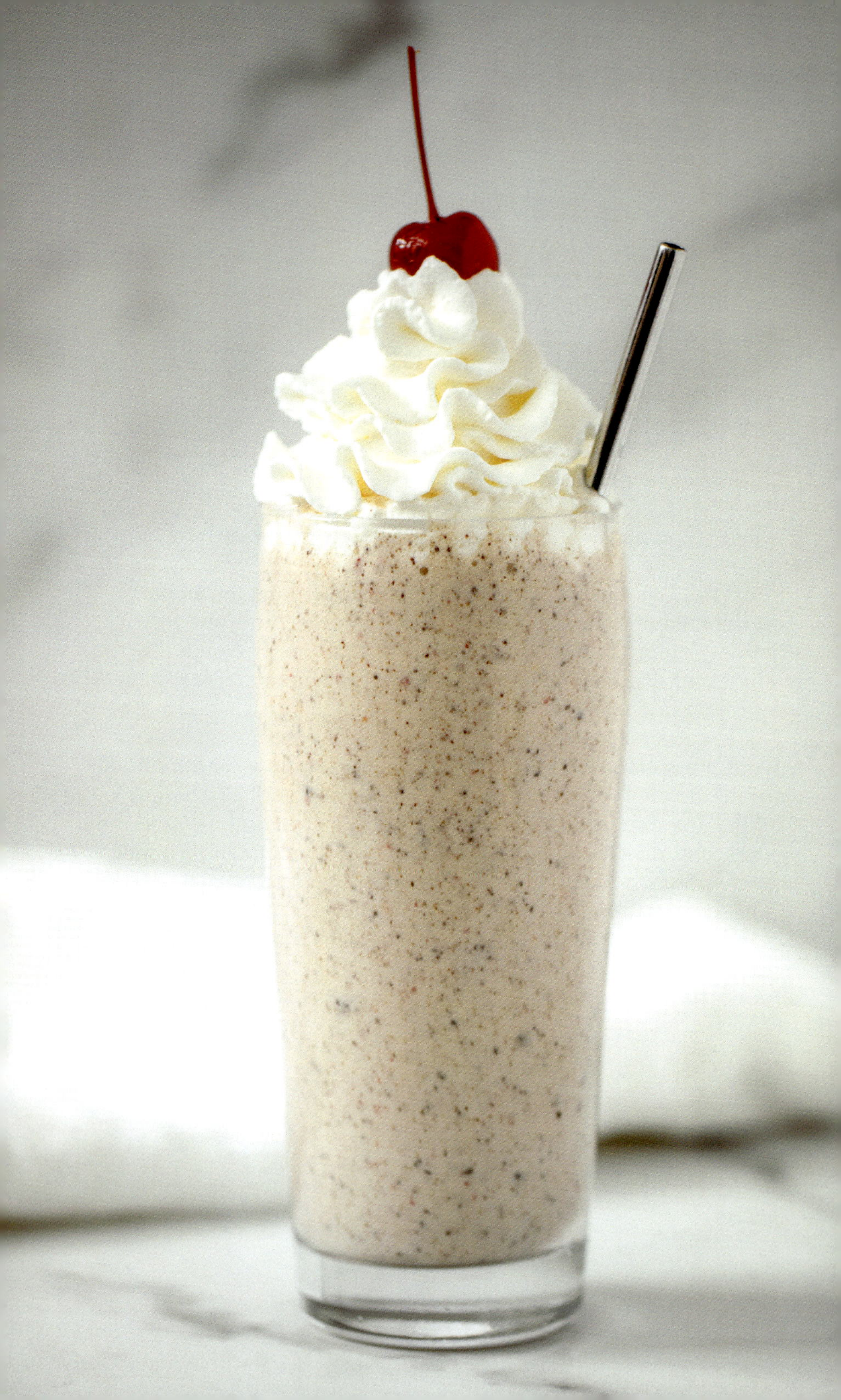

BANANA SPLIT SHAKE*

Makes 1 serving
415 calories / 17F / 36C / 30P

---

1 cup unsweetened almond milk
¼ cup plain, nonfat Greek yogurt
50g frozen bananas
50g frozen strawberries
1 serving CSE Strawberry Cheesecake
   or Simply Vanilla Protein Powder
1 Tbs. OffBeat Monkey Business Butter
10g dark chocolate chips
Toppings:
2 Tbs. spray whipped cream
1 maraschino cherry

1. Add all of the ingredients to a high-powered blender. Blend on high until smooth.

2. Pour into a cup, top with whipped cream and a maraschino cherry. Enjoy!

OffBeat Fam Recipe Submitted by Taylor Roller

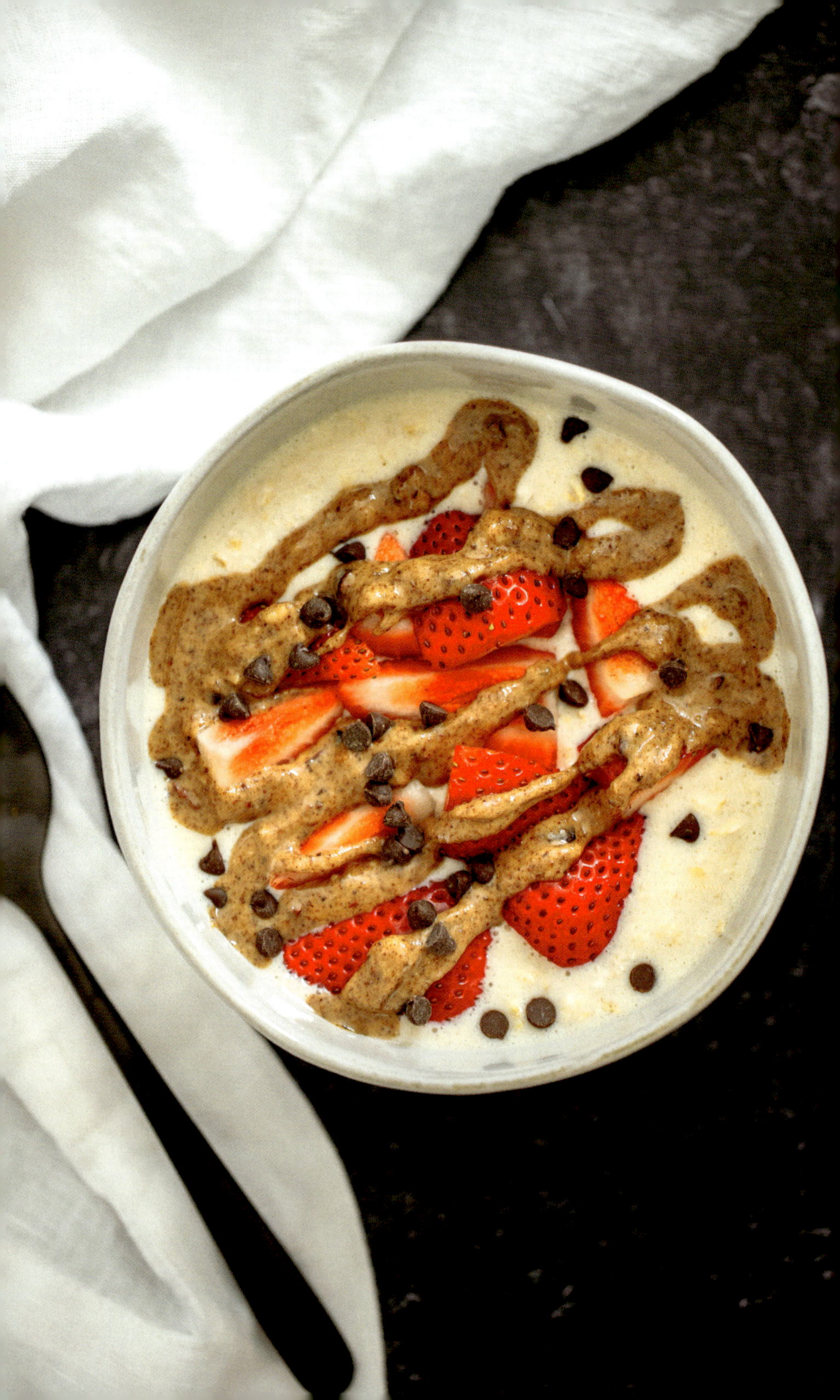

CHOCOLATE COVERED STRAWBERRY OVERNIGHT OATS
Makes 1 serving
410 calories 15F / 41C / 29P

⅓ cup old-fashioned rolled oats
½ cup almond milk
1 serving CSE Simply Vanilla Protein Powder
Toppings:
1 Tbs. OffBeat Monkey Business Butter
¼ cup strawberries
1 tsp. mini chocolate chips
2 Tbs. spray whipped cream

1. Mix together oats, almond milk, and protein powder. Store in the fridge overnight.

2. Top with Monkey Business Butter, strawberries, mini chocolate chips, and whipped cream. Enjoy!

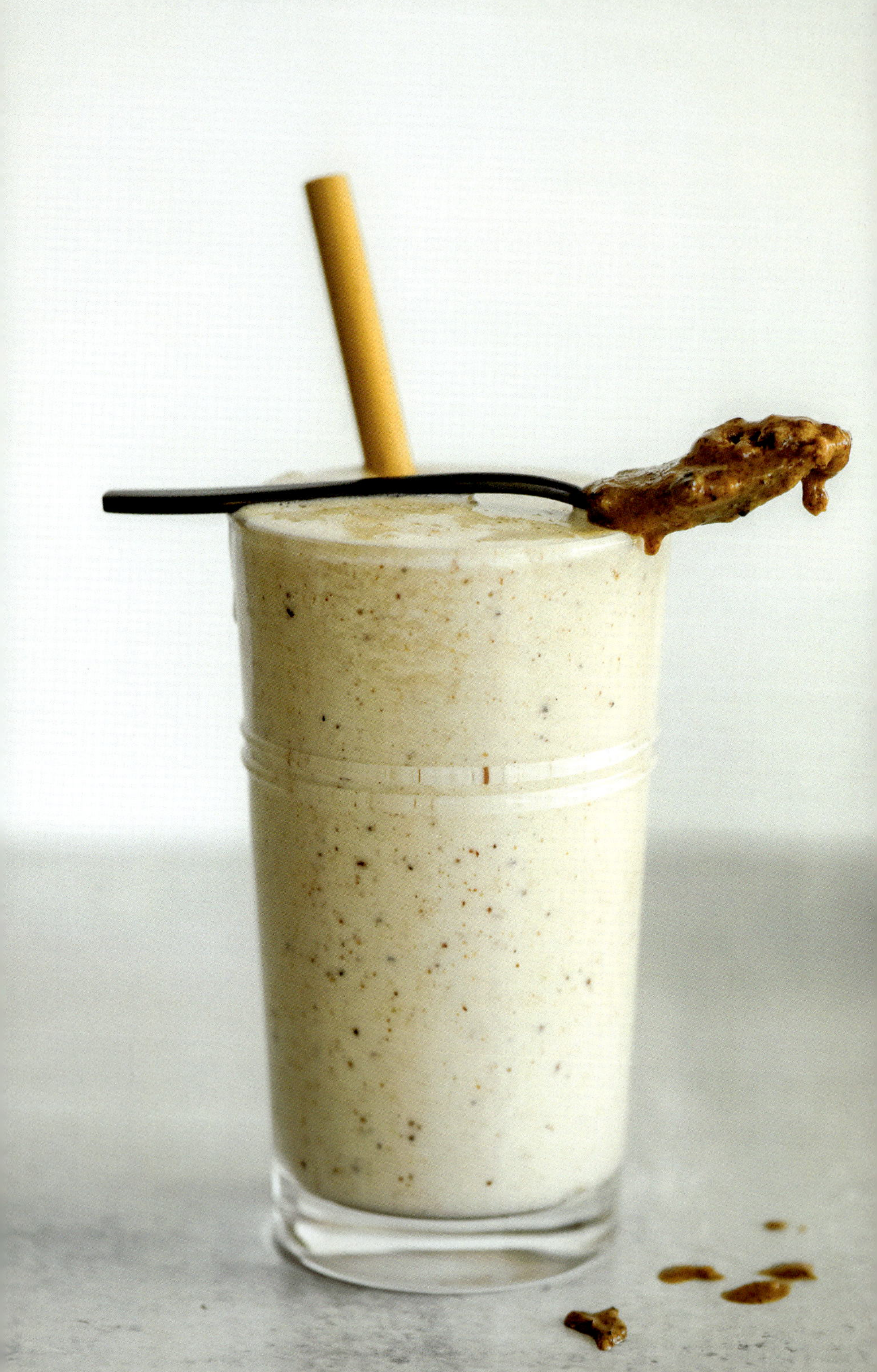

CHUNKY COCO-MONKEY SHAKE

Makes 1 serving
325 calories / 14.5F / 13.5C / 35P

---

1 cup unsweetened almond milk
21g OffBeat Monkey Business Butter
1 ½ servings CSE Coconut Cream Protein Powder
125g ice cubes

1. Place all of the ingredients in a high-powered blender. Blend on high until smooth.

2. Pour into a cup and enjoy!

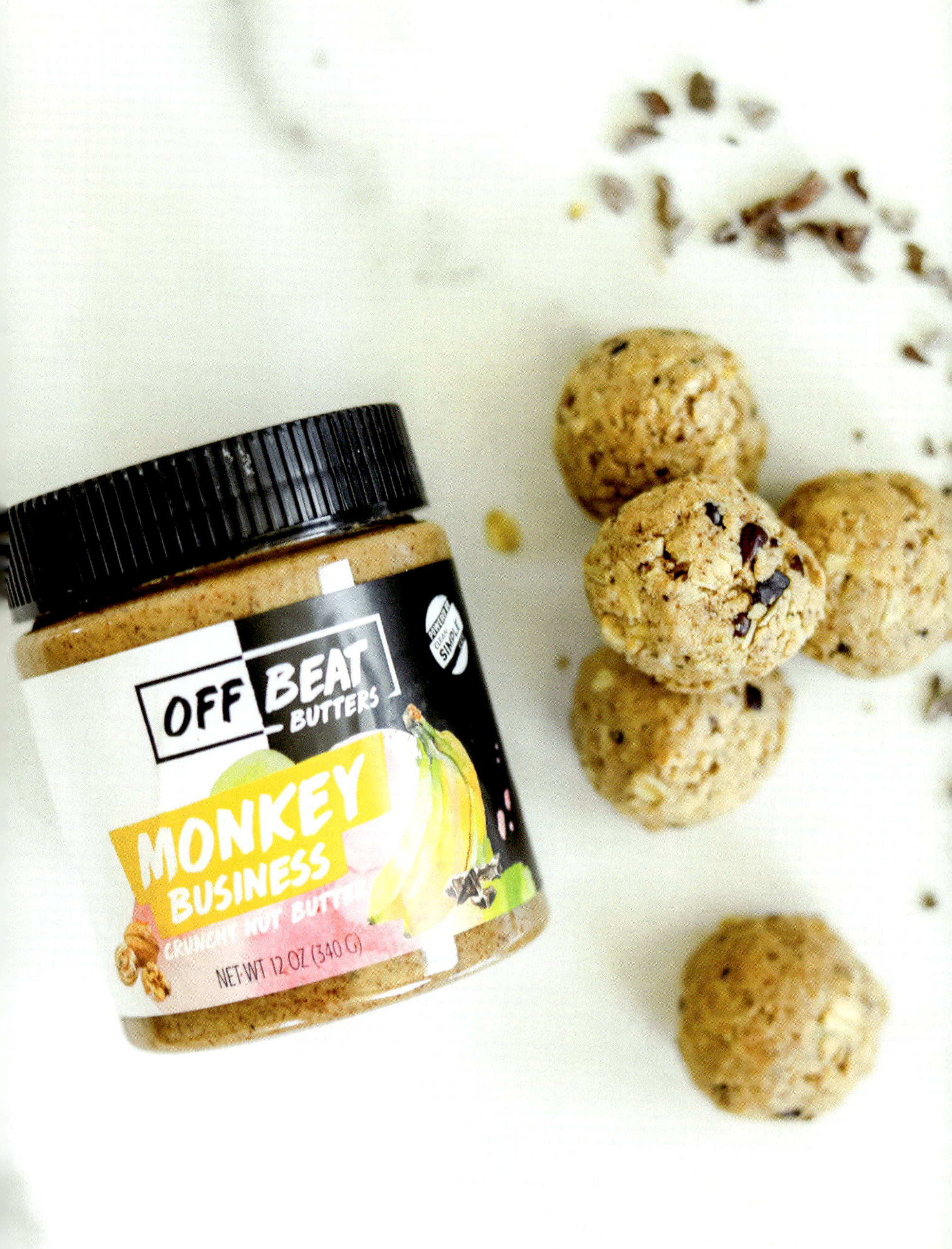

OFF BEAT BUTTERS
MONKEY BUSINESS
CRUNCHY NUT BUTTER
NET WT 12 OZ (340 G)

MONKEY BUSINESS BITES
Makes 28 servings
100 calories / 4F / 12C / 4P / per bite

1 cup OffBeat Monkey Business Butter
½ cup raw honey
2 servings CSE Bananas Foster, Coconut Cream,
   Simply Vanilla or Brownie Batter Protein Powder
1 cup old-fashioned rolled oats
Pinch coarse sea salt

1. Add all of the ingredients to a bowl and mix until well combined.

2. Using a small cookie scoop, scoop into balls and place in a container. Store in the fridge or freezer. Enjoy!

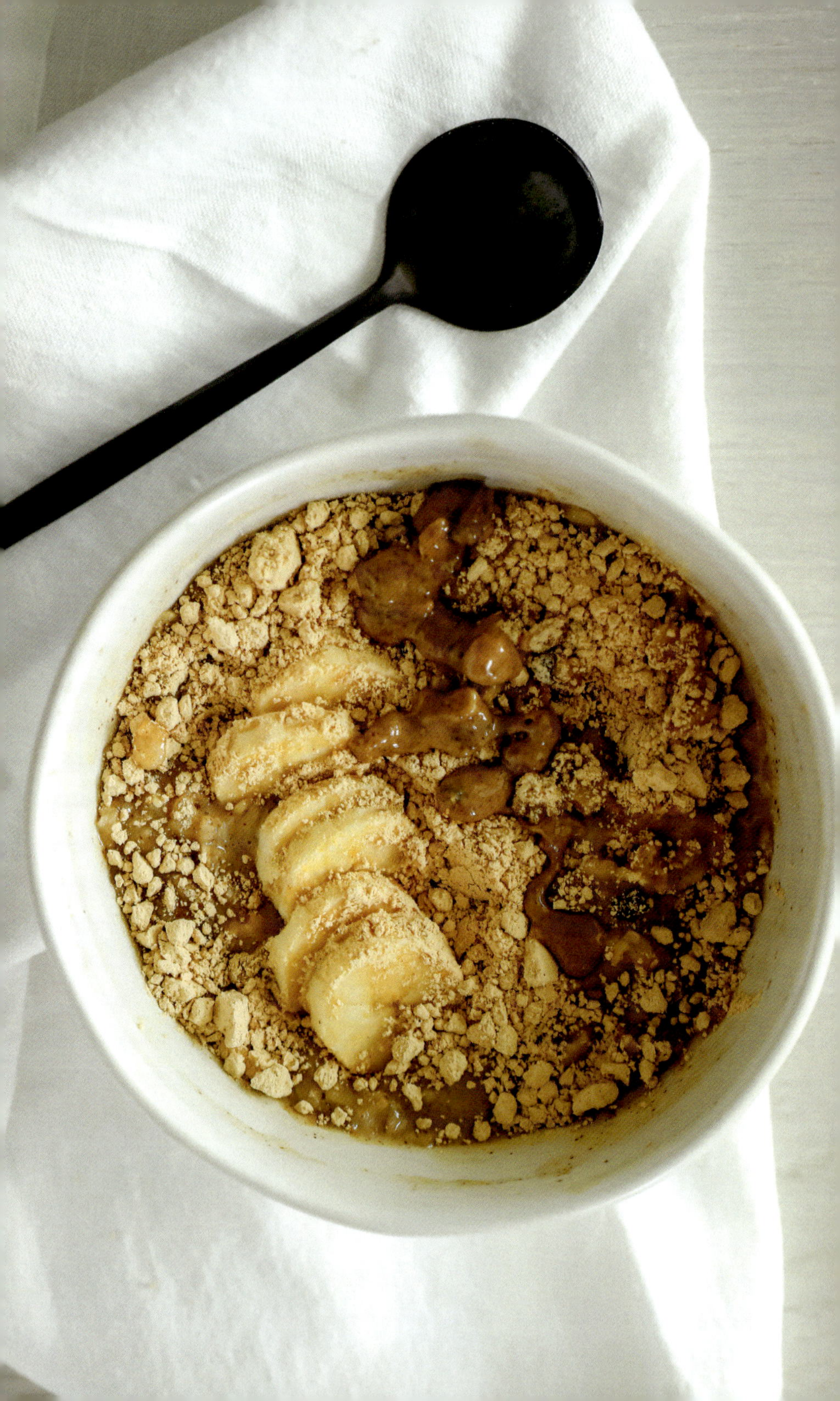

MONKEY BUSINESS OATS

Makes 1 serving
350 calories / 11F / 36C / 27P

⅓ cup old-fashioned rolled oats
½ cup water
1 Tbs. (14g) OffBeat Monkey Business Butter
¾ serving (27g) CSE Bananas Foster Protein Powder
Toppings:
20g banana slices
1½ Tbs. (12g) powdered peanut butter

1. Add the oats and water to a microwave-safe bowl. Microwave for 1-2 minutes.

2. Stir in the Monkey Business Butter. Let cool for a couple minutes, then stir in the protein powder.

3. Top with banana slices and powdered peanut butter. Enjoy!

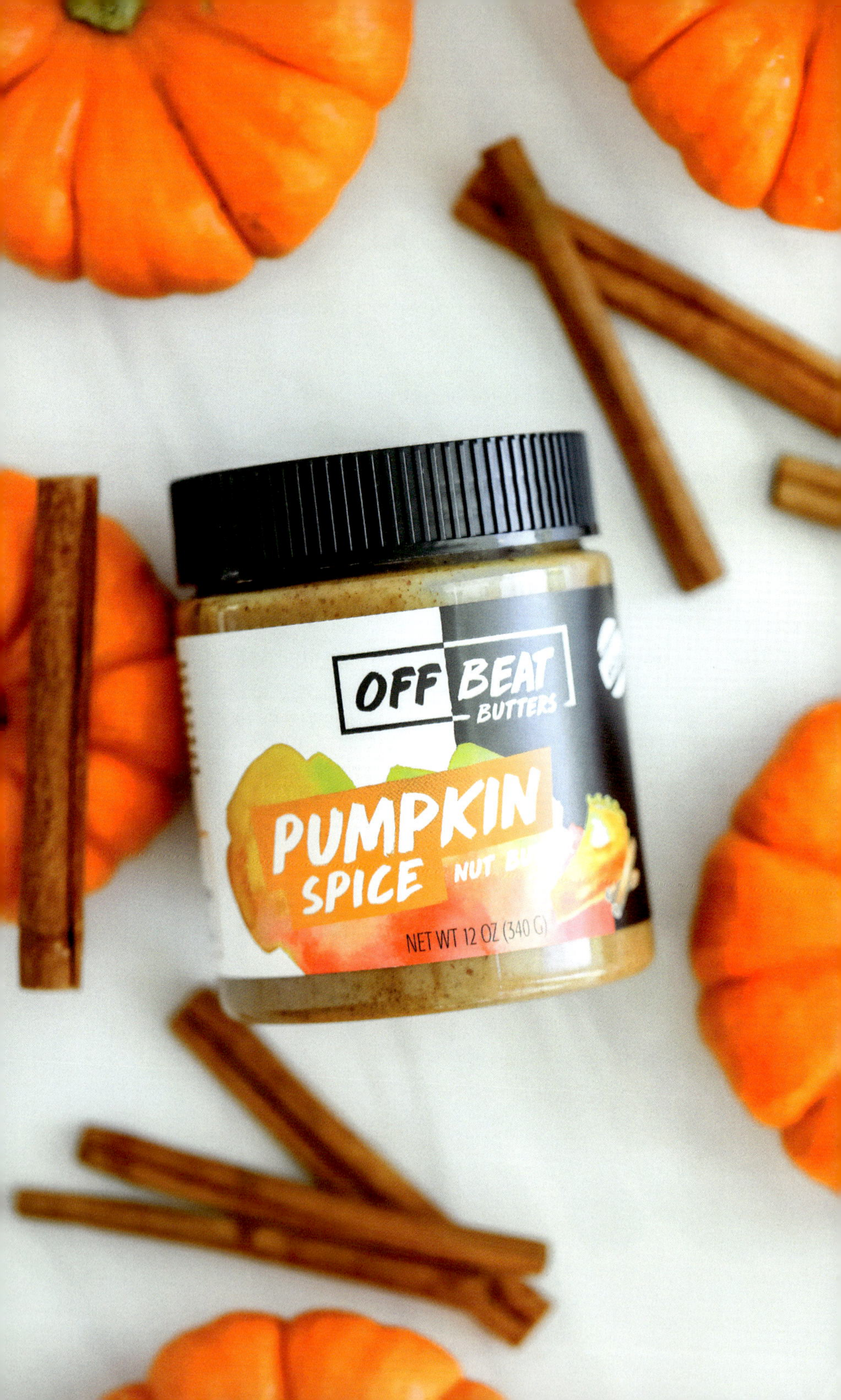

OFF BEAT
BUTTERS
PUMPKIN
SPICE
NUT BUTTER
NET WT 12 OZ (340 G)

AT THIS POINT,
MY BLOOD
TYPE IS
PUMPKIN SPICE

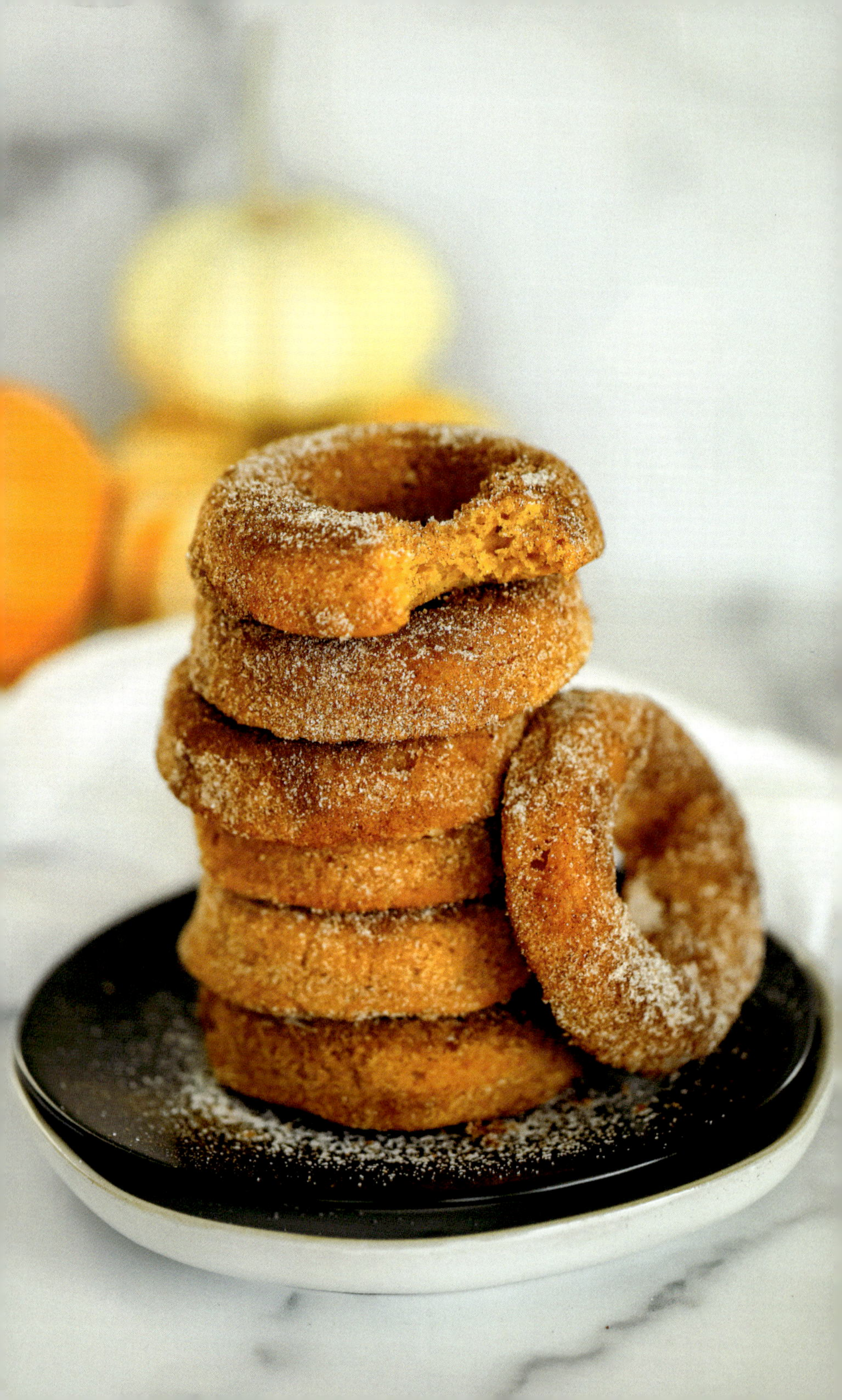

CINNAMON SUGAR PUMPKIN DONUTS
Makes 24 Servings
160 calories / 6F / 24C / 3P / per serving

¼ cup coconut oil
¼ cups OffBeat Pumpkin Spice Butter
1 cup raw honey
1 serving CSE Pumpkin Pie
   or Simply Vanilla Protein Powder
3 eggs
1 tsp. vanilla extract
1 ½ cups canned pumpkin
½ tsp. sea salt
½ Tbs. baking powder
8 oz. whole wheat pastry flour
¼ cup grass-fed, unsalted butter
½ cup white granulated sugar
1 Tbs. ground cinnamon

1. Heat the oven to 350 degrees.

2. Add the melted coconut oil, Pumpkin Spice Butter, honey and protein powder to a large bowl. Beat together until smooth. Beat in the eggs, vanilla and canned pumpkin. Set aside.

3. In a separate bowl, combine the sea salt, baking powder and flour. Add the dry ingredients to the wet ingredients and beat on low speed until well combined.

4. Scrape all of the batter into a large zip top plastic bag or piping bag. Cut off the corner and pipe the mixture into a greased donut pan, filing each one about ¾ of the way full. Bake at 350 degrees for 10-12 minutes.

5. Let the donuts cool in the pan for about 5 minutes, then transfer to a wire rack. Melt the butter and combine the sugar and cinnamon in a bowl. Baste both sides of each donut with melted butter and then dip into the cinnamon sugar mixture and place back on the wire rack. Best when eaten warm. Enjoy!

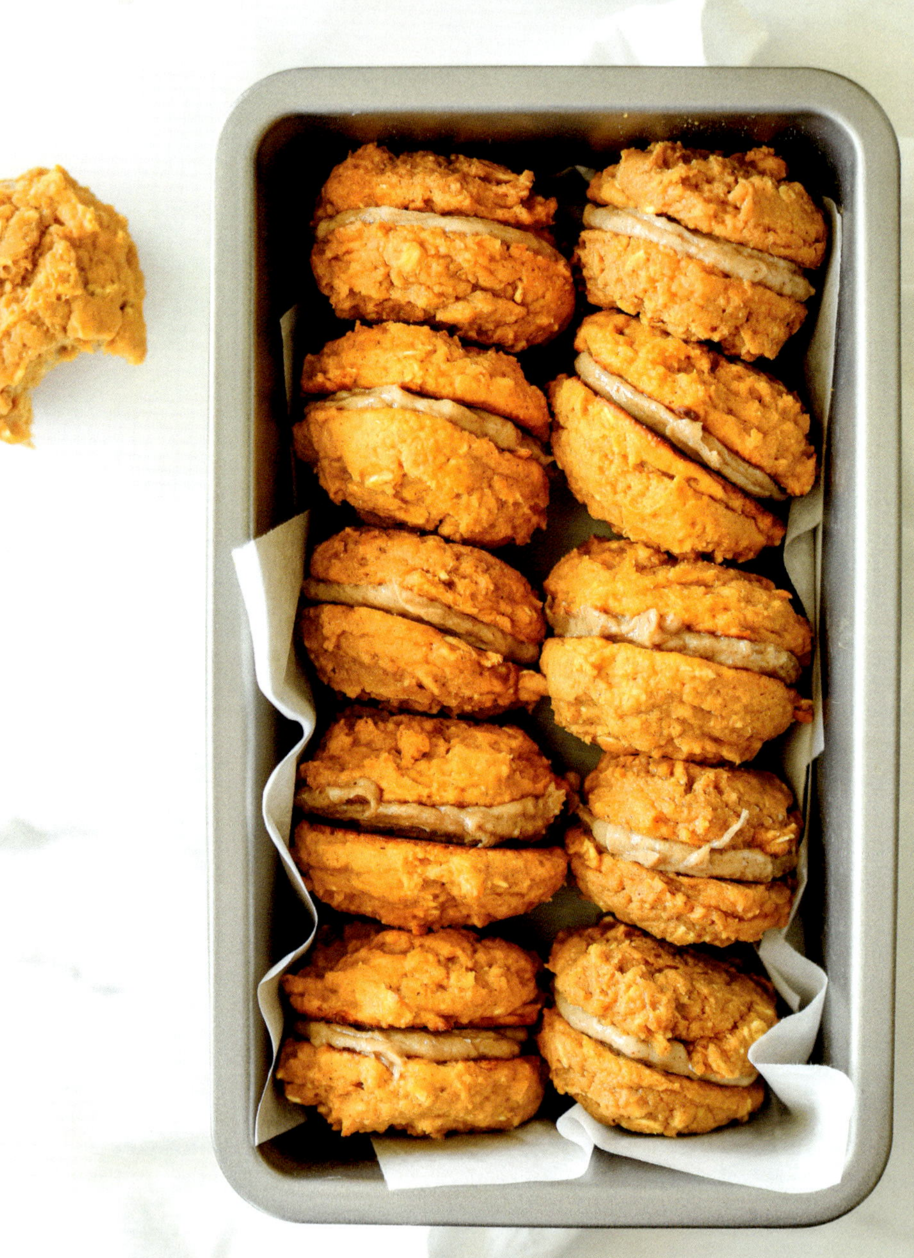

MINI PUMPKIN SPICE WHOOPIE PIES *

Makes 26 servings
150 calories / 7F / 15C / 7P / per cookie sandwich

Cake:
432g Cinnamon Oat Kodiak Cakes Mix
2 tsp. pumpkin pie spice
1 serving CSE Pumpkin Pie Protein Powder
½ tsp. baking powder
½ cup almond milk
1 (15 oz.) canned pumpkin puree
2 large eggs
⅓ cup coconut oil, melted
Frosting:
4oz. Neufchâtel cheese, softened
½ cup OffBeat Pumpkin Spice Butter
¼ cup raw unfiltered honey

1. Take Neufchâtel cheese, almond milk, and eggs out of fridge and bring to room temperature.

2. Preheat oven to 350 degrees. Line cookie sheet with parchment paper.

3. Mix dry cake ingredients together in a large bowl.

4. Add wet cake ingredients to dry ingredients.

5. Mix together well, using an immersion blender or blender and blend until smooth.

6. Using a small cookie scoop (½-inch diameter), scoop batter onto cookie sheets. Bake for 11-13 minutes. Let cool, then remove from cookie sheet.

7. While cookies are baking and/or cooling, add softened Neufchâtel cheese, Pumpkin Spice Butter, and honey to a small bowl and mix until smooth. Weigh frosting and divide by the number of whoopie pies that you have (two halves per pie).

8. Once sandwich parts are cool, pair with another of similar size and shape. Scoop the frosting onto one side of the whoopie pie sandwich and place the other half on top. Continue until all whoopie pies are assembled.

OffBeat Fam Recipe Submitted by Liz Skokan

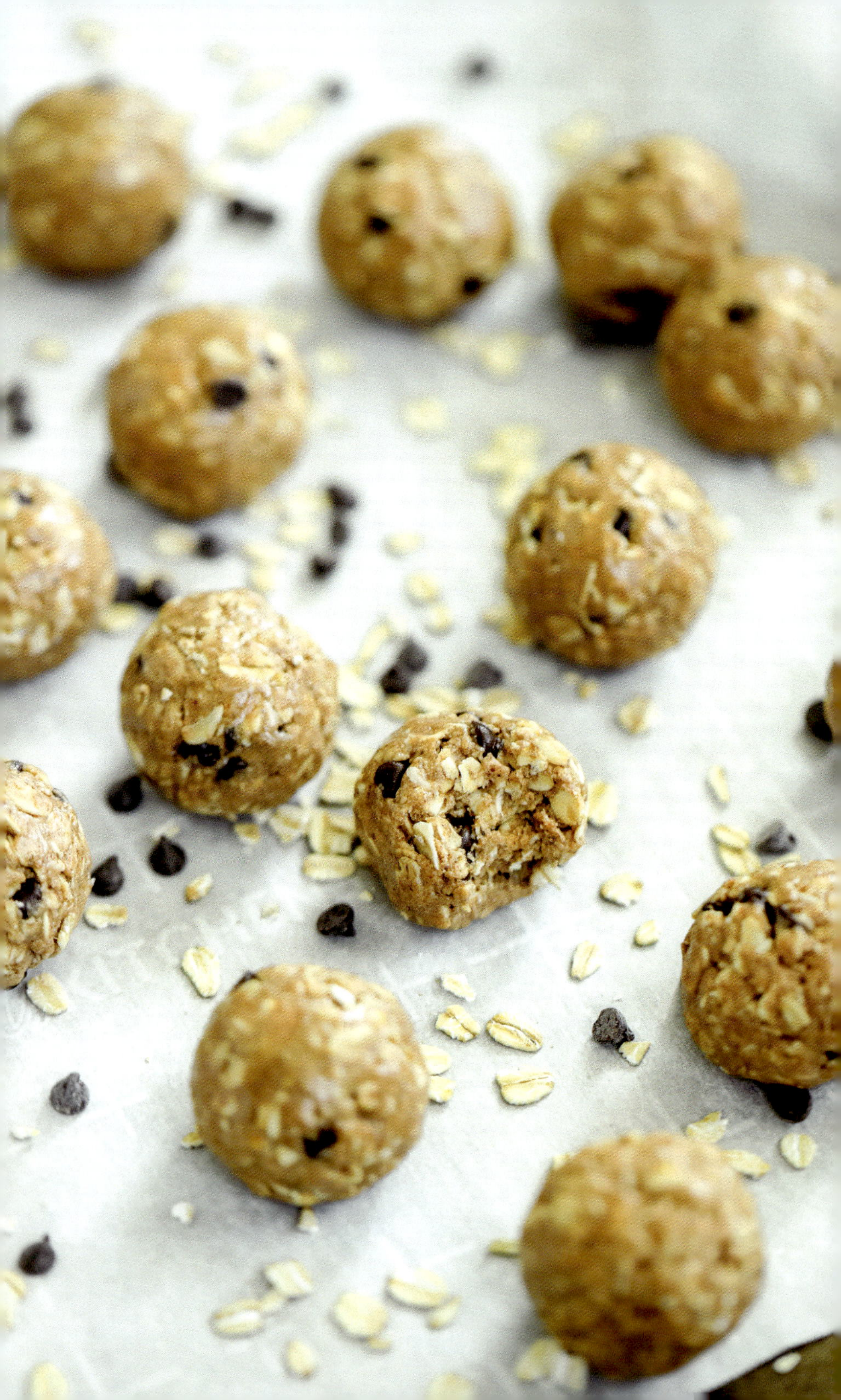

PUMPKIN CHOCOLATE CHIP COOKIE BITES

Makes 20 servings
125 calories / 6F / 15C / 3P / per bite

---

1 cup OffBeat Pumpkin Spice Butter
½ cup raw honey
1 serving CSE Pumpkin Pie
   or Simply Vanilla Protein Powder
1½ cups old-fashioned rolled oats
2 Tbs. mini chocolate chips
1 tsp. vanilla extract
Dash sea salt

1. Add all of the ingredients to a large bowl and mix until well combined.

2. Using a small cookie scoop, scoop into rounded balls (about 30g per ball). Place in a container and store in the fridge or freezer. Enjoy!

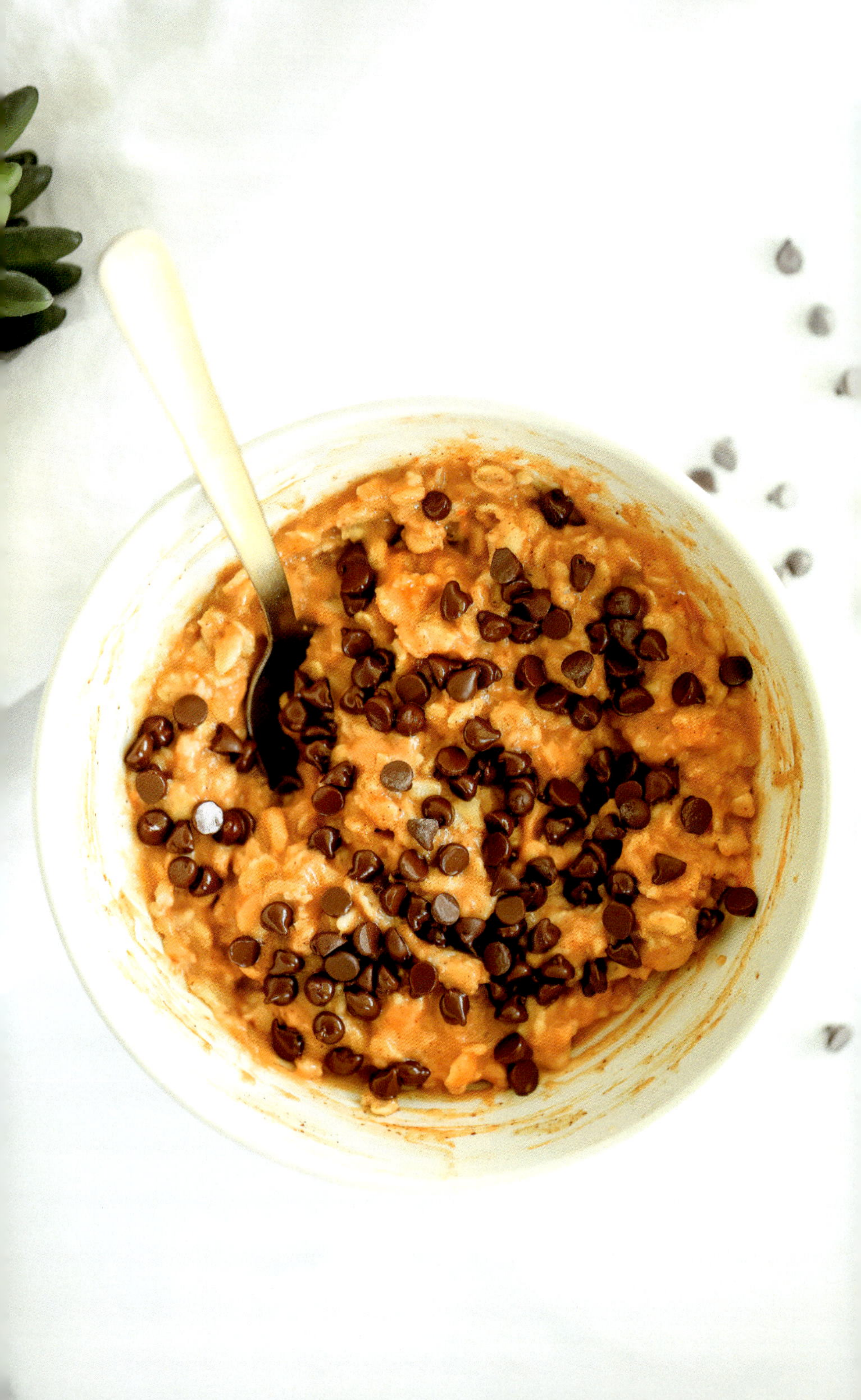

PUMPKIN CHOCOLATE CHIP COOKIE OATMEAL
Makes 1 serving
355 calories / 12F / 35C / 26.5P

⅓ cup old-fashioned rolled oats
½ cup water
3 Tbs. (46g) egg whites
1 Tbs. (14g) OffBeat Pumpkin Spice Butter
¾ (24g) serving CSE Pumpkin Pie Protein Powder
Dash sea salt
Vanilla stevia drops, optional to taste
Topping:
1 Tbs. (15g) mini chocolate chips

1. Add the oats, water, and egg whites to a microwave-safe bowl. Whisk until the egg whites are well combined. Microwave for 1-2 minutes.

2. Add the Pumpkin Spice Butter and stir until well combined. Let cool for a couple minutes. Stir in the protein powder, salt, stevia and a little almond milk if the oatmeal is too thick.

3. Sprinkle the chocolate chips over the top. Enjoy!

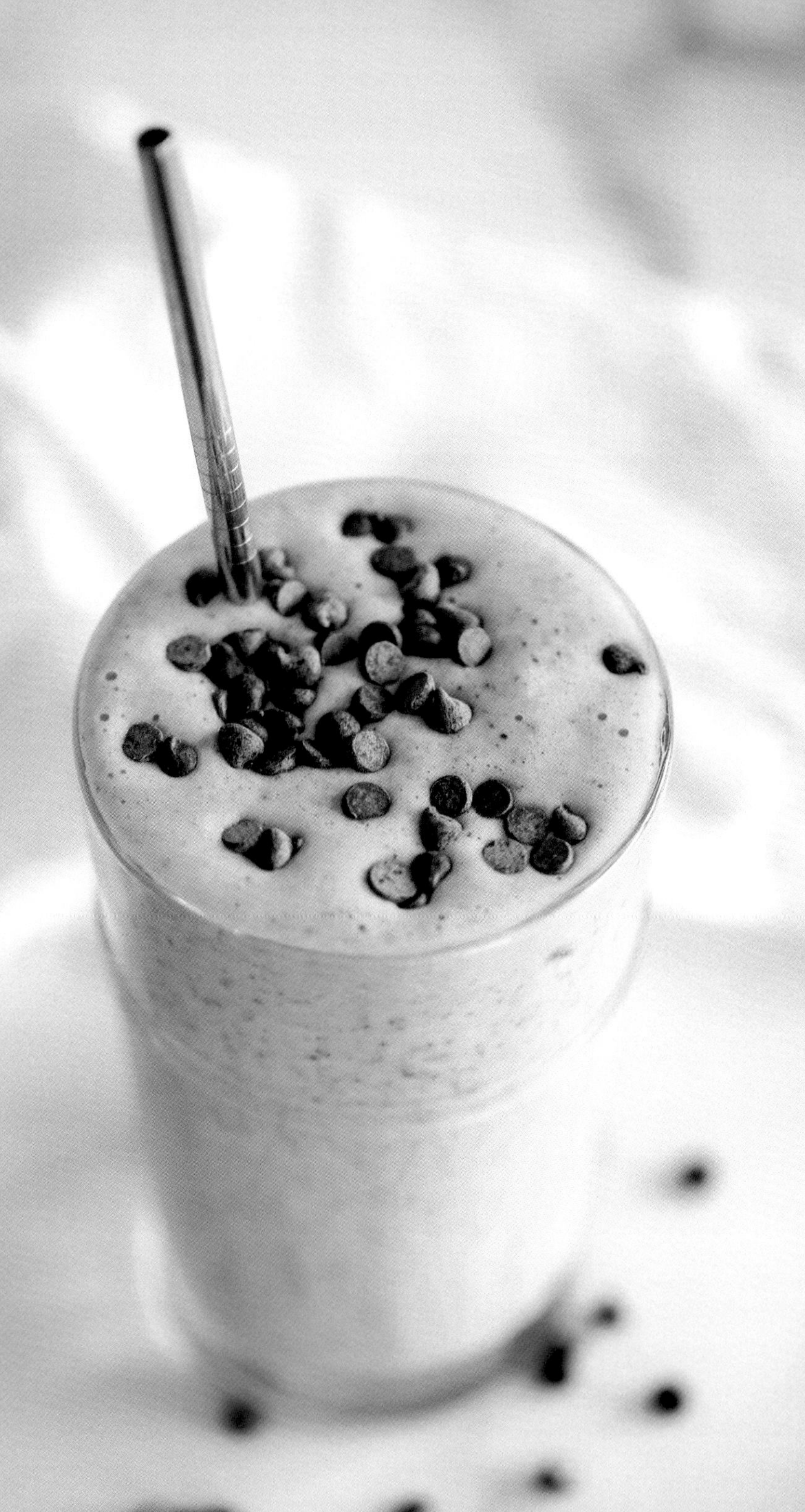

PUMPKIN CHOCOLATE SPECKLED SHAKE

Makes 1 serving
250 calories / 9F / 23.5C / 18.5P

---

1 cup unsweetened almond milk
¾ serving CSE Pumpkin Pie Protein Powder
2 Tbs. canned pumpkin
40g frozen banana slices
½ Tbs. (7g) OffBeat Pumpkin Spice or Cinnamon Bun Butter
½ Tbs. (7g) mini chocolate chips
6-8 (120g) ice cubes

1. Add all of the ingredients to a high-powered blender. Blend until smooth.

2. Pour into a cup. Enjoy!

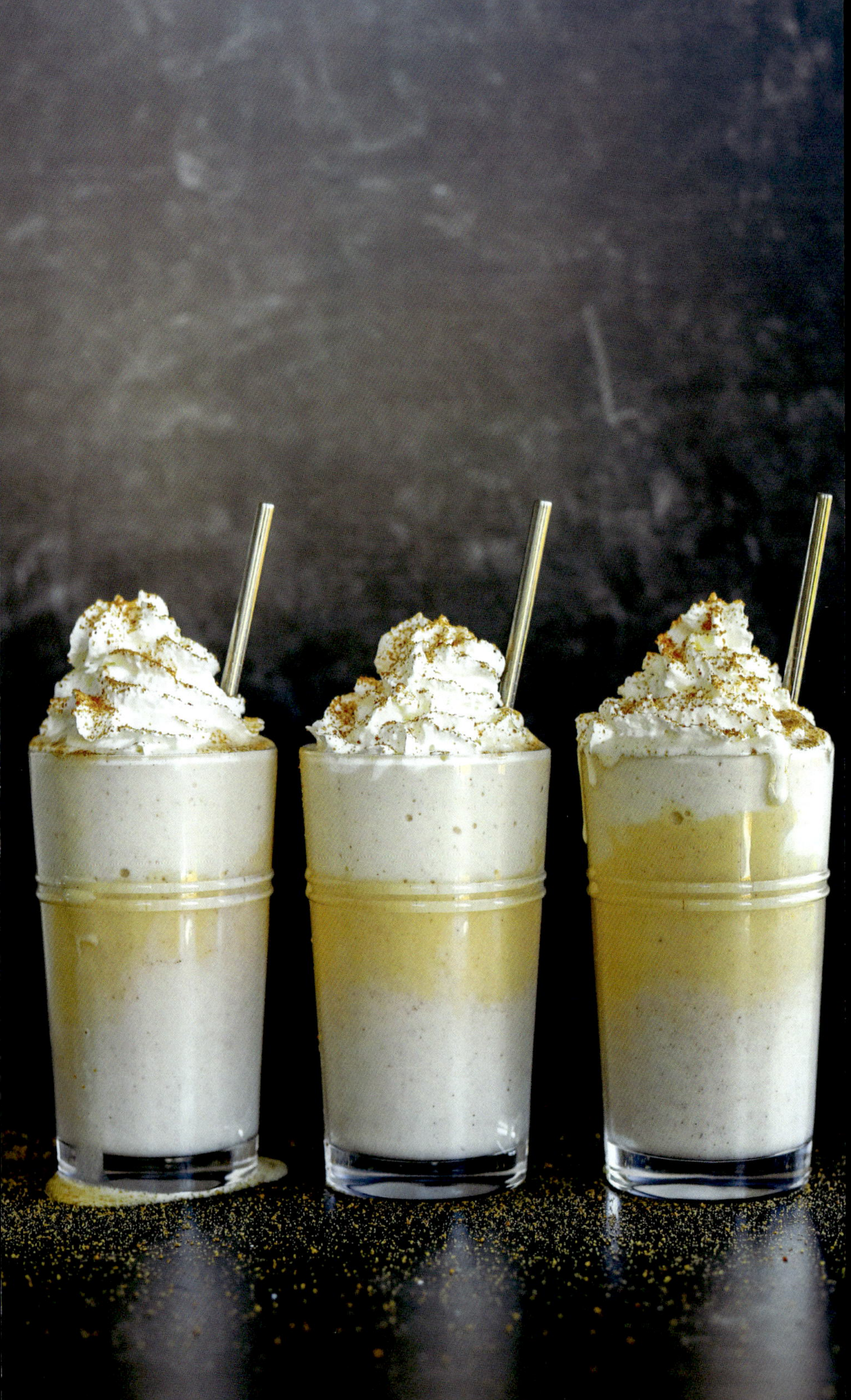

PUMPKIN CINNAMON ROLL SHAKE

Makes 3 servings
320 calories / 10F / 34C / 24P / per serving

Cinnamon Roll Layer:

1 cup unsweetened almond milk
1 serving CSE Cinnamon Roll Protein Powder
1 Tbs. OffBeat Cinnamon Bun Butter
100g frozen banana slices
6-8 (120g) ice cubes

Pumpkin Layer:

1 cup unsweetened almond milk
1 Serving CSE Pumpkin Pie Protein Powder
1 Tbs. OffBeat Pumpkin Spice Butter
100g frozen banana slices
6-8 (120g) ice cubes

Vanilla Layer:

1 cup unsweetened almond milk
1 serving CSE Simply Vanilla Protein Powder
1 Tbs. OffBeat Salted Caramel Butter
100g frozen banana slices
6-8 (120g) ice cubes

Toppings:

6 Tbs. spray whipped cream
¾ tsp. coconut sugar

1. Blend each shake separately in a blender and add ⅓ of each shake to each cup.

2. Top each with two tablespoons of spray whipped cream and sprinkle with ¼ teaspoon of coconut sugar.

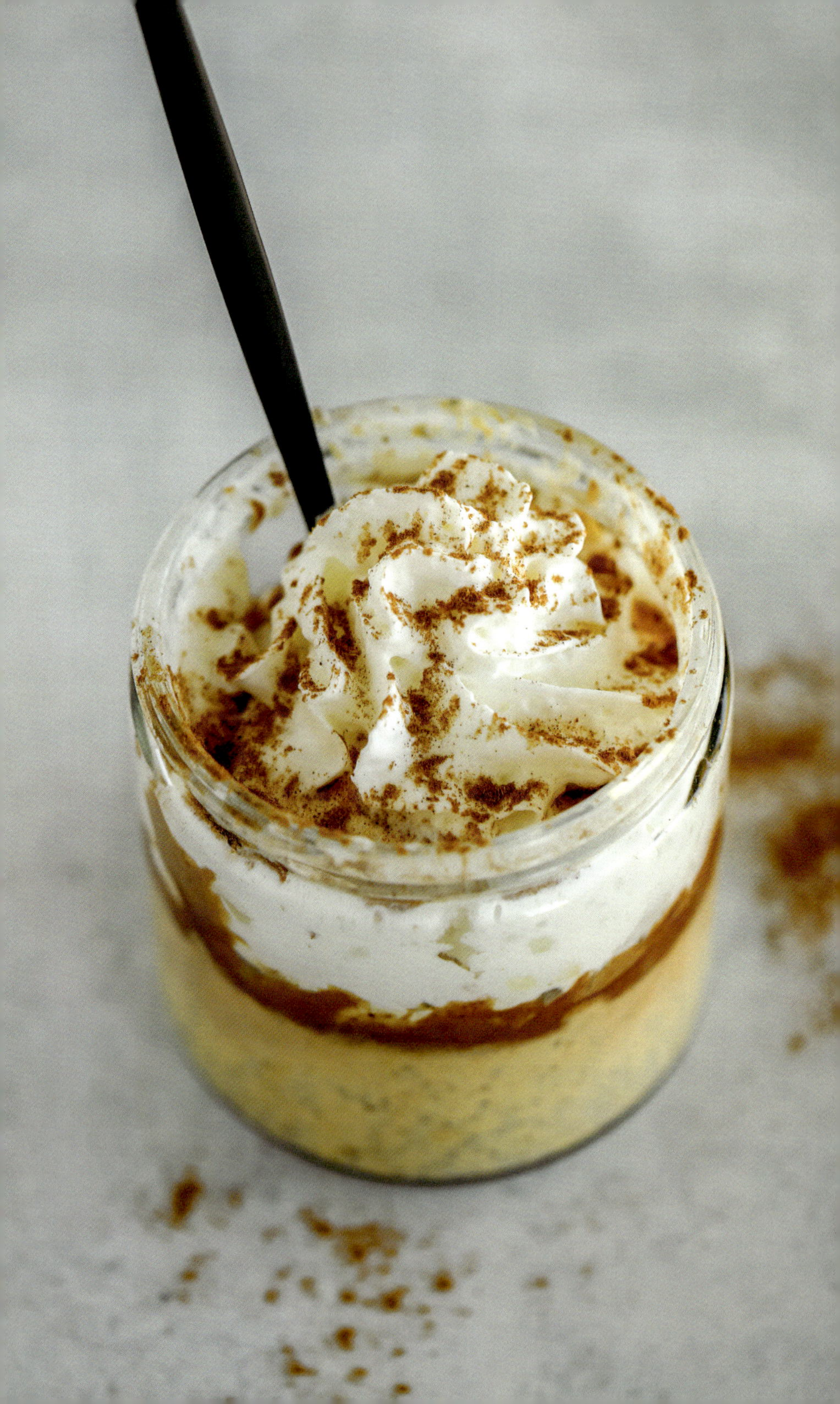

PUMPKIN PIE CHIA PUDDING
Makes 1 serving
350 Calories / 13F / 34C / 24P

¼ cup unsweetened almond milk
¼ cup plain non-fat Greek yogurt
1 Tbs. pumpkin, canned
2 Tbs. chia seeds
½ serving CSE Pumpkin Pie Protein Powder
1 serving vanilla Stevia drops, optional
½ Tbs Offbeat Pumpkin Spice Butter
Toppings:
60g bananas
4 Tbs. Spray Whipped Cream
1 dash pumpkin pie spice

1. Add the almond milk, yogurt, pumpkin puree, chia seeds, protein powder and stevia drops (if desired) to a glass jar. Whisk together until well combined.

2. Drizzle the Pumpkin Spice Butter over the top. Cover and store in the fridge overnight.

3. Top with sliced bananas, whipped cream and pumpkin pie spice. Enjoy cold.

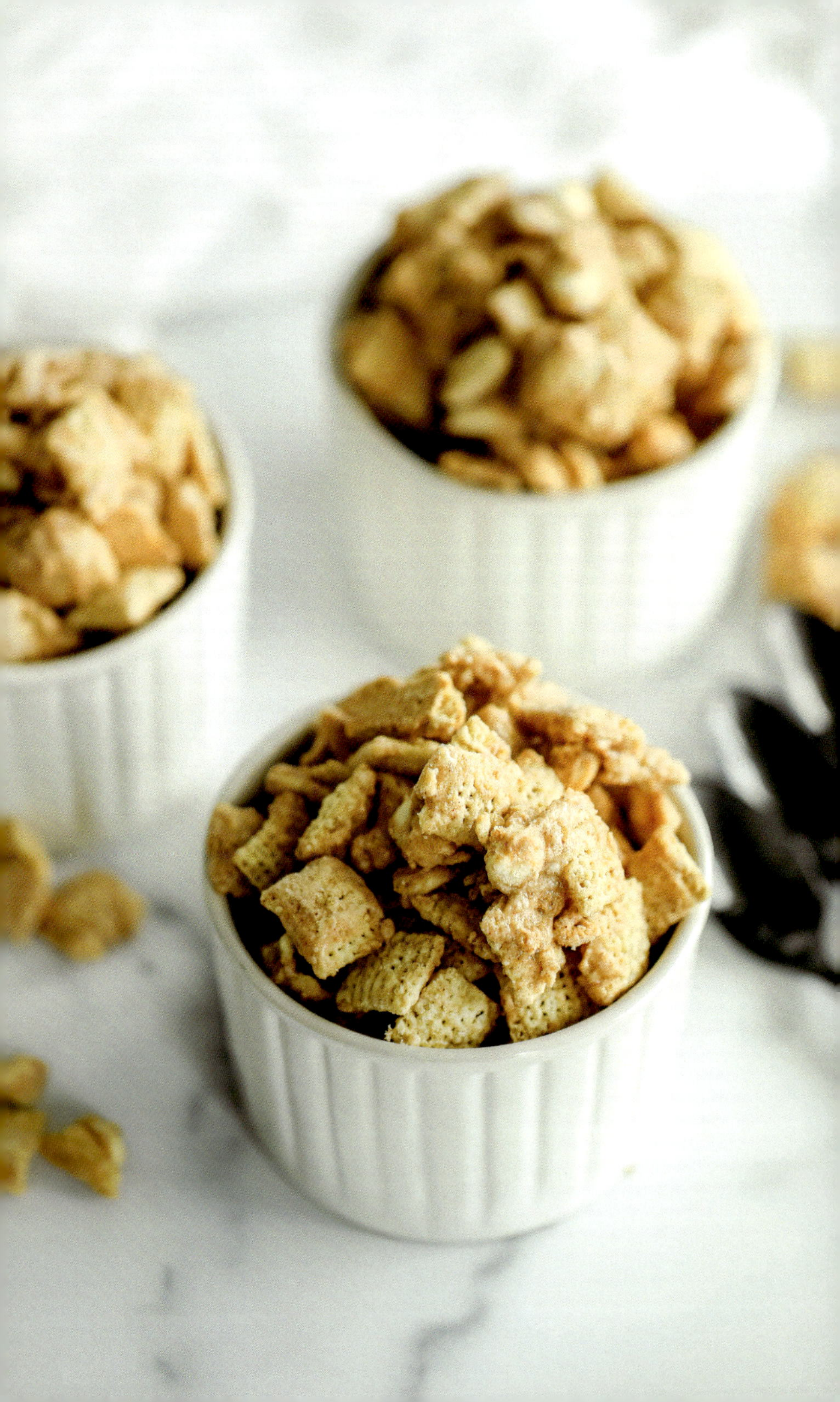

PUMPKIN PIE PUPPY CHOW

Makes 12 servings
310 calories / 15F / 38C / 8P / per serving

---

7 cups Chex Rice cereal
1 cup graham cracker crumbs
1 cup white chocolate chips
¼ cup grass-fed butter
½ cup OffBeat Pumpkin Spice Butter
¼ cup raw honey
Dash sea salt
Dash cinnamon
2 servings CSE Pumpkin Pie Protein Powder

1. Pour the cereal, graham cracker crumbs and ½ cup of the chocolate chips into a large bowl; set aside.

2. Add the butter to a small saucepan over low heat. Once melted, add the Pumpkin Spice Butter, honey, ½ cup white chocolate chips, sea salt and cinnamon. Stir constantly until completely melted. Remove from heat and let cool for a couple minutes. Stir in one serving of protein powder.

3. Pour the hot mixture over the top of the dry mixture in the bowl. Stir until well coated. Sprinkle with another serving of protein powder. Stir and serve. One serving is approximately one cup or 75 grams.

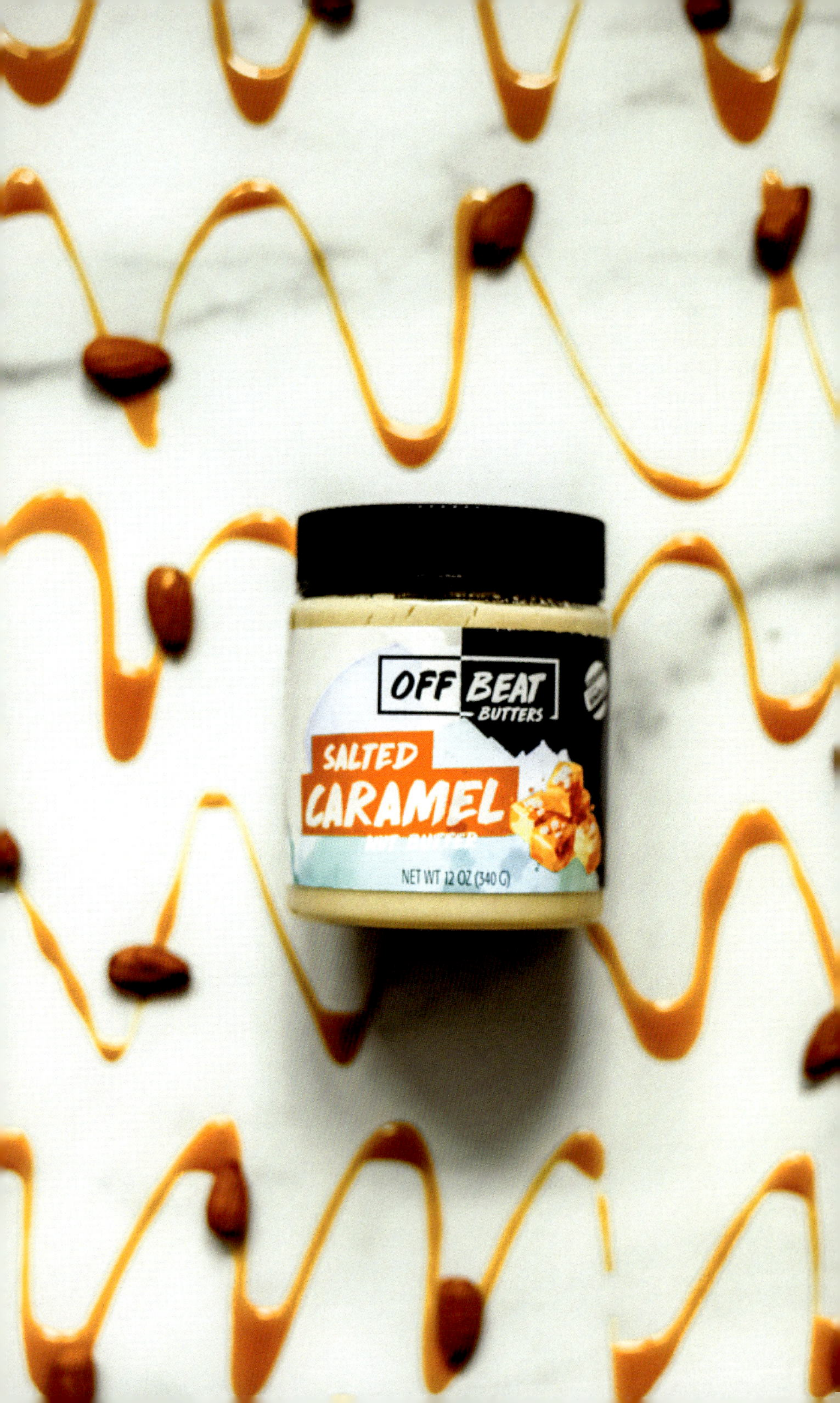
OFF BEAT
BUTTERS
SALTED
CARAMEL
NET WT 12 OZ (340 G)

A BAD DAY WITH SALTED CARAMEL BUTTER IS BETTER THAN A GOOD DAY WITHOUT

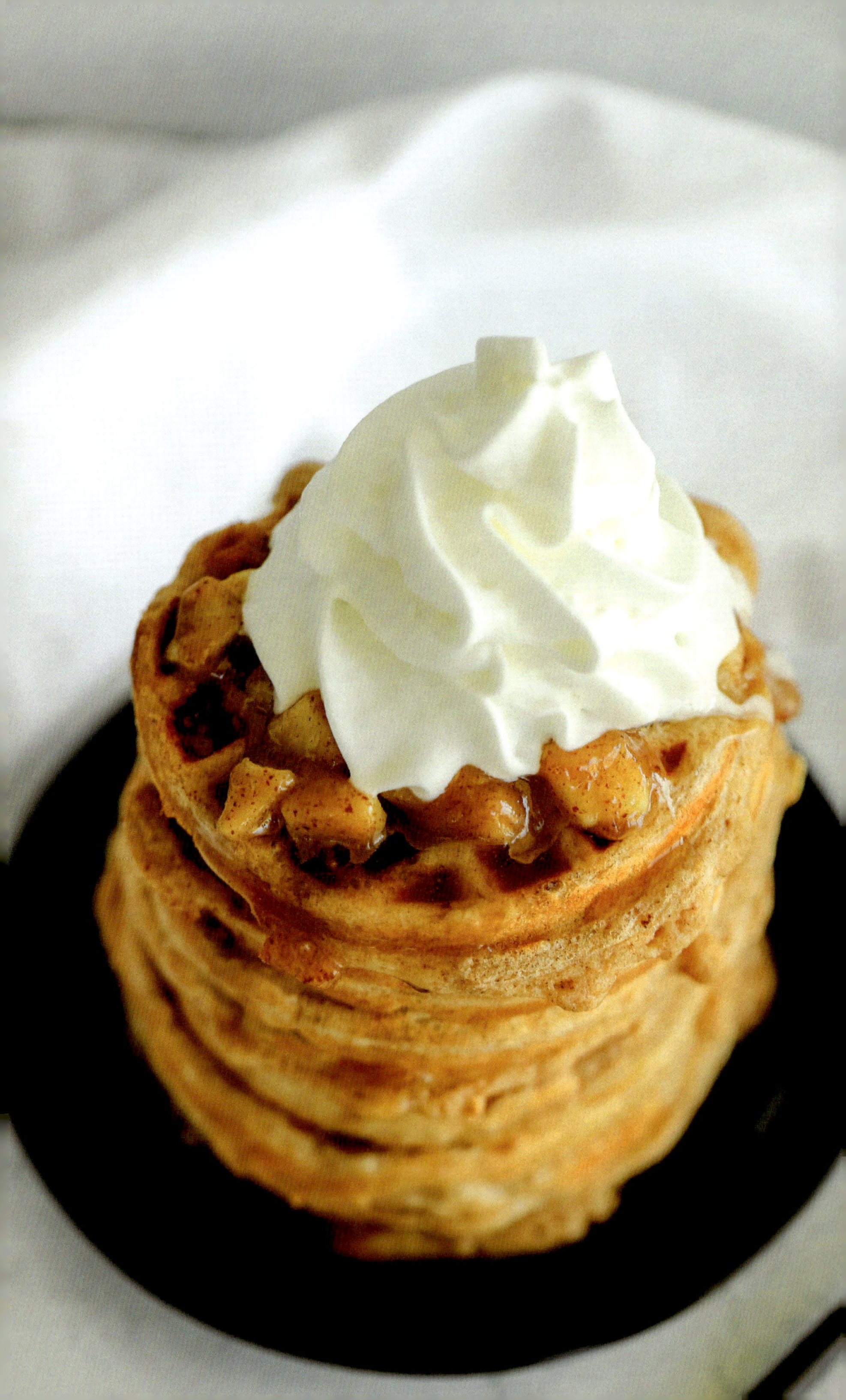

CARAMEL APPLE PIE WAFFLES

Makes 4 servings
350 calories / 11.5F / 38C / 24.5P / per serving

100g apples
80g OffBeat Salted Caramel Butter
2 Tbs. raw honey
1 ⅓ cups Kodiak Cinnamon Oat Power Cakes Mix
½ cup nonfat, plain Greek yogurt
1 ¼ cups liquid egg whites
Toppings:
8 Tbs. spray whipped cream
4 servings zero calorie syrup of choice

1. Peel and chop the apples into tiny pieces.

2. Heat a frying pan over low heat. Spray the pan with cooking spray, then add the apples, Salted Caramel Butter and honey. Stir until the apples are well coated. Cook until the apples are soft and the butter and honey are melted. Remove from heat, cover and set aside.

3. Heat a waffle iron.

4. Add the Kodiak Cakes Mix, Greek yogurt and egg whites to a bowl. Whisk together until smooth. Fold the caramel apple mixture into the batter. You can also save the caramel apple mixture and use it as a topping for the waffles after they're cooked. Spray the waffle iron with cooking spray, then add the batter and cook. Repeat with the remaining batter.

5. Weigh all the waffles and divide the weight by four to get the amount needed to fill one serving. Top each serving with two tablespoons of whipped cream and syrup. Enjoy!

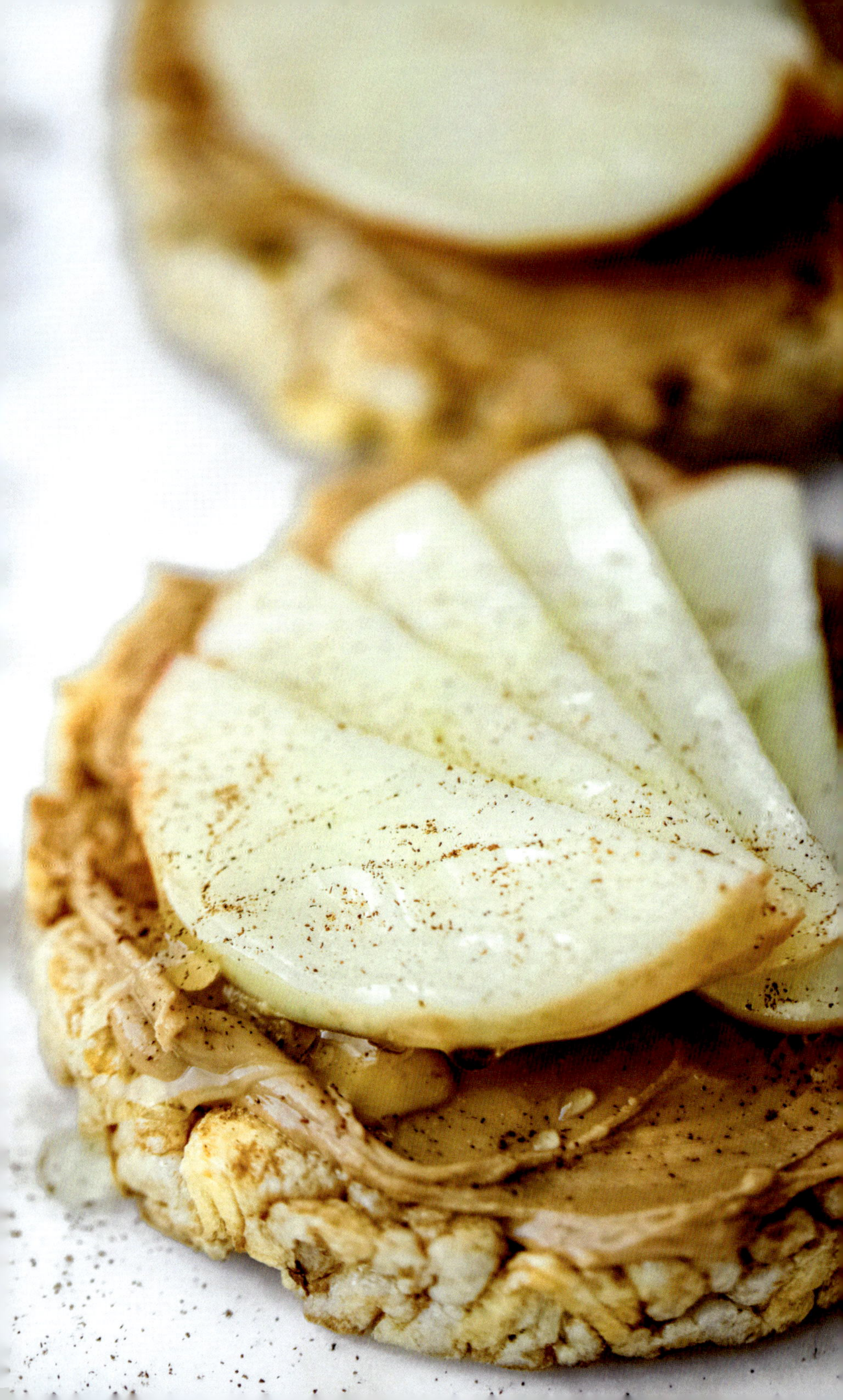

CARAMEL APPLE RICE CAKE SNACK
Makes 1 serving
180 calories / 7F / 28C / 3.5P

---

1 caramel rice cake
50g sliced apples
1 Tbs. OffBeat Salted Caramel
 or Cinnamon Bun Butter
1 tsp. honey

1. Add the Salted Caramel Butter to the rice cake (Quaker or Kroger are our favorites!).

2. Top with apple slices and drizzle with honey.

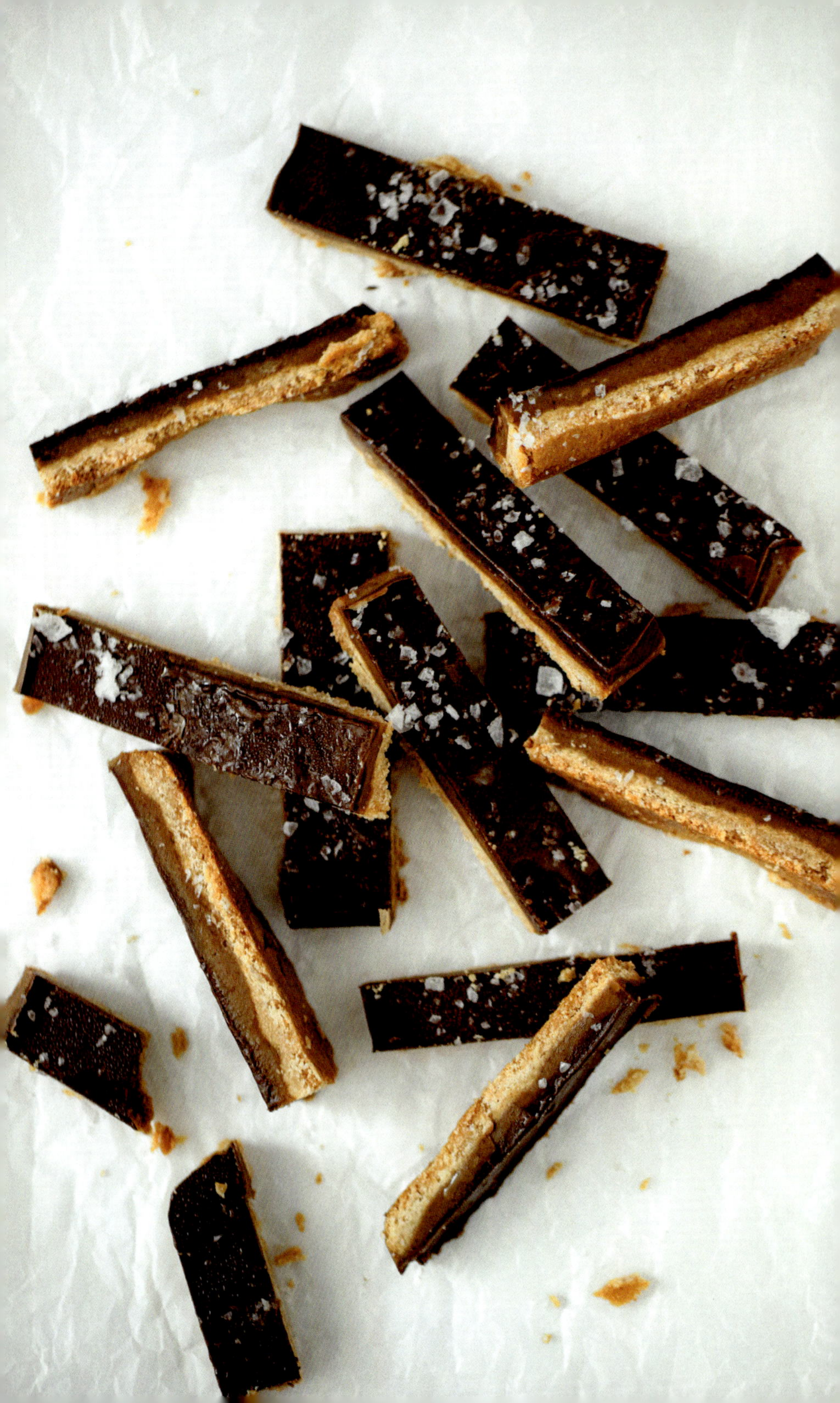

CHOCO CARAMEL CRUNCH BARS*
Makes 32 servings
110 calories / 8.5F / 8C / 1.5P / per serving

Shortbread Layer:
½ cup coconut flour
½ cup almond flour
⅓ cup coconut oil
3 Tbs. honey, melted
Caramel Layer:
½ cup OffBeat Salted Caramel Butter
¼ cup coconut oil

1 tsp. vanilla extract
¼ cup maple syrup
Chocolate Layer:
½ cup chocolate chips
1 ½ Tbs. coconut oil
½ tsp. flaky sea salt, optional

1. Preheat oven to 350 degrees. Combine coconut and almond flours with melted coconut oil & warmed honey in a large bowl. Stir until thoroughly combined.

2. Line an 8x8 pan with parchment paper and pack down shortbread mixture into the base.

3. Bake for 10-12 minutes, or until starting to turn golden brown. Remove once done and let cool completely.

4. Combine Salted Caramel Butter, coconut oil, vanilla, maple syrup and sea salt in a saucepan over the stove on medium-low heat and heat until completely liquified, whisking together about 2-3 minutes. Remove from heat and cool completely.

5. Put chocolate chips into a small bowl and add coconut oil. Warm in microwave for 30 second intervals, stirring in between, until completely liquified. Or, heat over the stove.

6. Once shortbread and caramel have completely cooled, pour caramel sauce over the base layer, spreading out evenly. Set in the freezer until it hardens (about 1-2 hours).

7. Remove from the freezer and pour and evenly spread chocolate over the top. Sprinkle flaky sea salt and set back in the fridge for 5-10 minutes to harden.

8. Once chilled, remove from the pan and slice into ½-inch strips and then slice each strip in half. Enjoy!

OffBeat Fam Recipe Submitted by Jenn Orr

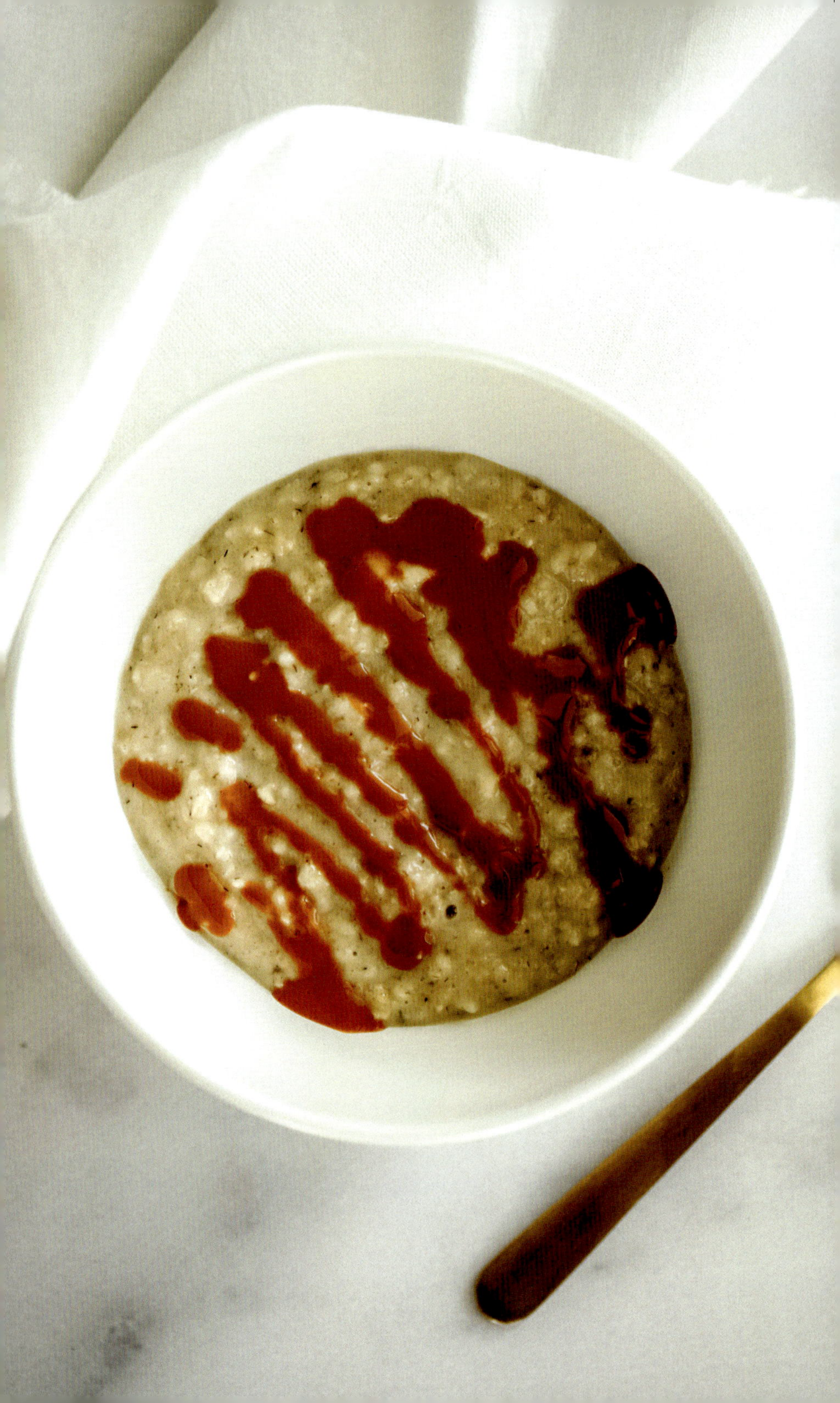

DOUBLE CARAMEL APPLE OATMEAL

Makes 1 serving
340 calories / 10F / 37C / 26P

⅓ cup old-fashioned rolled oats
½ cup water
3 Tbs. (46g) liquid egg whites
50g chopped apples
1 Tbs. (14g) OffBeat Salted Caramel Butter
¾ serving CSE Caramel Toffee Protein Powder
Toppings:
Dash cinnamon
Drizzle of Walden Farms Caramel Syrup, optional

1. Add the oats, water, egg whites, and chopped apples to a microwave-safe bowl. Whisk until the egg whites are well combined. Microwave for 1-2 minutes.

2. Stir in the Salted Caramel Butter. Let cool for a couple minutes, then stir in the protein powder.

3. Top with a dash of cinnamon and caramel sauce, if desired.

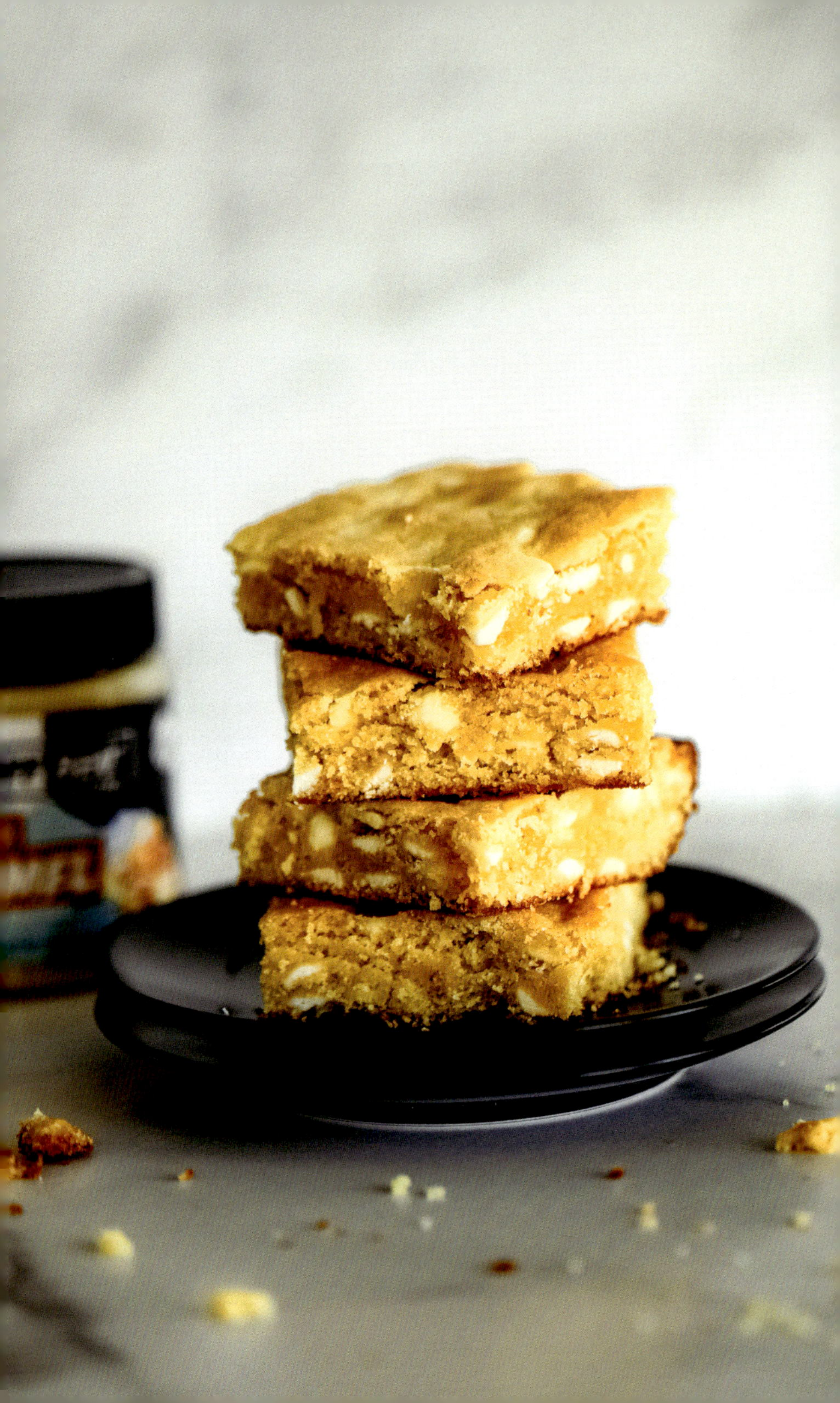

GRANDMA'S DESSERT BARS*

Makes 20 bars
279 calories / 16F / 32C / 3.5P / per bar

---

1 box yellow cake mix
½ cup grass-fed butter
1 cup OffBeat Salted Caramel Butter
2 large eggs
⅓ cup water
1 ½ cups white chocolate chips

1. Preheat the oven to 375 degrees.

2. Add half of the cake mix, butter, Salted Caramel Butter, eggs and water together in a large bowl.

3. Beat until smooth. Stir in remaining cake mix and white chocolate chips.

4. Spray a 9x13 baking pan with cooking spray.

5. Pour the batter into the pan and spread out evenly. Bake for 20-22 minutes or until golden brown.

OffBeat Fam Recipe Submitted by Amy Newton

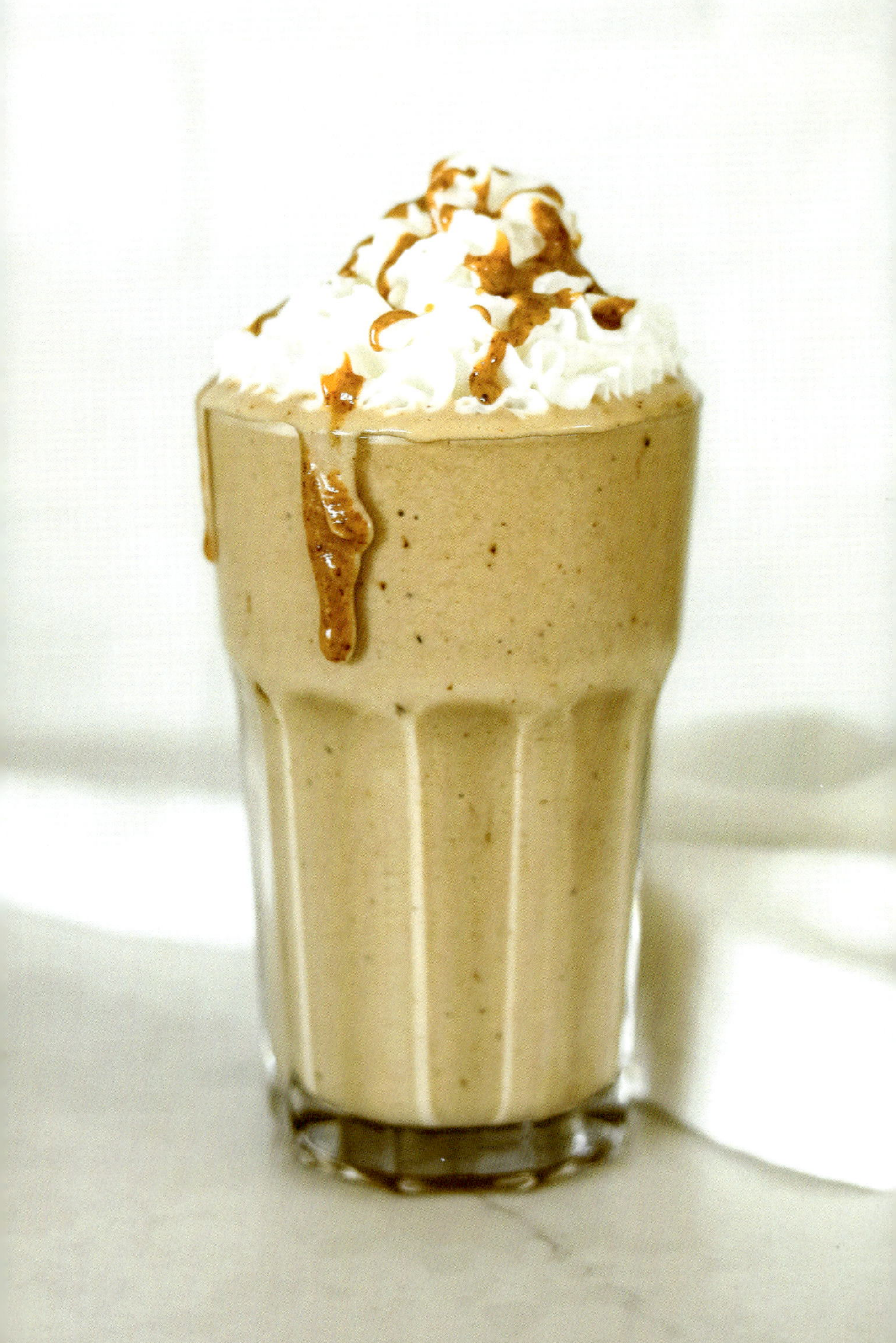

ROOT BEER FLOAT SHAKE*

Makes 1 serving
320 calories / 13F / 28C / 23P

---

1 cup unsweetened cashew milk
½ cup Halo Top Vanilla Bean Ice Cream
¾ serving (25g) CSE Simply Vanilla Protein Powder
½ Tbs. OffBeat Salted Caramel Butter
1 tsp. root beer extract
6-8 ice cubes
Topping:
2 Tbs. spray whipped cream

1. Add all ingredients to a high-powered blender, and blend on high until smooth.

2. Pour into a cup, top with whipped cream and enjoy!

OffBeat Fam Recipe Submitted by Karen Heasley

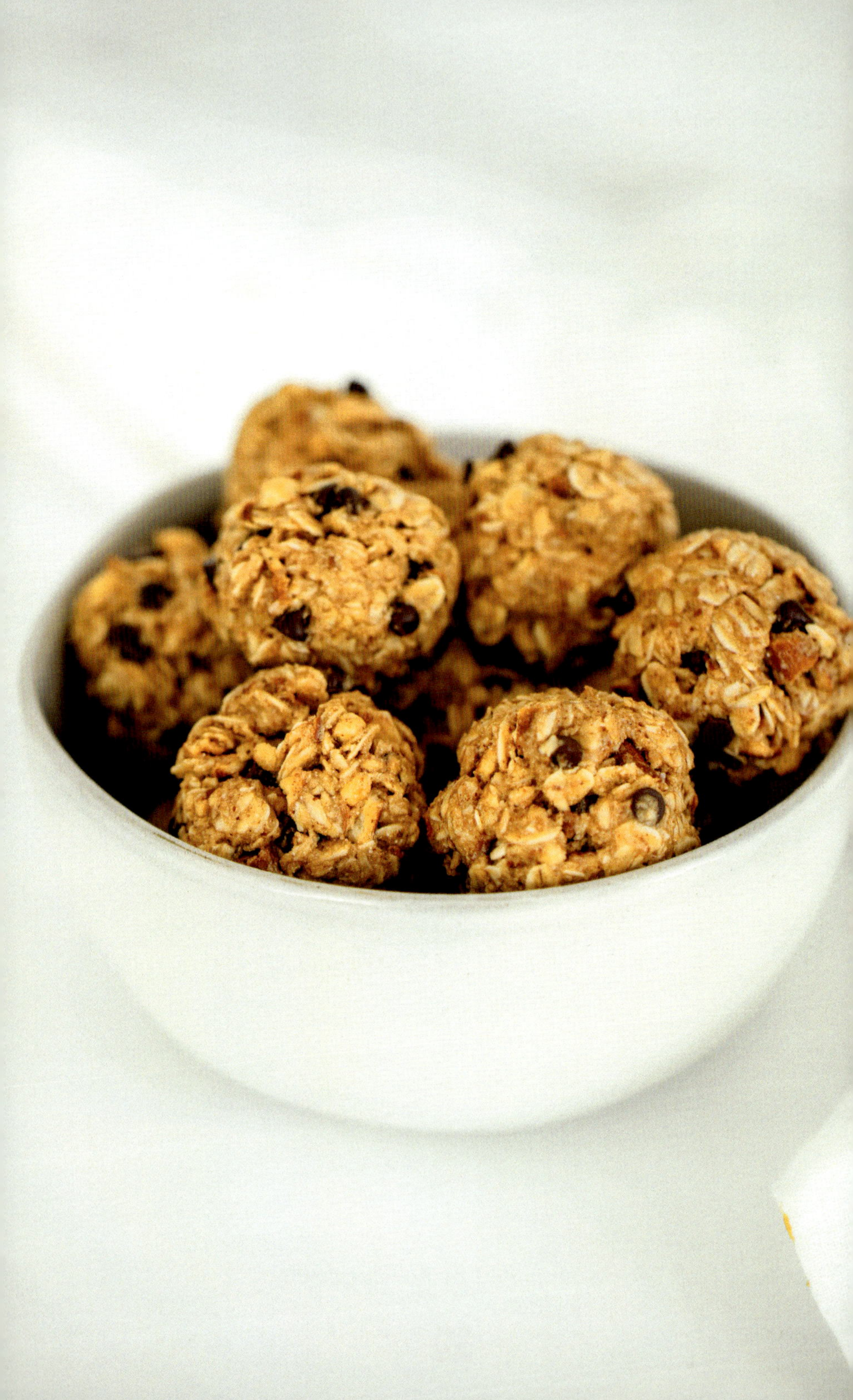

SALTED CARAMEL & PRETZEL GRANOLA BITES*

Makes 32 servings
85 calories / 3F / 12.5C / 3P / per bite

½ cup OffBeat Salted Caramel Butter
½ cup honey
1 Tbs. coconut oil, melted
Dash salt
¼ tsp. vanilla
1 serving CSE Caramel Toffee Protein
1 ¾ cups GF quick oats
28g GF pretzels, broken into pieces
2 Tbs. semi-sweet mini chocolate chips

1. Mix the Salted Caramel Butter, honey, and coconut oil together in a stand mixer until smooth.

2. Add salt and vanilla. Mix again.

3. Add protein powder, oats, pretzel pieces and chocolate chips. Mix well, scrapping down sides as needed.

4. Place 25g of mix into silicone square ice cube trays OR make into balls. Chill for 30 minutes. Remove from tray and store in an airtight container.

OffBeat Fam Recipe Submitted by Kim Rogers

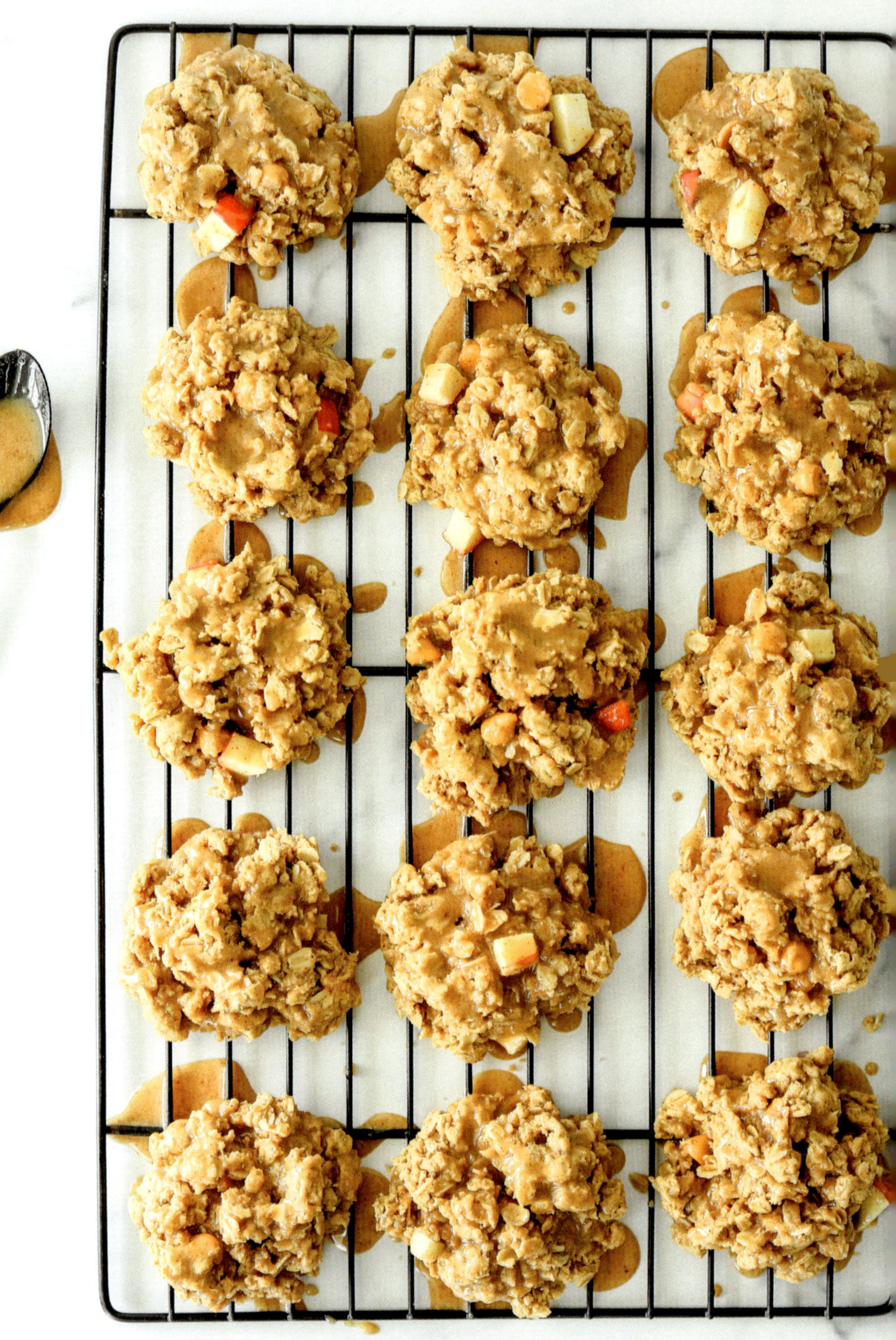

SALTED CARAMEL APPLE CRISP COOKIES*

Makes 24 cookies
258 calories / 12F / 34C / 4.5P / per cookie

¾ cup OffBeat Salted Caramel Butter
¾ cup sugar
¾ cup brown sugar
½ cup butter, softened
2 eggs
1 ½ tsp. vanilla
½ tsp. salt
1 ½ cups flour
1 tsp. baking soda
½ tsp. apple pie spice
1 ½ cups old-fashioned rolled oats
1 ½ cups crisp rice cereal
1 cup dried apples, chopped
Cinnamon chips (or vanilla or toffee baking pieces to liking)
Glaze drizzle
2 Tbs. OffBeat Salted Caramel Butter, melted
1 cup powdered sugar
Hot water to "drizzle consistency"

1. Preheat the oven to 365 degrees.

2. Cream together the Salted Caramel Butter, butter and sugars. Add eggs and vanilla.

3. Mix in dry ingredients and apples and chips.

4. Using a medium cookie scoop, (1 ½-oz. size), scoop onto greased cookie sheet and bake for 10-12 minutes; do not over-bake.

5. After cooled, whisk glaze ingredients and drizzle (good without glaze as well).

OffBeat Fam Recipe Submitted by Kallie Browne

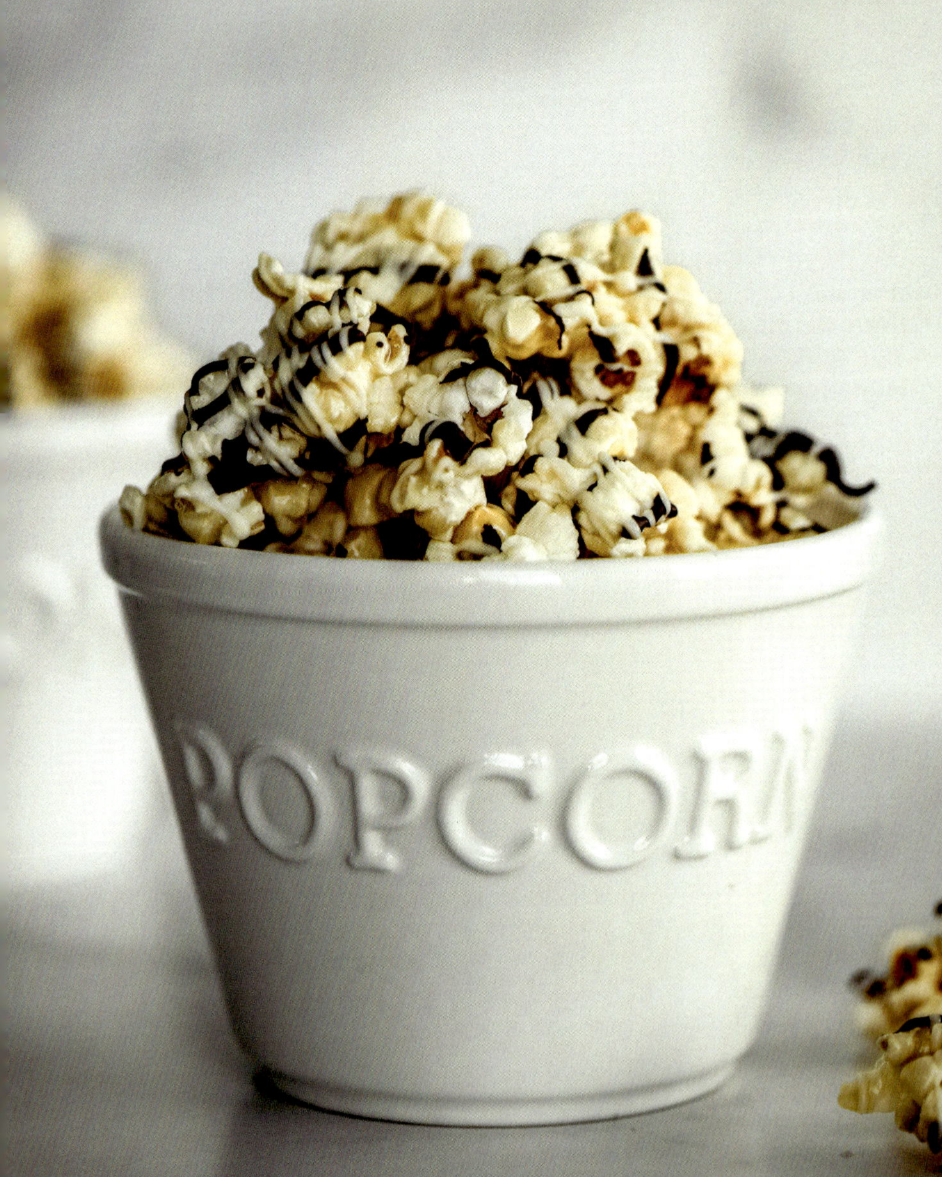

SALTED CARAMEL CORN
Makes 8 servings
265 calories / 11F / 38C / 4P / per serving

---

12 cups air-popped popcorn
½ cup OffBeat Salted Caramel Butter
½ cup raw honey
1 tsp. vanilla
¼ cup dark chocolate chips
¼ cup white chocolate chips
Dash sea salt

1. Add the Salted Caramel Butter, honey and vanilla to a sauce pan and heat on low. Stir constantly until melted together and smooth.

2. Place the popcorn in a large bowl. Pour the mixture over the top and stir until well coated. Dump onto a large baking sheet lined with parchment paper.

3. Place the chocolate chips in two separate bowls. Melt the chocolate chips in the microwave for 30 seconds at a time, stirring in between until smooth.

4. Pour each flavor of chocolate into a separate zip top bag and cut a small hole in the corner. Drizzle over the popcorn and then sprinkle sea salt over the top. Let the chocolate harden, then dig in!

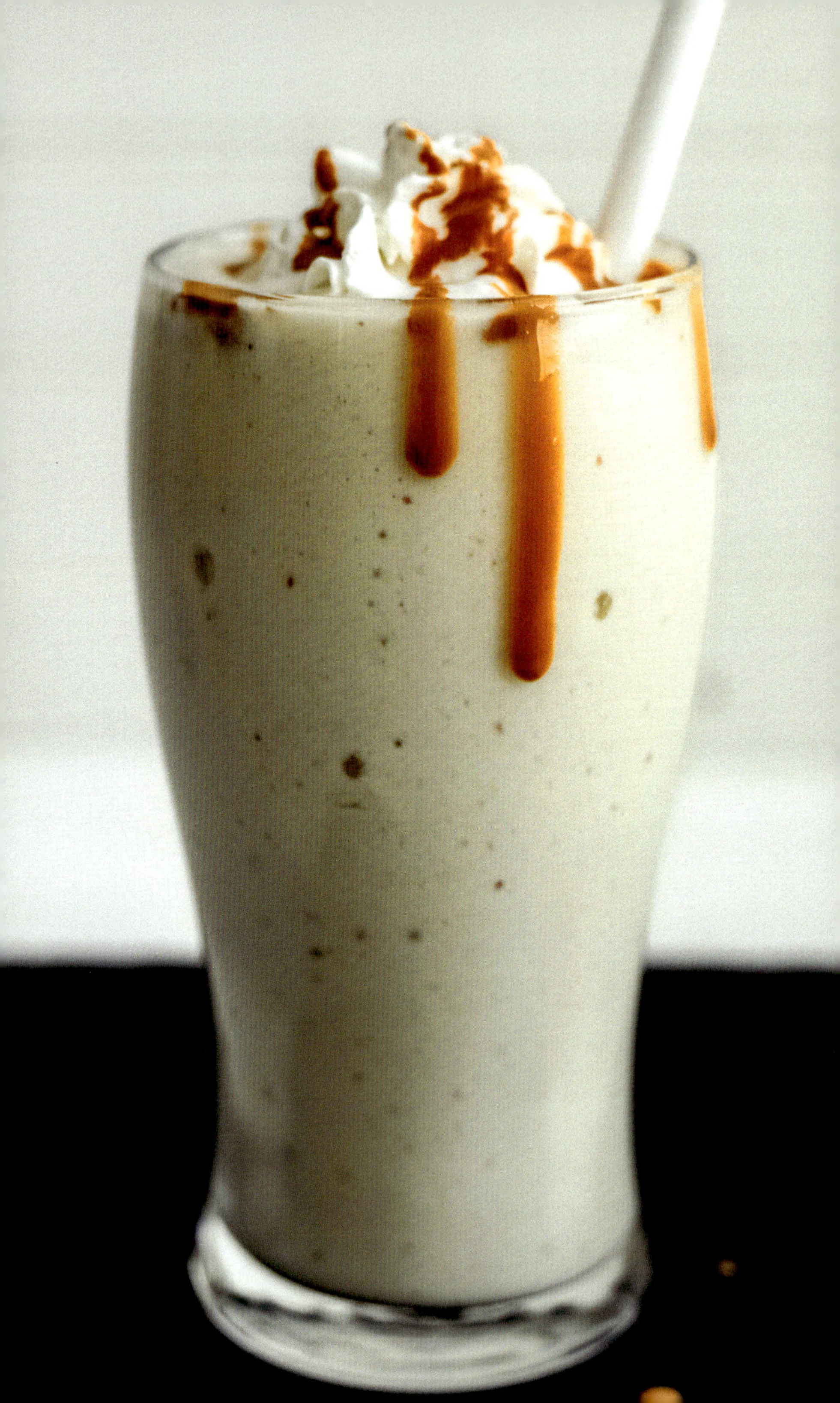

SALTED CARAMEL MILKSHAKE
Makes 1 serving
345 calories / 12.5F / 30C / 28.5P

1 cup unsweetened cashew milk
1 serving CSE Caramel Toffee Protein Powder
1 Tbs. OffBeat Salted Caramel Butter
½ cup Halo Top Creamery Sea Salt Ice Cream
¼ tsp. xanthan gum
140g ice cubes
Optional Toppings:
2 Tbs. spray whipped cream
Walden Farms Caramel syrup

1. Add the cashew milk, protein powder, Salted Caramel Butter, ice cream, xanthan gum and ice to a high-powered blender. Blend until smooth.

2. Serve topped with spray whipped cream and caramel syrup.

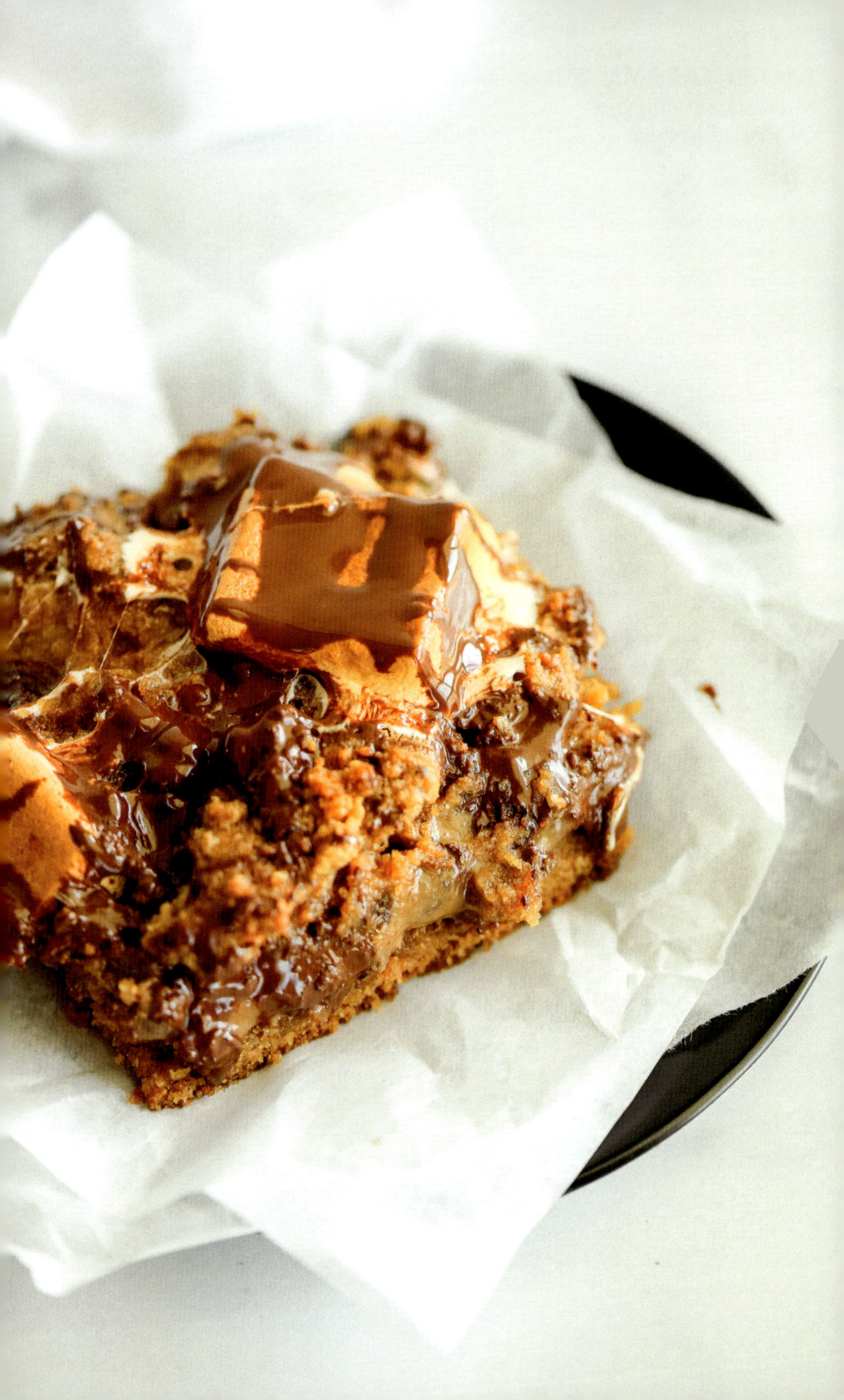

SALTED CARAMEL NUT BUTTER S'MORES BARS*

Makes 15 bars
515 calories / 23F / 68.5C / 8P / per bar

Cookie Base:.
1 cup unsalted butter; softened
½ cup light brown sugar
½ cup coconut sugar
½ cup Lakanto Monkfruit
  Sweetener
2 large eggs
1 tsp. vanilla
2 cups white whole wheat flour
2 cups crushed graham cracker
  crumbs
1 tsp. baking powder
¼ tsp. sea salt
1 cup dark chocolate chips

1 (4.5 oz.) package
  Smashmallows® Cookie
  Dough or Toasted Vanilla
Caramel Butter Layer:
5-6 oz. soft caramel
2 Tbs. fat-free milk
1 cup OffBeat Salted Caramel
  Butter
Topping:
¼ cup dark chocolate chips,
  melted

1. Preheat the oven to 350 degrees. Line a 9x13 inch pan with enough parchment paper to hang over the edge.

2. Beat butter, light brown sugar, coconut sugar, and monkfruit sweetener together for 1-2 minutes until creamed. Beat in the eggs and vanilla until well combined.

3. Add flour, graham cracker crumbs, baking powder, and sea salt on low speed and mix well. Press a little more than half of the dough evenly on the bottom of the pan with parchment paper.

4 In a microwave-safe bowl, combine the soft caramel and milk and microwave it for 1 minute Stir and if not melted and smooth, microwave for another 30 seconds. Stir in the Salted Caramel Butter until well combined.

5. Pour caramel/nut butter mixture on cookie dough and spread evenly on top. Sprinkle the chocolate chips over caramel/nut butter mixture. Then put the remaining cookie dough over the top in small pieces, followed by the Smashmallows® in the empty areas.

6. Bake for 30-35 minutes or until soft and golden brown. Let cool fully before serving. Enjoy!

**OffBeat Fam Recipe Submitted by Krista Larsen*

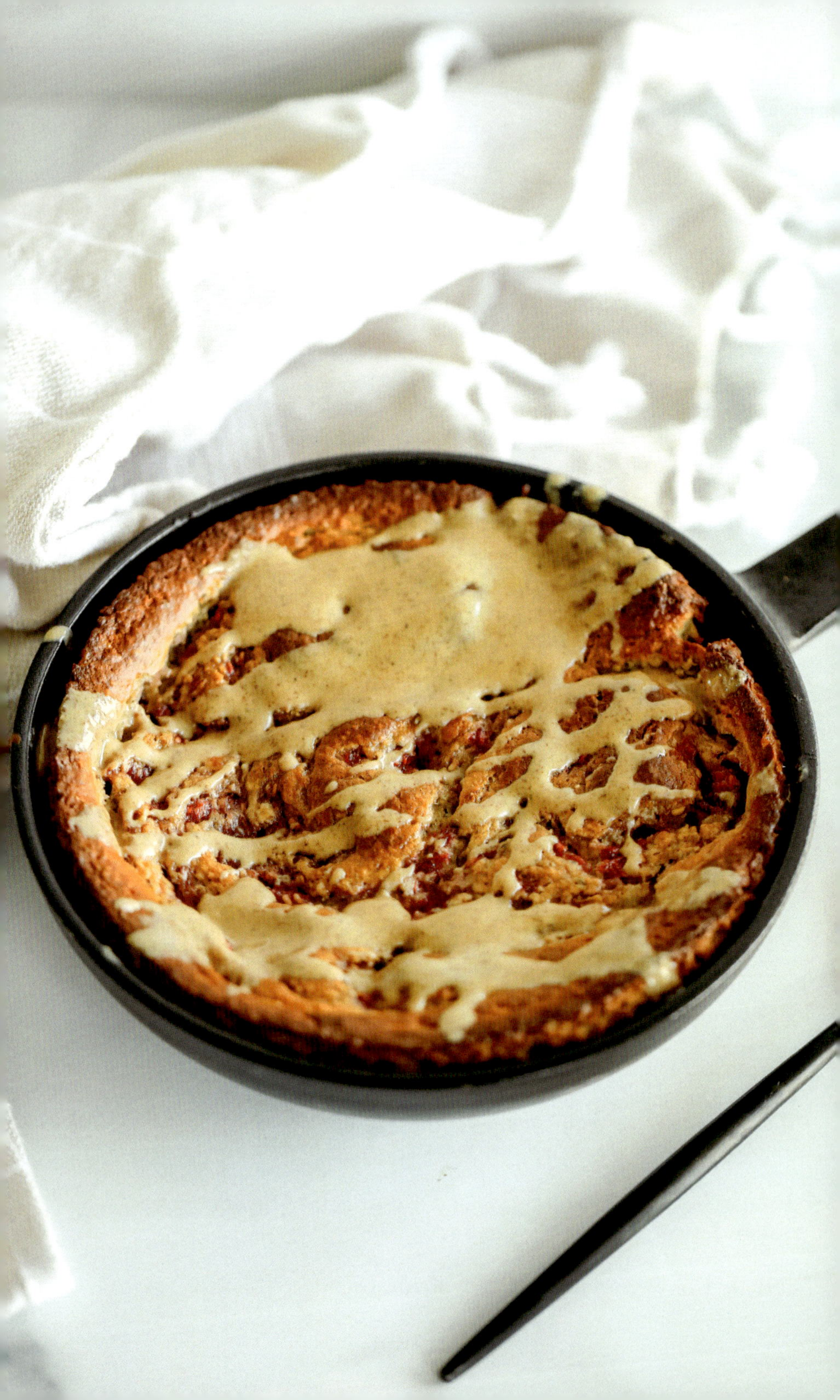

SALTED CARAMEL PB&J BAKED OATMEAL*
Makes 1 serving
575 calories / 18.5F / 70C / 33P

½ cup old-fashioned rolled oats
½ cup unsweetened almond milk
½ (60g) banana
1 Tbs. OffBeat Salted Caramel Butter
1 tsp. baking powder
1 Tbs. chia seeds
½ tsp. vanilla extract
Dash sea salt
1 serving CSE Caramel Toffee
   or Simply Vanilla Protein Powder
Toppings:
4-5 raspberries
2 tsp. pure maple syrup
½ Tbs. OffBeat Salted Caramel Butter

1. Preheat oven to 400 degrees.

2. Add all the oatmeal ingredients together in a blender or food processor, adding protein last.

3. Spray an oven-safe bowl or ramekin with cooking spray and pour the blended mix in.

4. Make the berry jam by heating the maple syrup & mashed raspberries over low heat for 2-3 minutes.

5. Swirl the berry jam on top of the oatmeal mixture.

6. Bake 25-30 minutes at 400 degrees until desired consistency.

7. Drizzle with Salted Caramel Butter and enjoy!

OffBeat Fam Recipe Submitted by Courtney Harp

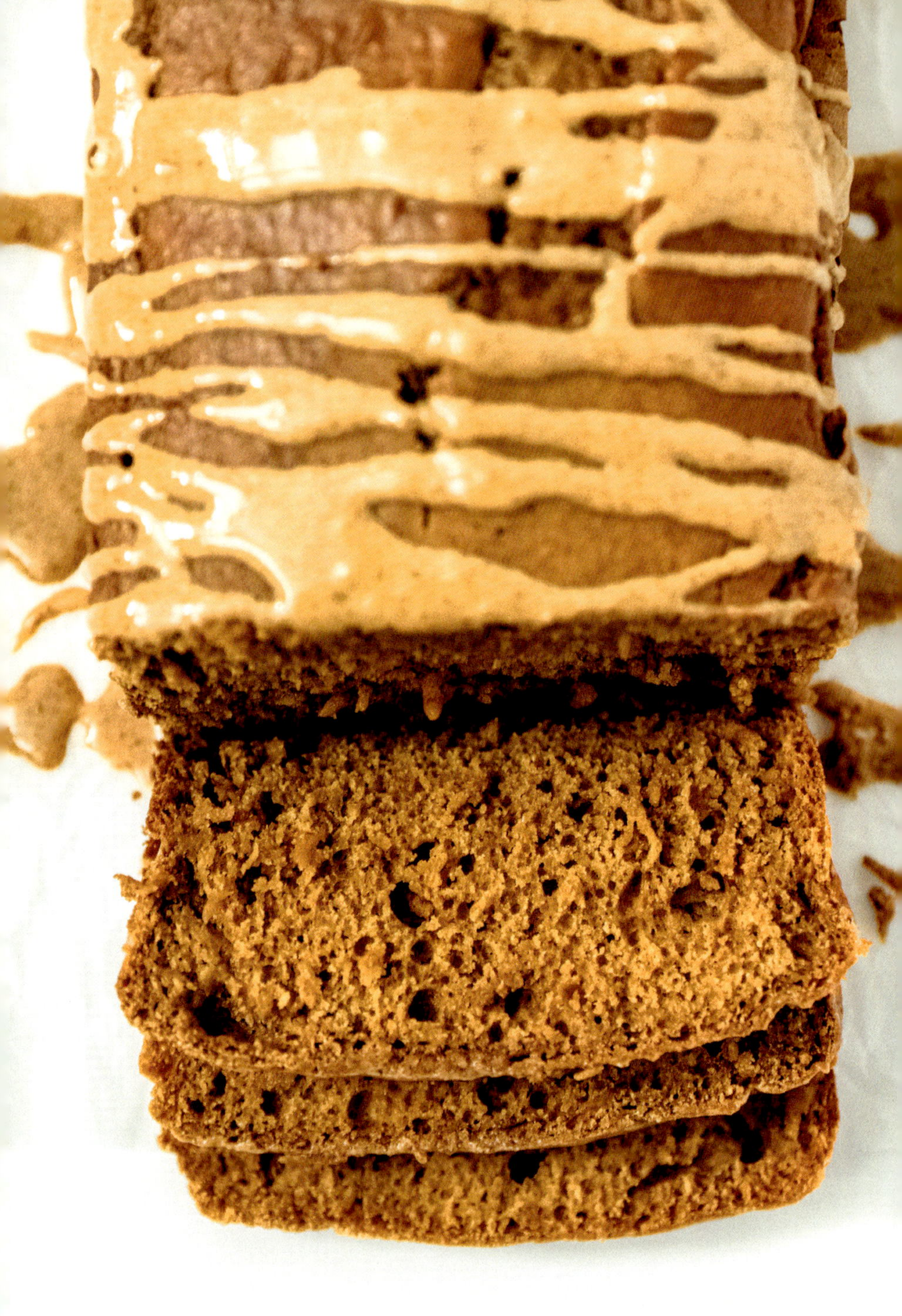

SALTED CARAMEL PUMPKIN BREAD

Makes 20 servings

177 calories / 2.5F / 35C / 4.5P / per serving

15 oz. canned pumpkin
3 eggs
¾ cup raw honey
¾ cup coconut sugar
½ cup unsweetened applesauce
½ cup nonfat, plain Greek yogurt
2 Tbs. fresh orange juice
½ Tbs. molasses
1 tsp. vanilla extract
3 cup white whole wheat flour
2 tsp. cinnamon
½ tsp. nutmeg
½ tsp. cloves
1 tsp. baking powder
1 tsp. baking soda
½ tsp. sea salt
¼ cup OffBeat Salted Caramel Butter

1. Preheat oven to 350 degrees.

2. Beat the pumpkin, eggs, honey, coconut sugar, applesauce, Greek yogurt, orange juice, molasses, and vanilla together in a large bowl. Mix until well combined; set aside.

3. In a separate bowl, stir the flour, cinnamon, nutmeg, cloves, baking powder, baking soda, and sea salt together. Add the wet ingredients to the dry ingredients and stir until just combined.

4. Grease two, 9x5, glass loaf pans. Pour the batter evenly into the two pans.

5. Bake for 40 minutes. Remove from the oven and cover loosely with foil. Bake an additional 10 minutes and let cool.

6. Top with Salted Caramel Butter. Enjoy!

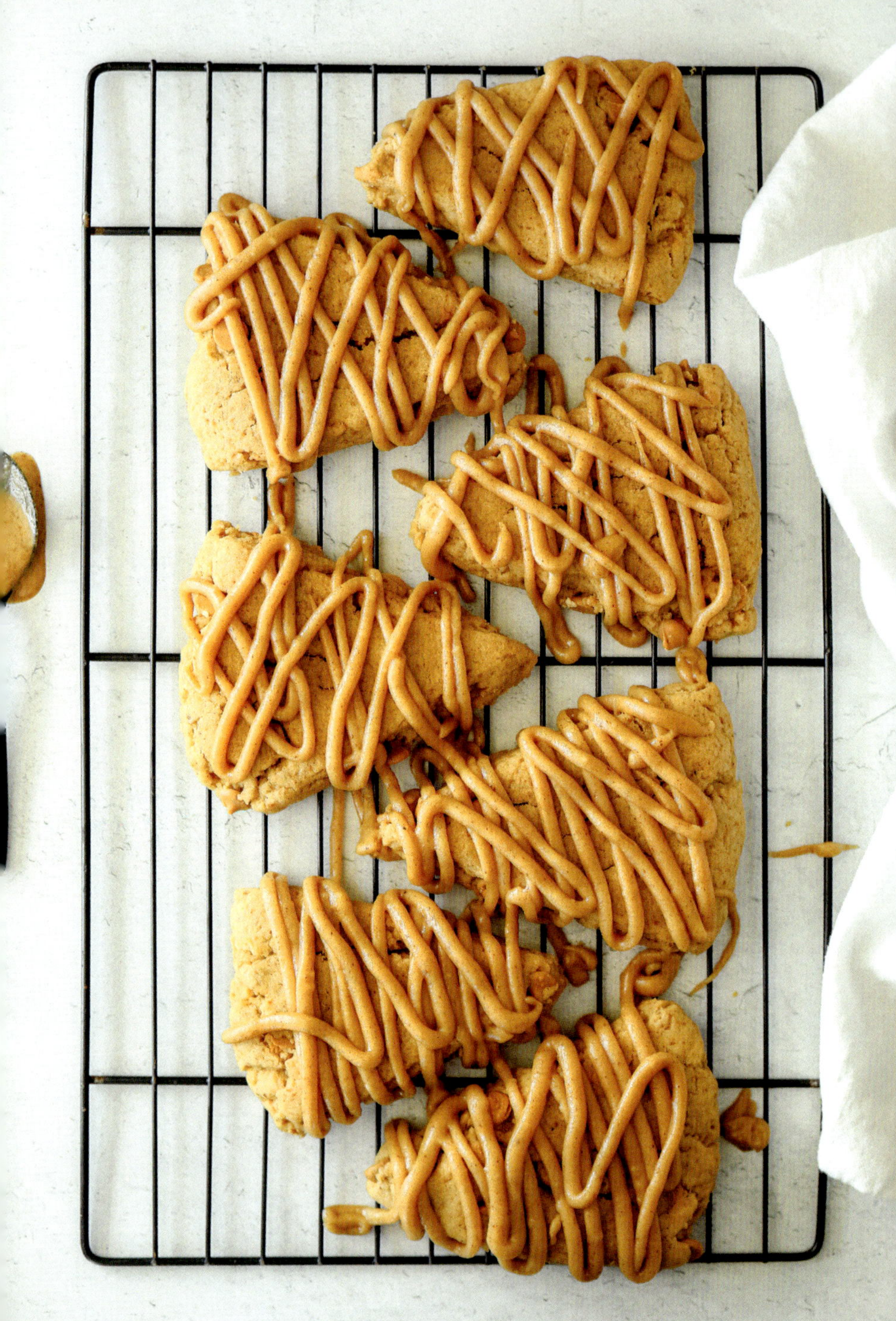

SALTED CARAMEL SCONES WITH BROWN BUTTER GLAZE*

Makes 8 servings
530 calories / 26F / 66C / 8P / per serving

---

2 cups all-purpose flour
½ cup coconut sugar
1 Tbs. baking powder
Dash sea salt
½ cup unsalted butter, cold and
    cubed
1 large egg
⅓ cup OffBeat Salted Caramel Butter
¼ cup Greek yogurt (or sour cream)
2 tsp. vanilla bean paste
½ cup sea salt caramel chips
    (such as Hershey's)

Glaze:
3 Tbs. grass-fed butter
2 tsp. vanilla bean paste
2 Tbs.OffBeat Salted Caramel
Butter
1 cup powdered sugar or
    powdered Swerve sweetener
2-3 Tbs. low-fat milk
Toppings:
Flaky sea salt

1. Preheat oven to 400 degrees and line a baking sheet with parchment paper.

2. In a medium-sized bowl, mix the flour, coconut sugar, baking powder, and salt.

3. Using a pastry cutter, cut in the cold butter to form small pea-sized chunks. In a separate bowl, whisk the egg, Salted Caramel Butter, sour cream (or yogurt) and vanilla bean paste. Stir the wet ingredients into the dry and fold in the caramel chips.

4. Turn dough onto baking sheet, then pat and shape into an 8-inch round disk.

5. Cut into eight triangles and pull a couple of inches apart. Bake for 12 minutes. While baking, make the glaze. In a small saucepan, brown the butter by melting on medium heat until it begins to foam and brown specks form on the bottom.

6. Immediately turn off the heat. Once butter has cooled, whisk in the remaining glaze ingredients. Drizzle the glaze over the cooled scones and sprinkle with flaky sea salt. Enjoy!

OffBeat Fam Recipe Submitted by Whitney Houlin

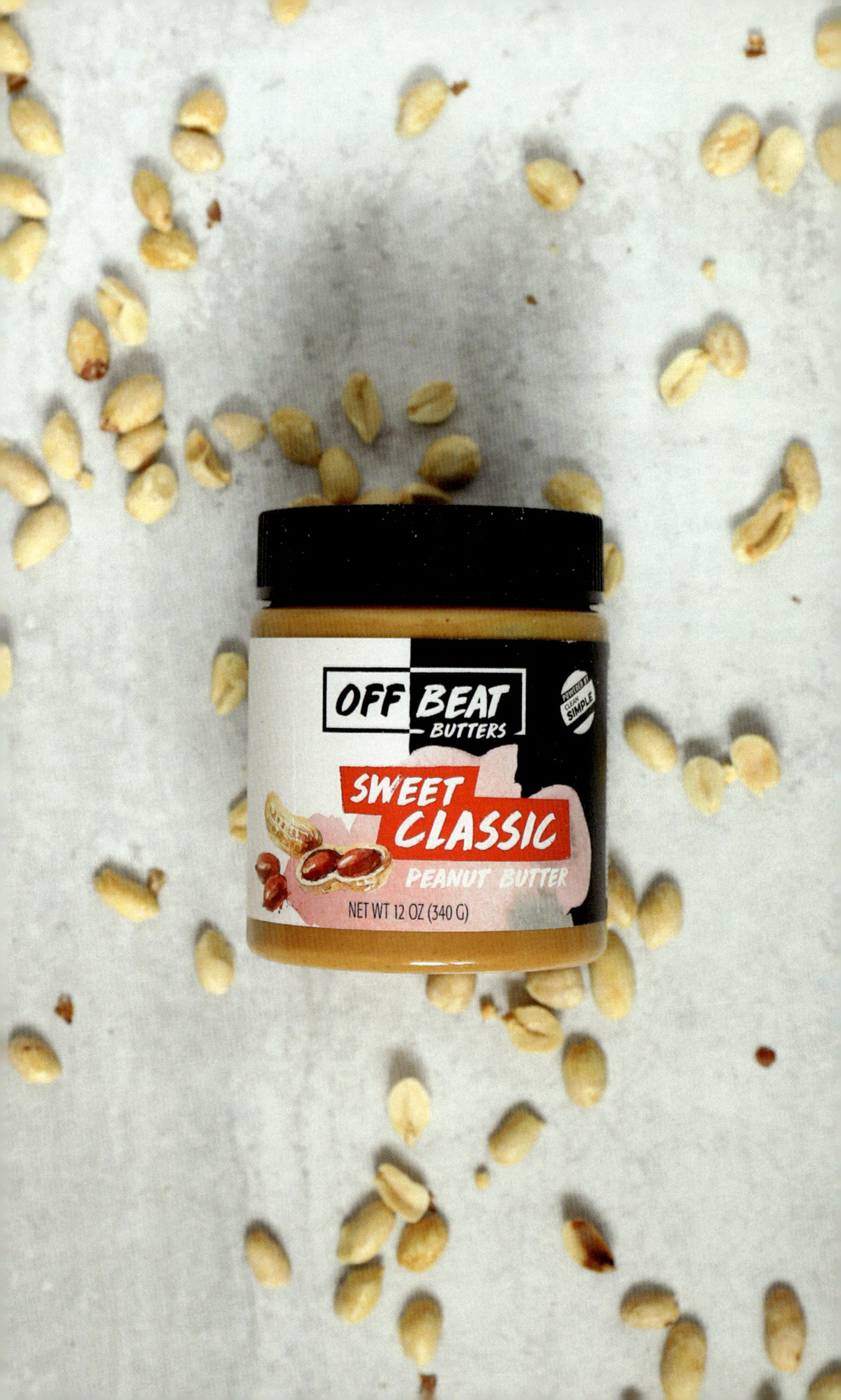

OFF BEAT
BUTTERS
POWERED BY CLEAN SIMPLE
SWEET CLASSIC
PEANUT BUTTER
NET WT 12 OZ (340 G)

PEANUT BUTTER IS THE GLUE THAT HOLDS THIS BODY TOGETHER

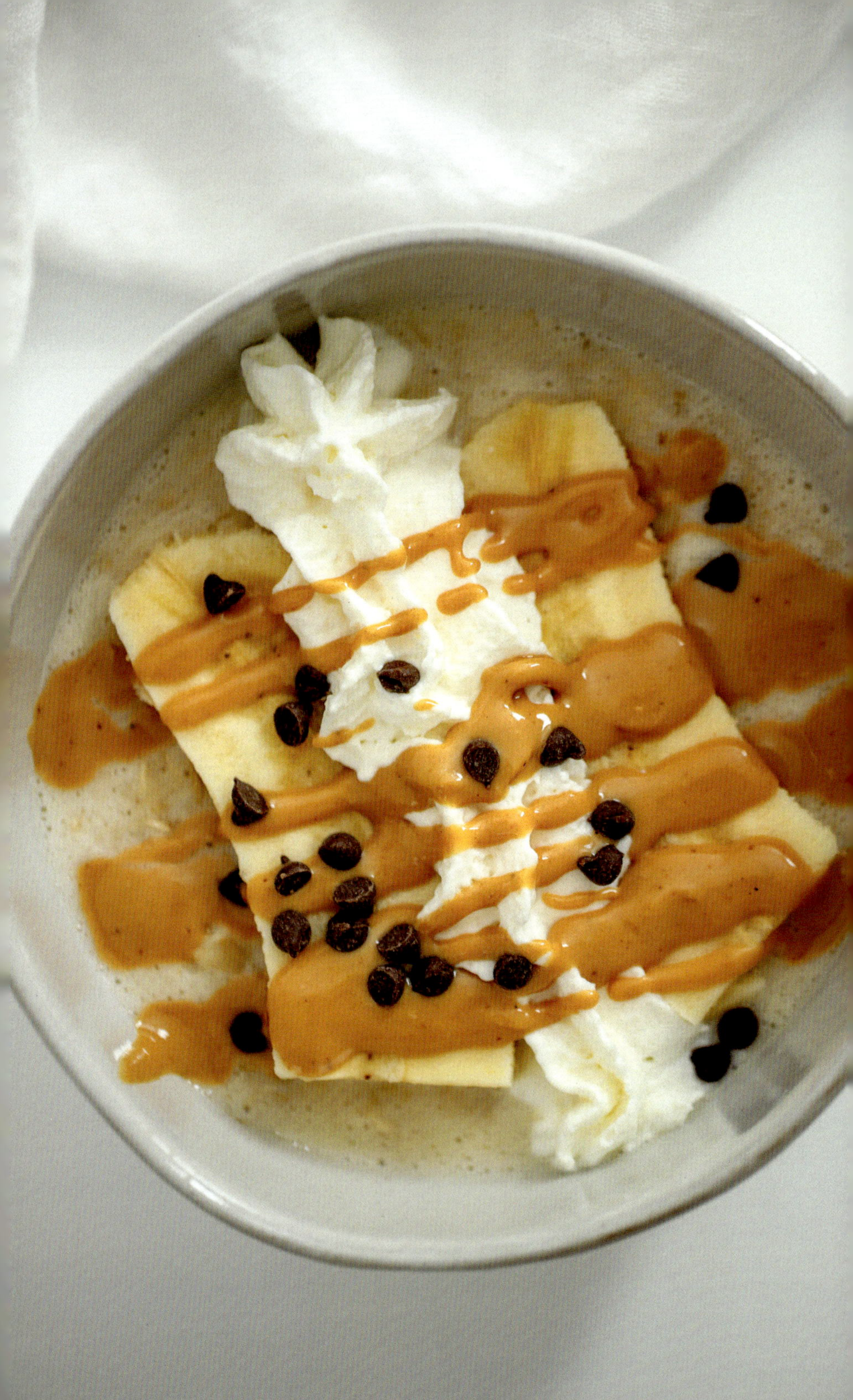

BANANA SPLIT OATS
Makes 1 serving
375 calories / 44C / 11F / 26P

⅓ cup old-fashioned rolled oats
½ cup water
2 tsp. OffBeat Sweet Classic Peanut Butter
1 serving CSE Simply Vanilla Protein Powder
Toppings:
20g thinly sliced bananas
2 Tbs. spray whipped cream
10g dark chocolate chips
Dash sea salt

1. Add the oats, and water to a microwave-safe bowl. Microwave for 1-2 minutes.

2. Stir in Sweet Classic Peanut Butter. Let cool for a couple minutes, then stir in the protein powder.

3. Top with sliced bananas, spray whipped cream, dark chocolate chips, and a dash of sea salt.

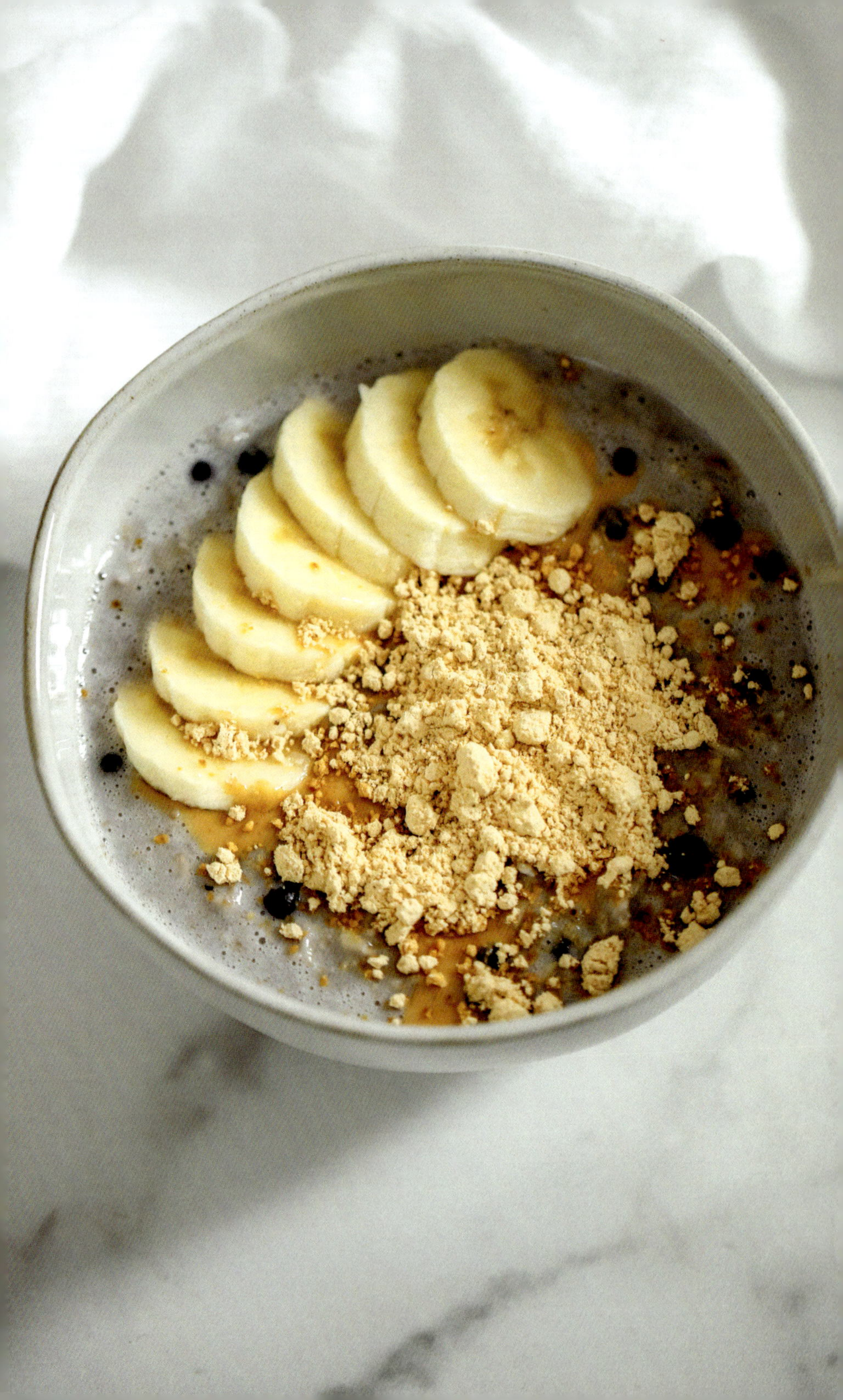

BLUEBERRY PB OATMEAL
Makes 1 serving
365 calories / 9F / 42C / 29.5P

⅓ cup old-fashioned rolled oats
½ cup water
46g liquid egg whites
½ cup frozen blueberries
10g OffBeat Sweet Classic Peanut Butter
¾ serving CSE Simply Vanilla Protein Powder
Toppings:
20g banana slices
1 Tbs. powdered peanut butter
4g OffBeat Sweet Classic Peanut Butter

1. Add the oats, water, egg whites, and blueberries to a microwave-safe bowl. Whisk until the egg whites are well combined. Microwave for 1-2 minutes.

2. Stir in the Sweet Classic Peanut Butter (10g). Let cool for a couple minutes, then stir in the protein powder.

3. Top with banana slices and powdered peanut butter. Drizzle the remaining nut butter over the top.

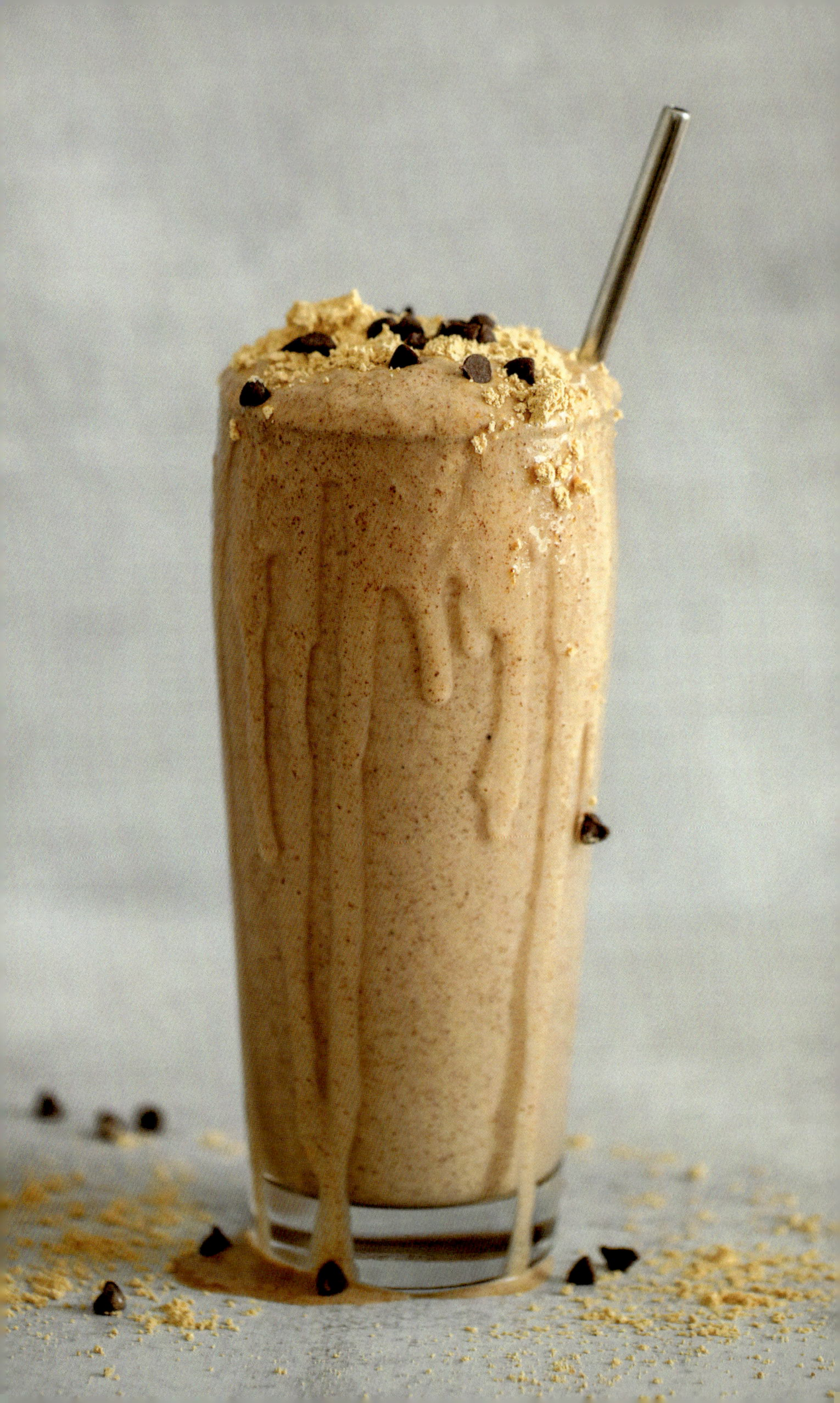

BUTTERFINGER SHAKE
Makes 1 serving
350 calories / 11.5F / 36C / 27P

---

1 cup unsweetened almond milk
¾ serving CSE Simply Vanilla Protein Powder
30g frozen banana slices
10g OffBeat Sweet Classic Peanut Butter
10g butterscotch pudding mix
10g semi-sweet chocolate chips
120g ice cubes
Topping:
16g powdered peanut butter

1. Add all the ingredients to a high-powered blender and blend until smooth.

2. Pour into a cup. Top with powdered peanut butter and gently fold into the shake. Enjoy!

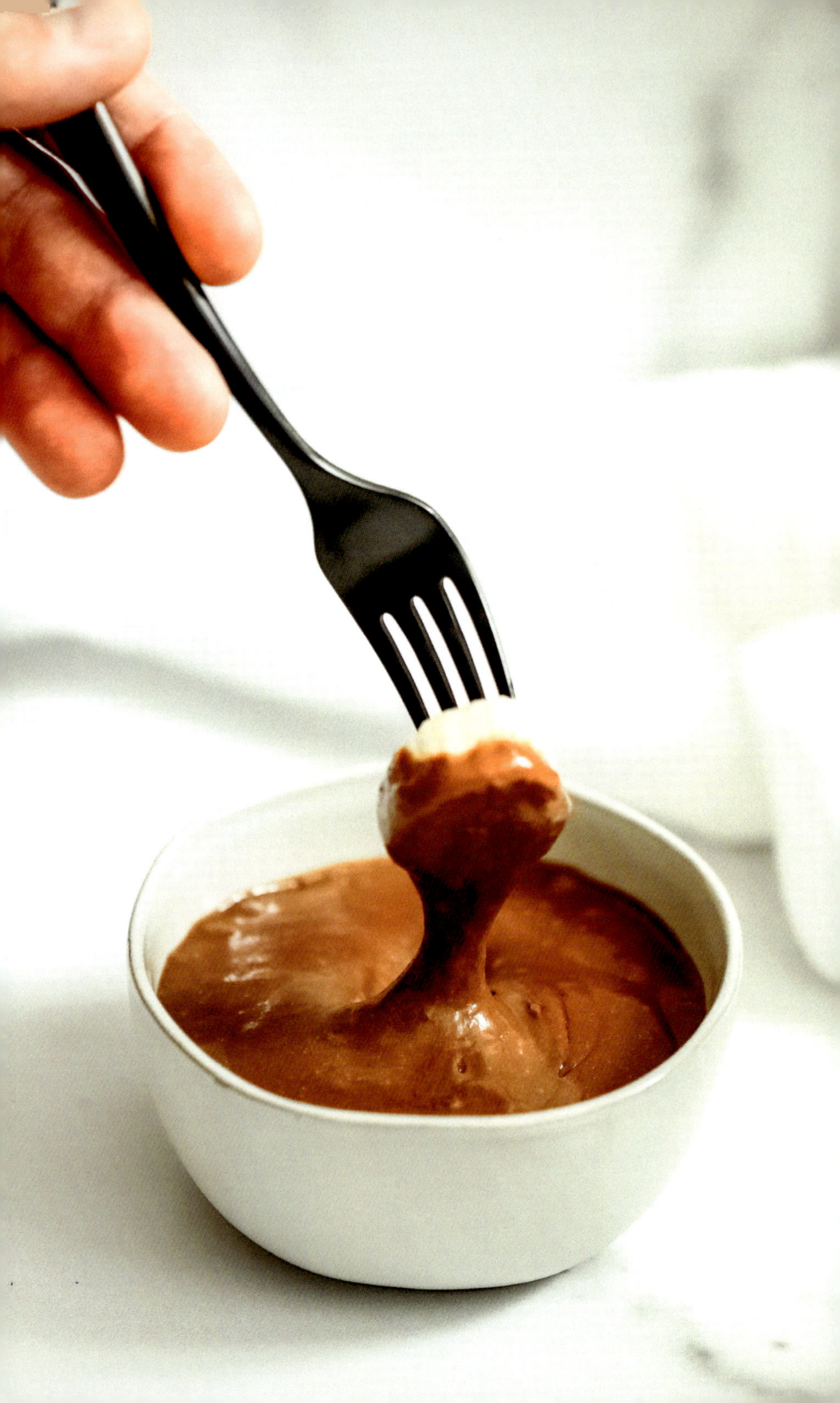

CHOCOLATE ELVIS DIP*
Makes 1 serving
260 calories / 11F / 43C / 27P

---

2 Tbs. CSE Brownie Batter Protein Powder
1 tsp. cocoa powder
2 Tbs. water
1 Tbs. OffBeat Sweet Classic Peanut Butter
1 tsp. honey
1 tsp. Greek yogurt
½ banana

1. Stir together protein powder, cocoa, and water until smooth.

2. Add the Sweet Classic Peanut Butter, honey, and Greek yogurt. Stir until thoroughly combined.

3. Slice the banana on top and enjoy with a spoon, or dip in the banana with a fork.

**OffBeat Fam Recipe Submitted by Brooke Dickert*

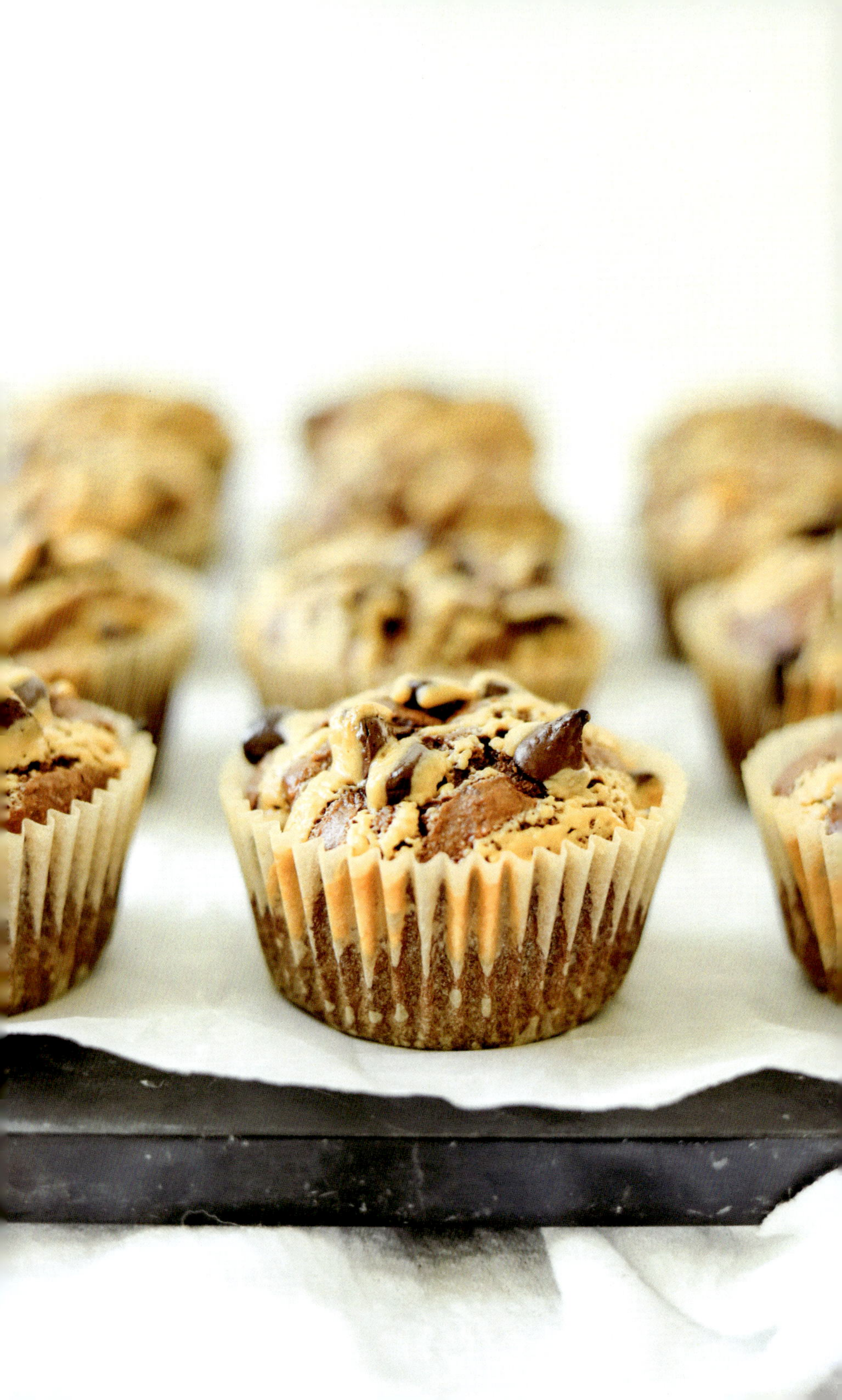

CHOCOLATE PB SWIRL MUFFINS

Makes 16 muffins
175 calories / 8F / 20C / 6P / per muffin

¾ cup bananas
¼ cup raw honey
¼ cup organic cane sugar
2 eggs
½ cup OffBeat Sweet Classic Peanut Butter
1 tsp. vanilla extract
½ cup old-fashioned rolled oats
½ cup white whole-wheat flour
¼ cup cocoa powder
1 Serving CSE Brownie Batter
   or Chocolate Peanut Butter Protein Powder
1 tsp. baking powder
½ tsp. baking soda
½ tsp. sea salt
½ cup dark chocolate chips
Topping:
16 tsp. OffBeat Sweet Classic Peanut Butter

1. Preheat oven to 350 degrees.

2. Mash the banana. Add the mashed banana, honey, sugar, eggs, Sweet Classic Peanut Butter, and vanilla extract into a large mixing bowl. Beat until smooth; set aside.

3. In a separate bowl, mix the oats, flour, cocoa, protein powder, baking powder, baking soda and sea salt together. Add to the wet ingredients and mix until just combined. Fold in the chocolate chips.

4. Add muffin liners to a muffin tin. Fill each muffin liner ¾ full with batter. Drizzle about one teaspoon of peanut butter over the top of each muffin. Place in the oven and bake for 10-12 minutes.

5. Let cool for a couple minutes and then remove each muffin from the muffin tin. Store extras in the fridge. Enjoy!

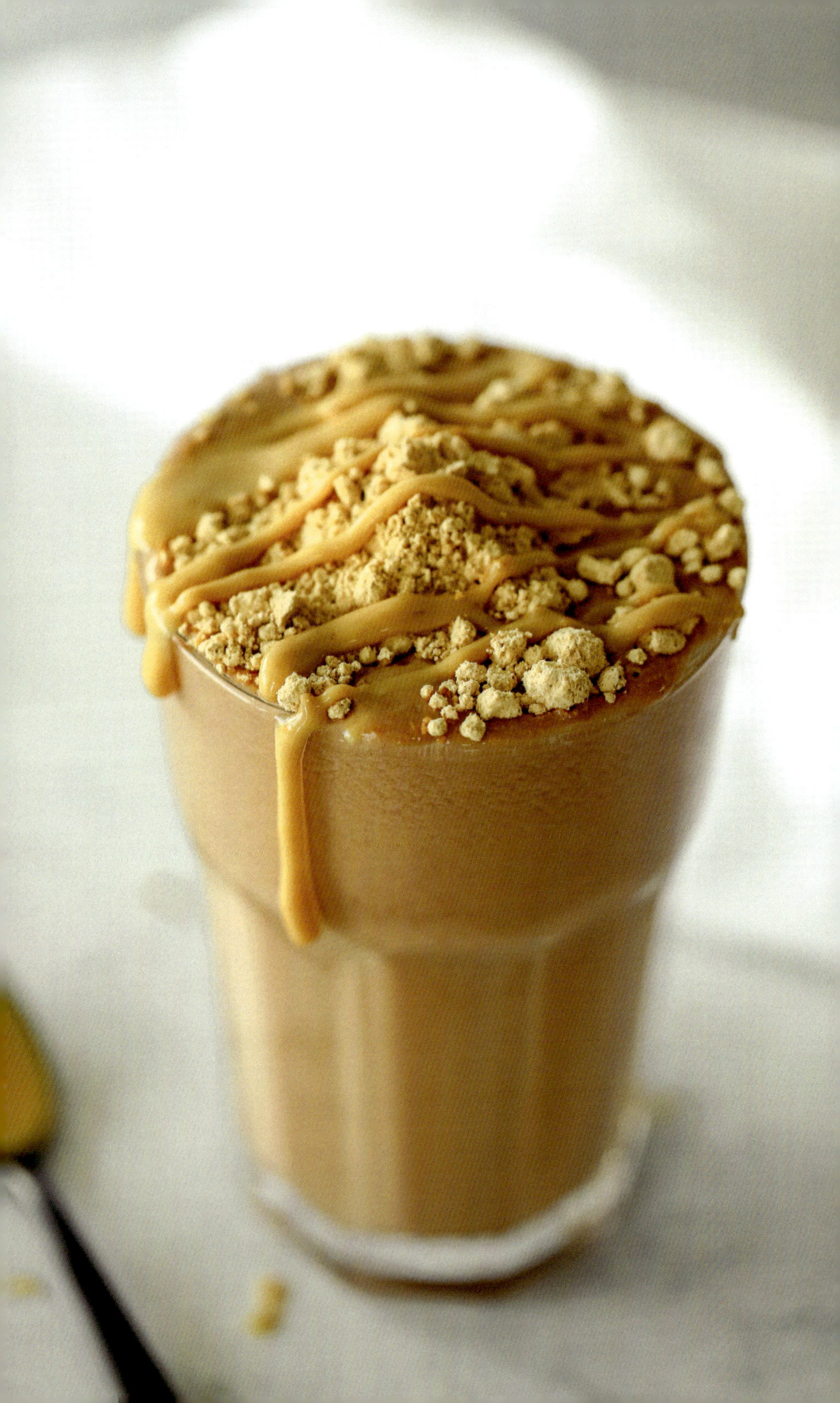

CHOCOLATE PEANUT BUTTER CUP SHAKE
Makes 1 serving
345 calories / 11F / 32C / 29.5P

---

1 cup unsweetened vanilla almond milk
1 serving CSE Chocolate Peanut Butter Protein Powder
1 Tbs. cocoa powder
14g OffBeat Sweet Classic Peanut Butter
60g frozen bananas
6-8 (120g) ice cubes
Topping:
1 Tbs. powdered peanut butter

1. Add all of the shake ingredients to a high-powered blender. Blend until smooth.

2. Pour into a cup. Top with powdered peanut butter and lightly fold into the shake. Enjoy!

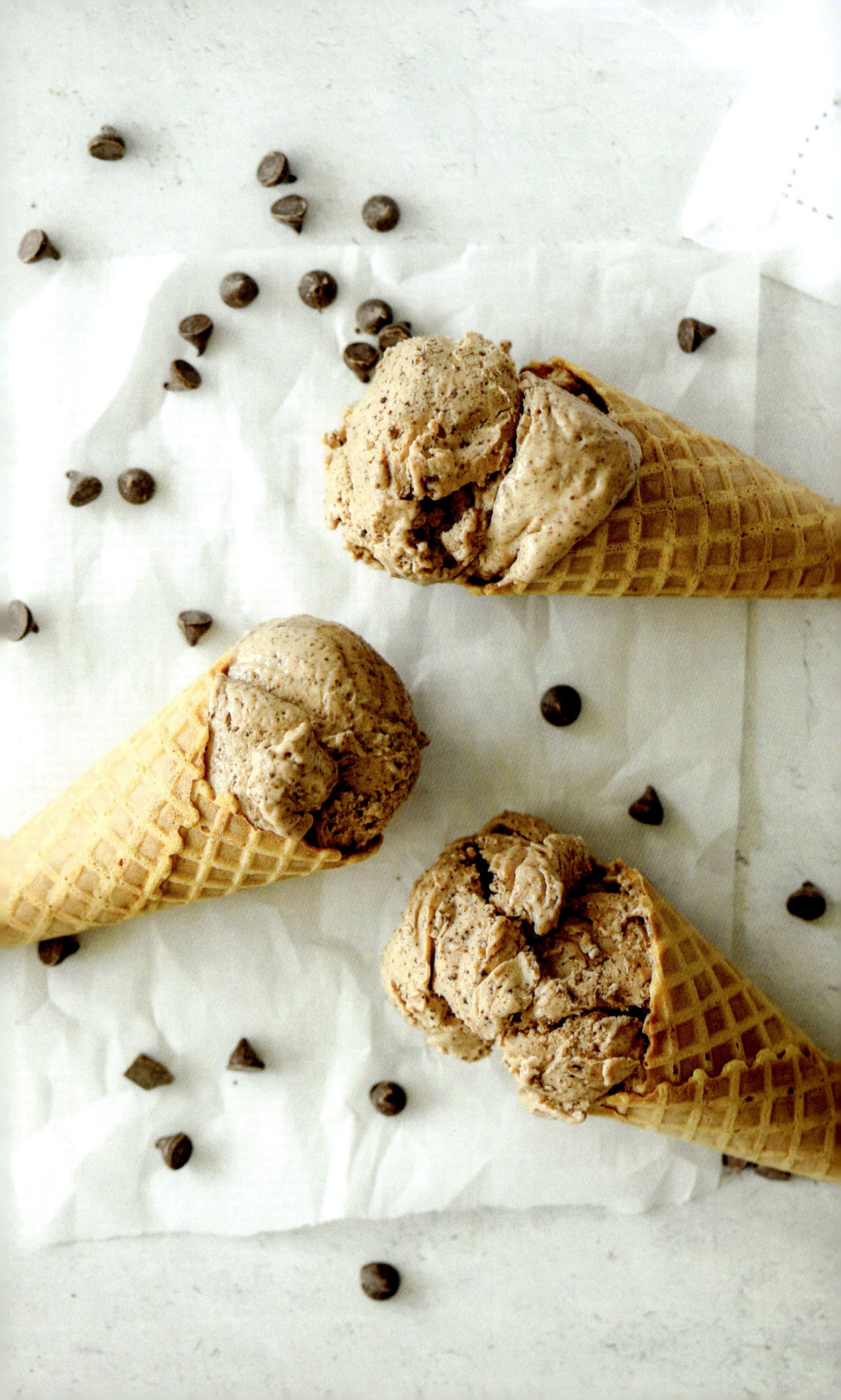

CHOCOLATE SPECKLED PB ICE CREAM
Makes 4 servings
300 calories / 11.5F / 35C / 15P / per serving

400g frozen banana slices
2 servings CSE Chocolate Peanut Butter Protein Powder
¼ cup OffBeat Sweet Classic Peanut Butter
   or Buckeye Brownie Peanut Butter
¼ cup unsweetened almond milk
3 Tbs. (45g) dark chocolate chips

1. Add all of the ingredients to a high-powered blender or food processor. Blend until thick and smooth. Scrape down the sides and stir in between blending, if needed.

2. Pour into a loaf pan lined with parchment paper. Freeze for 2+ hours. Use an ice cream scoop to serve the ice cream. Scoop into a bowl or a cone. Enjoy!

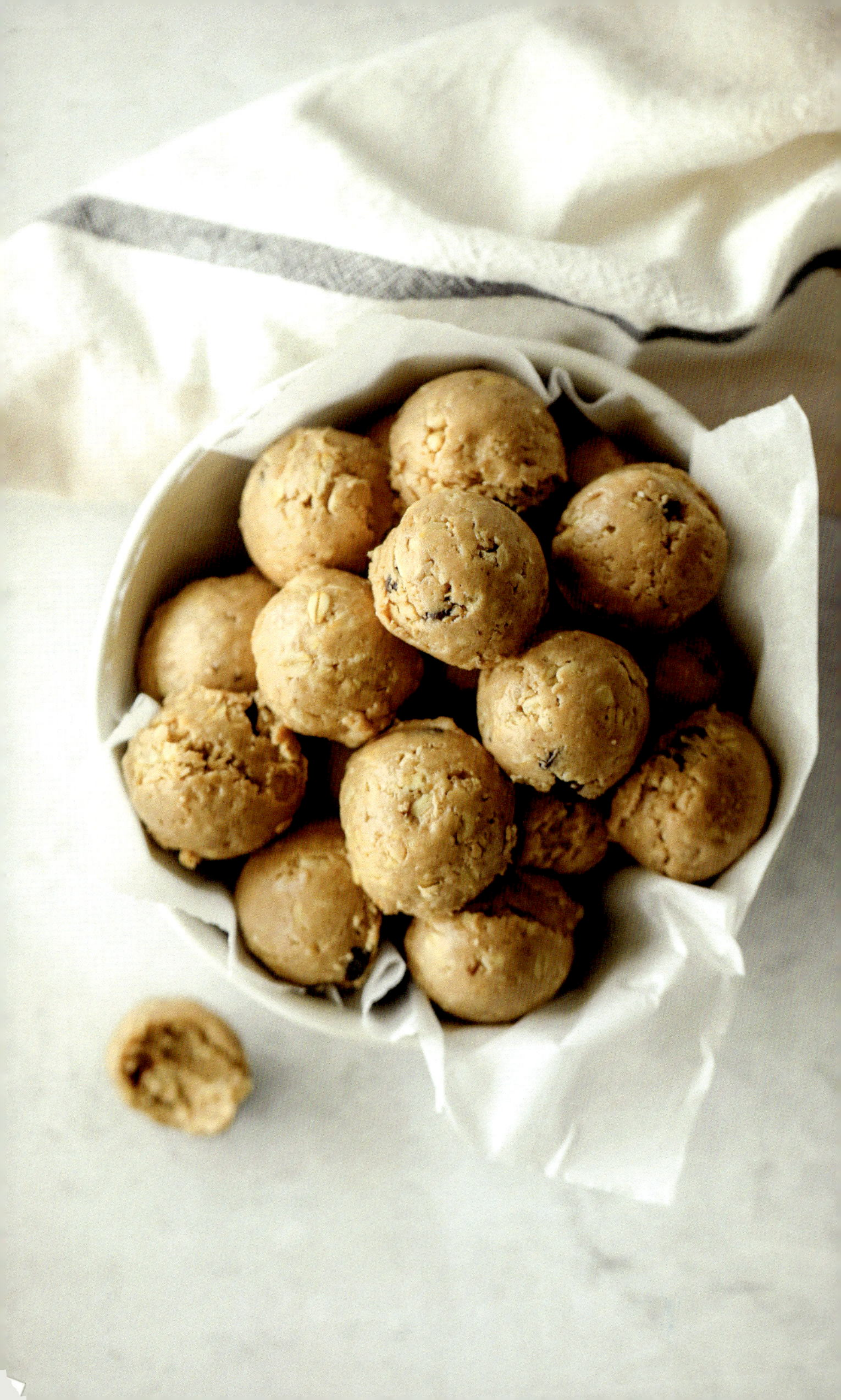

CRISPY CHOCOLATE PB BITES
Makes 25 servings
100 calories / 5F / 10C / 4P / per bite

---

1 cup OffBeat Sweet Classic Peanut Butter
½ cup raw honey
2 servings CSE Chocolate Peanut Butter Protein Powder
Dash sea salt
1 tsp. vanilla extract
1 cup old-fashioned rolled oats
1 cup crispy rice cereal
2 Tbs. (30g) mini dark chocolate chips

1. Add the Sweet Classic Peanut Butter, honey, protein powder, salt and vanilla to a large mixing bowl. Mix until well combined.

2. Add the remaining ingredients and mix well.

3. Using a small cookie scoop, scoop the dough into balls and place in a container. Store in the fridge or freezer. Enjoy!

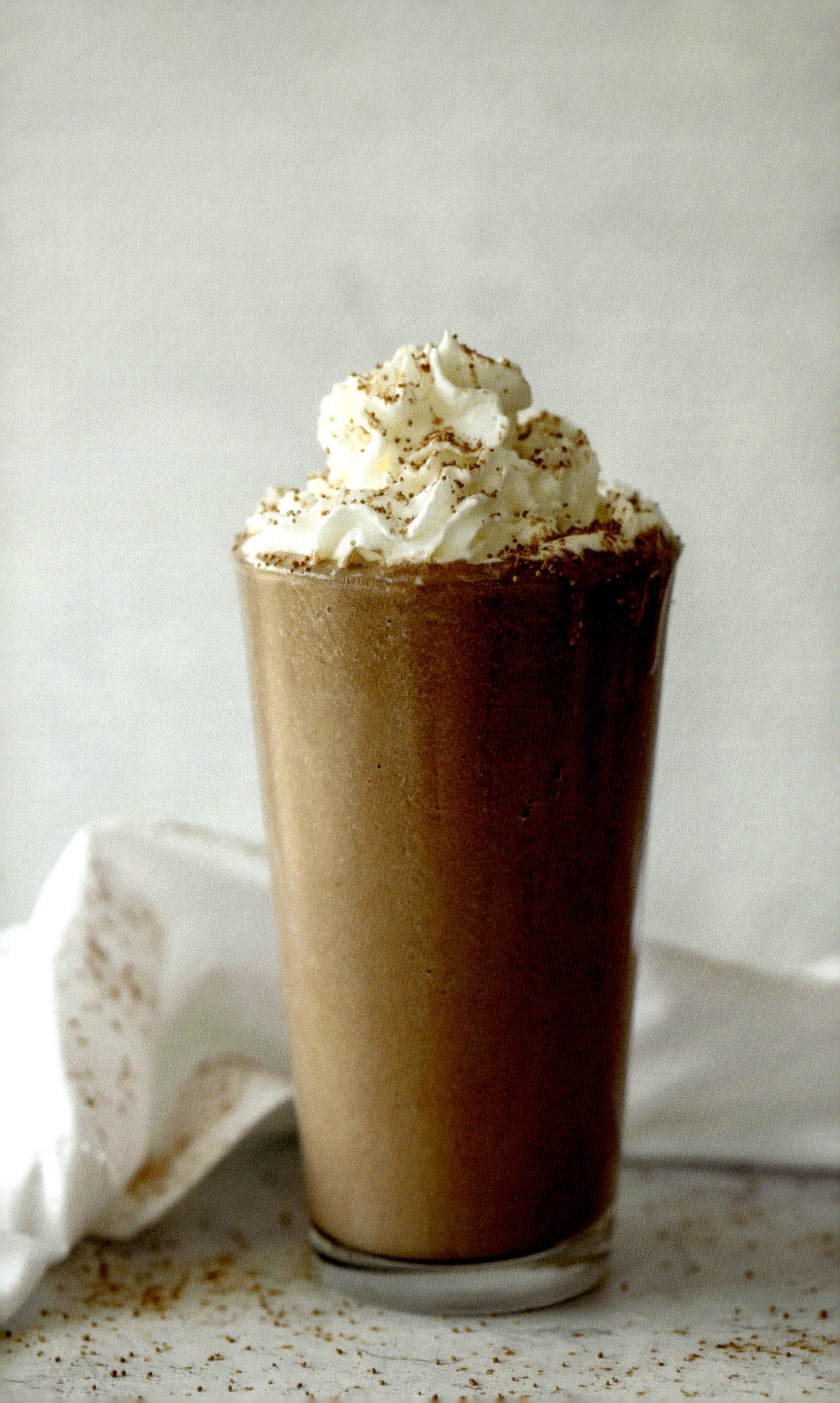

DARK CHOCOLATE PB SHAKE
Makes 1 serving
240 calories / 6F / 26C / 22.5P

1 cup dark chocolate almond milk
1 serving CSE Chocolate Peanut Butter Protein Powder
½ Tbs. OffBeat Sweet Classic Peanut Butter
6-8 (120g) ice cubes

1. Add all of the ingredients to a high-powered blender. Blend until smooth.

2. Pour into a cup. Enjoy!

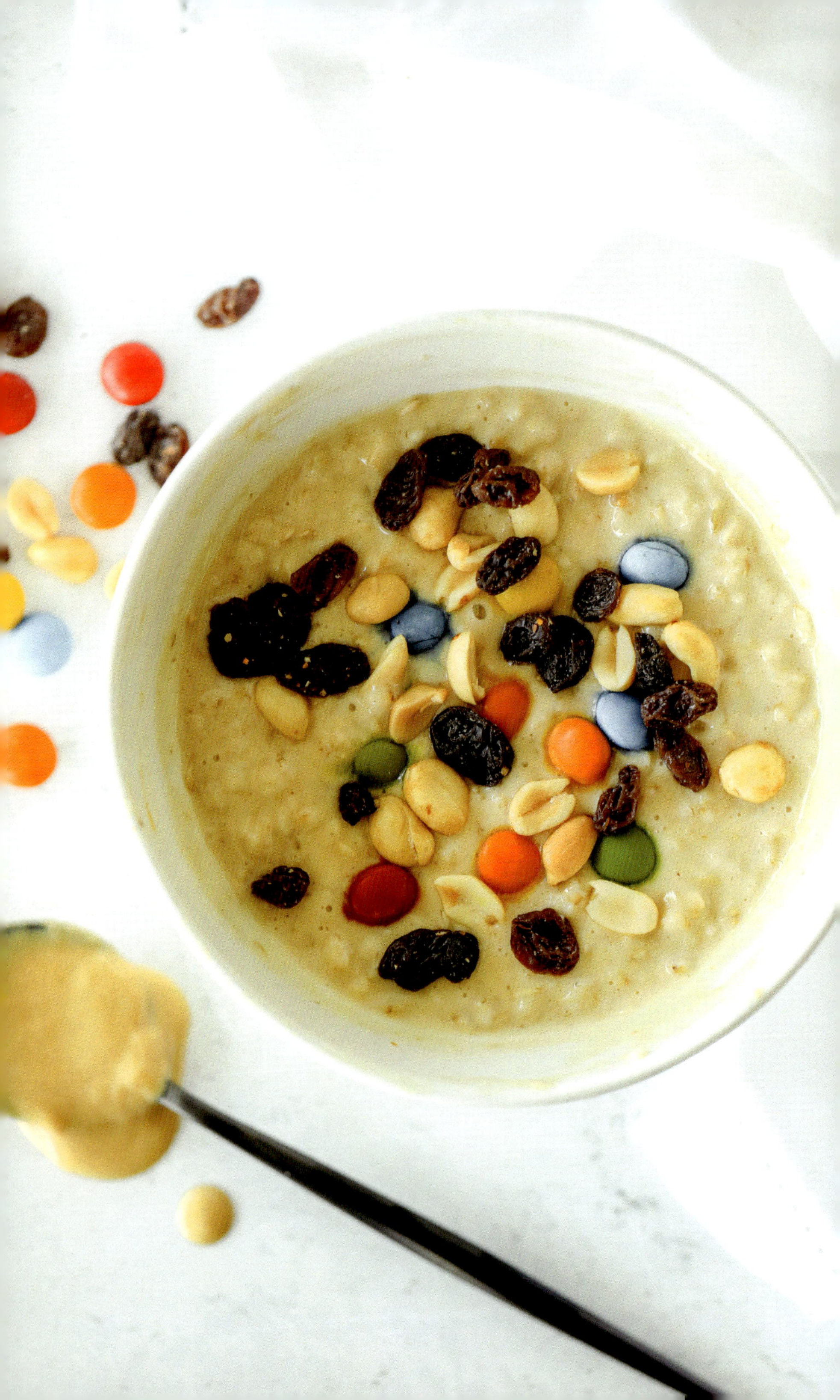

MONSTER COOKIE OATMEAL
Makes 1 serving
360 calories / 12F / 36C / 28P

⅓ cup old-fashioned rolled oats
½ cup water
46g liquid egg whites
1 Tbs. OffBeat Sweet Classic Peanut Butter
¾ serving CSE Simply Vanilla Protein Powder
Toppings:
10g Unreal Milk Chocolate Gems or M&M's
5g peanuts, chopped
5g raisins

1. Add the rolled oats, water and egg whites to a microwave-safe bowl. Microwave for 1-2 minutes.

2. Stir in the Sweet Classic Peanut Butter and let the oatmeal cool for a couple of minutes. Stir in the protein powder.

3. Top with the chocolate candies, peanuts and raisins. Enjoy!

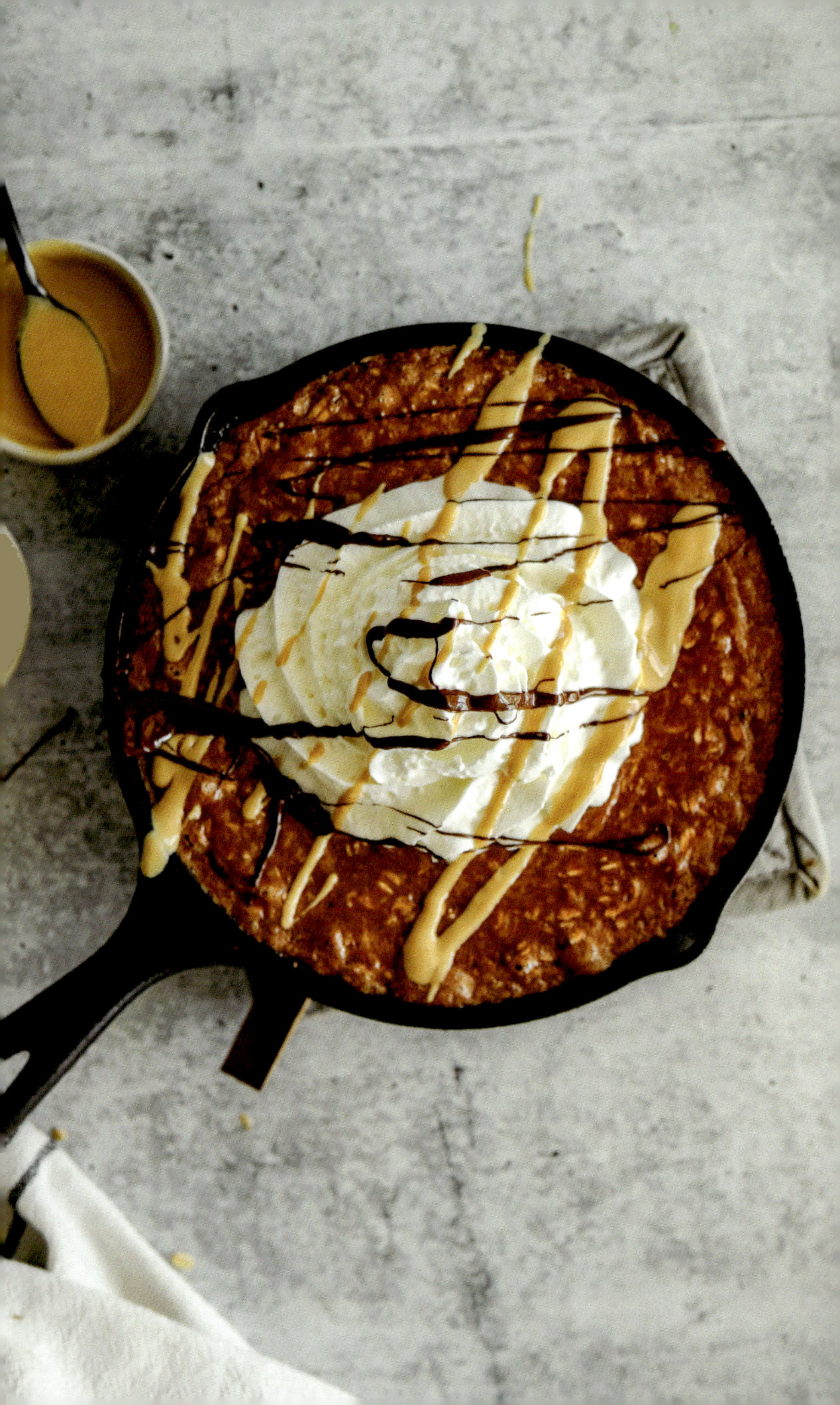

OOEY-GOOEY BREAKFAST BROWNIES
Makes 4 servings
350 calories / 13F / 37C / 25P / per serving

1½ cups old-fashioned rolled oats
3 servings CSE Brownie Batter
    or Chocolate Peanut Butter Protein Powder
1 Tbs. cocoa powder
1 dash sea salt
½ tsp. baking powder
¾ cup unsweetened almond milk
½ cup unsweetened applesauce
100g liquid egg whites
50g OffBeat Sweet Classic Peanut Butter
½ tsp. vanilla extract
Toppings:
8 Tbs. spray whipped cream
32g dark chocolate chips

1. Preheat oven to 350 degrees.

2. Add the oats, protein powder, cocoa powder, sea salt, and baking powder to a bowl. Stir together.

3. In a separate bowl, add the almond milk, applesauce, egg whites, Sweet Classic Peanut Butter, and vanilla. Whisk together until well combined.

4. Add the wet ingredients to the dry ingredients and stir until well coated.

5. Pour into a greased 8x8 baking dish or cast iron skillet of similar size (if you're feeling fancy). Bake for 10-12 minutes or to your desired doneness. Divide into four equal servings. Top each serving with two tablespoons of spray whipped topping and 8g chocolate chips (as is or melted). Enjoy!

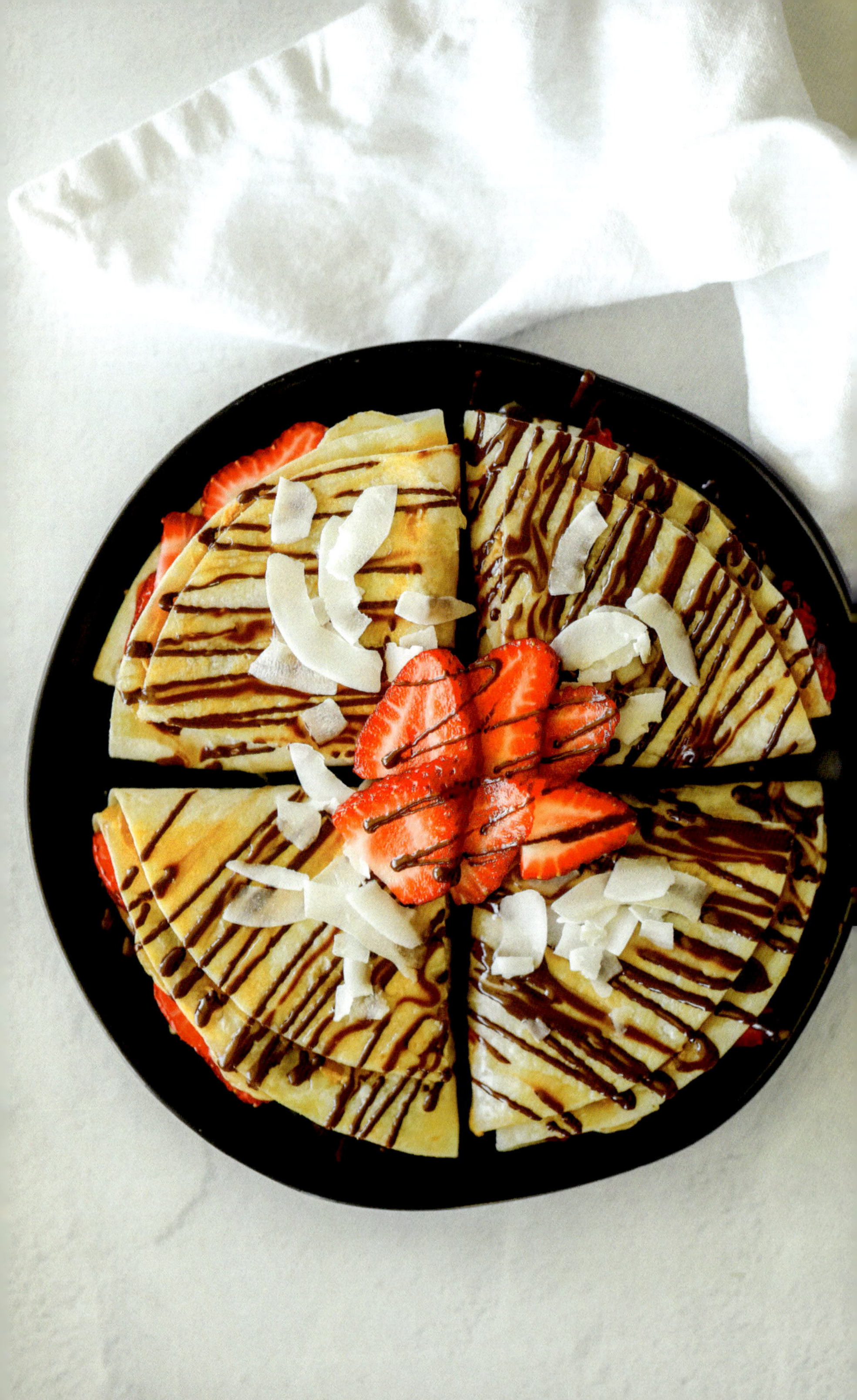

PB CHOCONUT BANANA STUFFED FOLDOVER
Makes 1 serving
250 calories / 12F / 31C / 8P

1 small La Tortilla Factory whole wheat tortilla (70 cal.)
30g bananas
20g fresh strawberries
½ Tbs. OffBeat Sweet Classic Peanut Butter
10g dark chocolate chips
5g unsweetened coconut, shredded
1 tsp. raw honey

1. Lay the tortilla flat on a cutting board. Place a knife in the center and make one slice in the tortilla out to the edge.

2. Place the sliced bananas in the bottom left corner of the tortilla, taking up ¼ of the entire tortilla, the coconut in the top left corner, the chocolate chips in the top right corner, and Sweet Classic Peanut Butter in the bottom right. Fold the corner with bananas up over the coconut. Then fold the left corner over the chocolate chips. Last, fold the top right corner down over the peanut butter, making a triangular shape.

3. Place the stuffed tortilla in a frying pan over medium heat. Once browned on one side, flip and brown on the other side.

4. Remove from the pan. Serve warm with sliced strawberries and honey drizzled over the top. Enjoy!

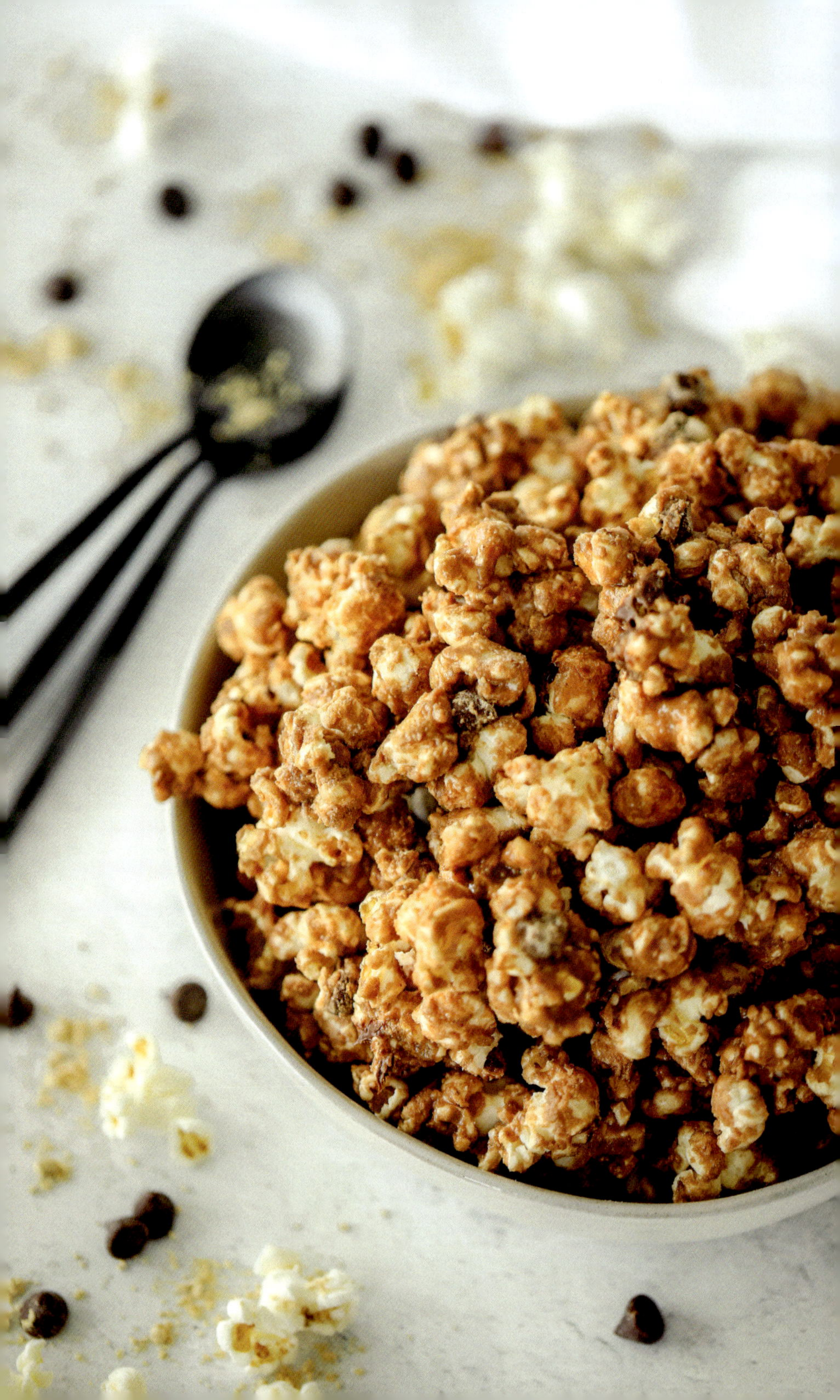

PEANUT BUTTER CUP POPCORN
Makes 8 servings
400 calories / 19.5F / 42.5C / 14P / per serving

---

12 (72g) cups air-popped popcorn
1 cup (8 oz.) OffBeat Sweet Classic Peanut Butter
¾ (6 oz.) cup raw honey
2 Tbs. grass-fed butter
1 tsp. vanilla extract
Pinch sea salt
1 Tbs. cocoa powder
1 serving CSE Chocolate Peanut Butter Protein Powder
Topping:
60g dark chocolate chips
¼ (32g) cup powdered peanut butter
1 serving CSE Chocolate Peanut Butter Protein Powder

1. Pop the popcorn kernels (about ⅓ cup) into a large bowl. Remove all unpopped kernels from the bowl. Set aside.

2. Add the Sweet Classic Peanut Butter, honey, butter and vanilla to a small saucepan over low-medium heat. Whisk until well combined and melted down. Remove from heat.

3. Add the sea salt, cocoa powder and protein powder to the pot with the peanut butter mixture. Stir until combined. Pour over the top of the popcorn while the sauce is still warm and stir until the popcorn is well coated.

4. Sprinkle the dark chocolate chips, powdered peanut butter and protein powder over the top of the popcorn. Stir until the popcorn is well coated and all the dry powder is incorporated. Weigh the entire batch and divide by eight to get the amount needed for one serving (about 85g per serving). Enjoy!

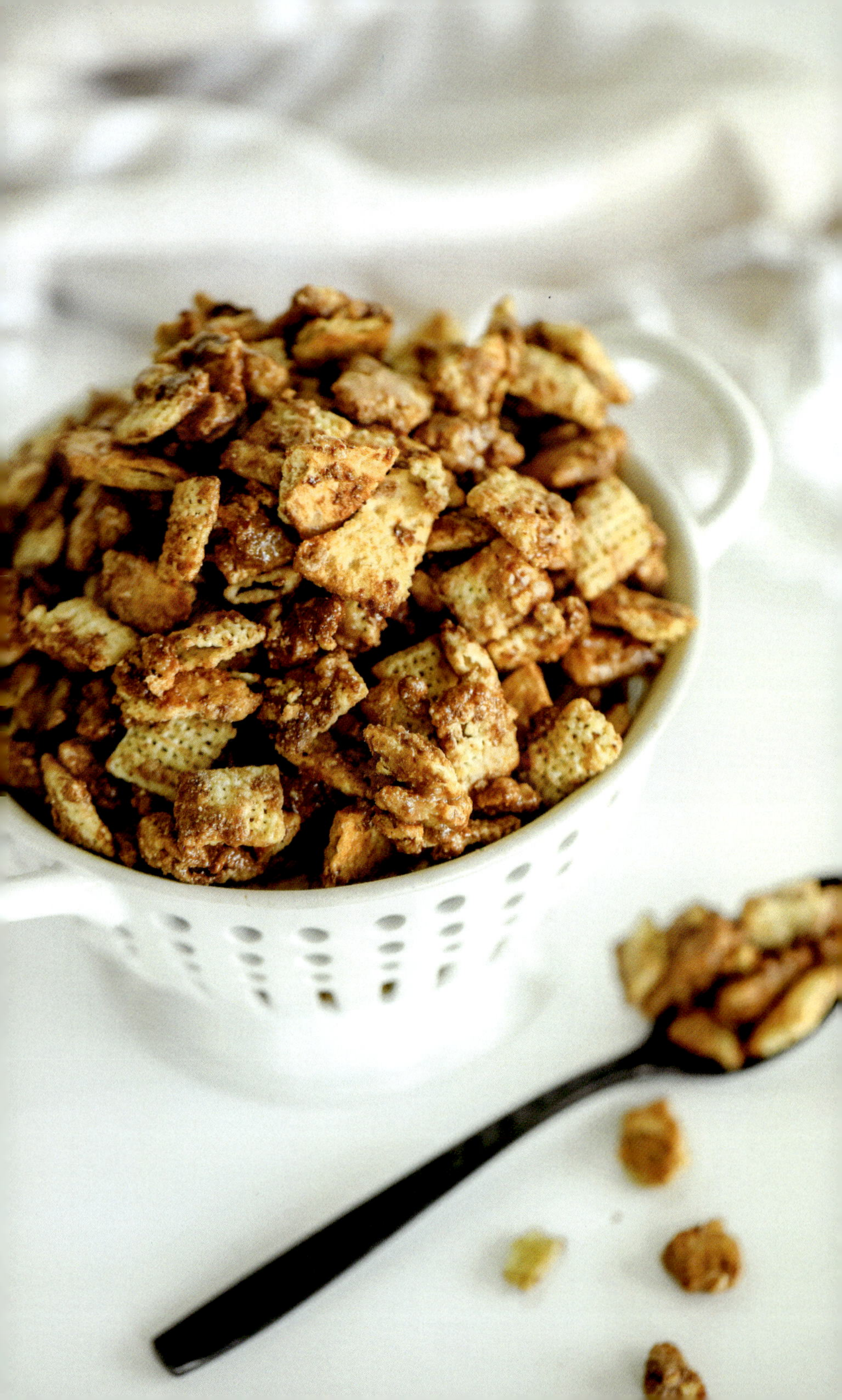

S'MORES PUPPY CHOW

Makes 12 servings
310 calories / 15F / 38C / 8P / per serving

---

7 cups Rice Chex cereal
5 graham cracker sheets (about 1 cup crumbled)
½ cup chocolate chips
¼ cup grass-fed butter
½ cup OffBeat Sweet Classic Peanut Butter
¼ cup raw honey
½ cup white chocolate chips
2 servings CSE S'mores Protein Powder

1. Pour the cereal, graham cracker crumbs and chocolate chips into a large bowl; set aside.

2. Add the butter to a small saucepan over low heat. Once melted, add the Sweet Classic Peanut Butter, honey and white chocolate chips. Stir constantly until completely melted. Remove from heat and let cool for a couple minutes. Stir in one serving of protein powder.

3. Pour the hot mixture over the top of the dry mixture in the bowl. Stir until well coated. Sprinkle with an additional serving of protein powder. Stir and serve. Enjoy!

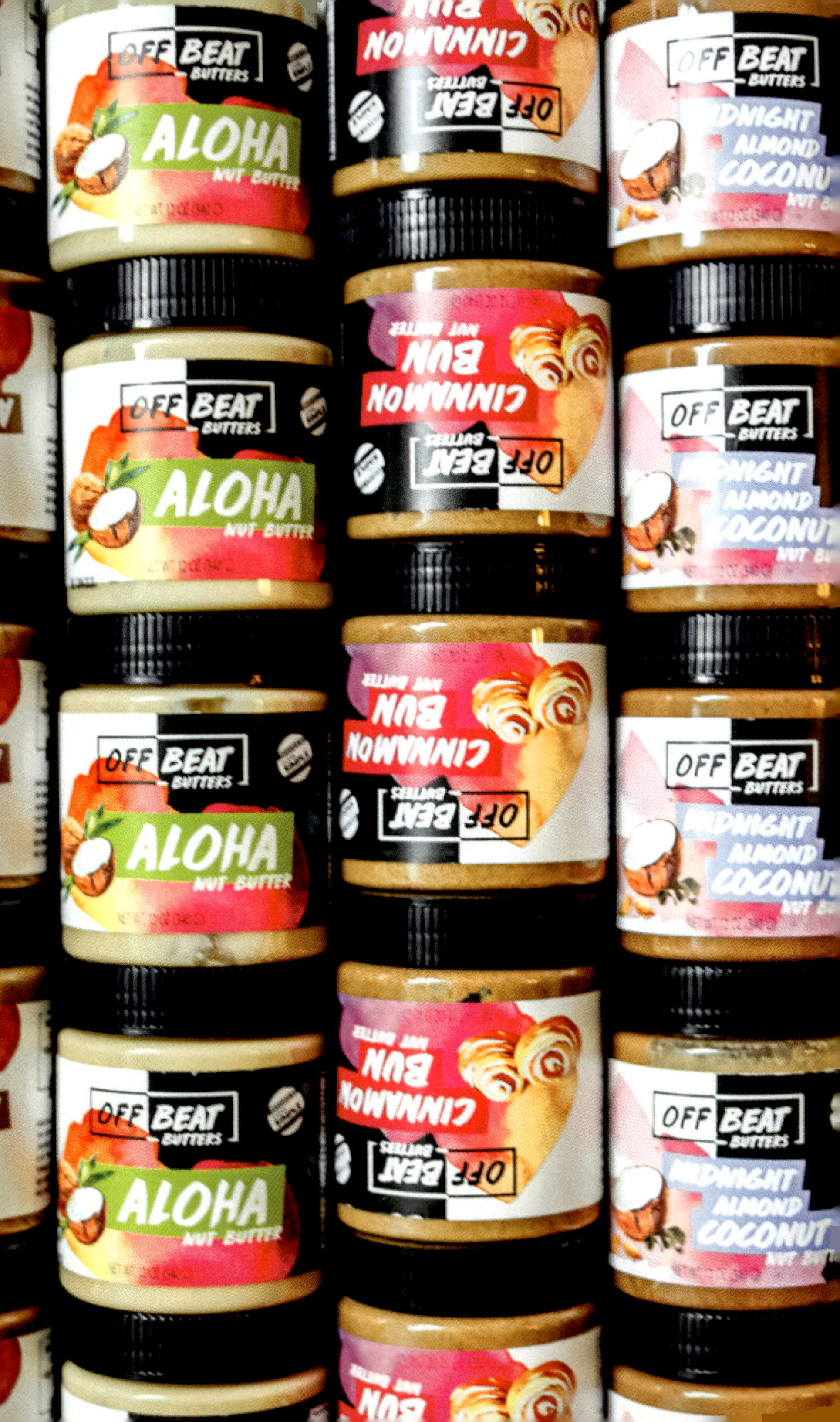
OFF BEAT BUTTERS
ALOHA
NUT BUTTER
CINNAMON BUN
OFF BEAT BUTTERS
OFF BEAT BUTTERS
MIDNIGHT ALMOND COCONUT
NUT BUTTER

A BALANCED DIET IS A JAR OF OFFBEAT BUTTER IN ONE HAND AND A SPOON IN THE OTHER

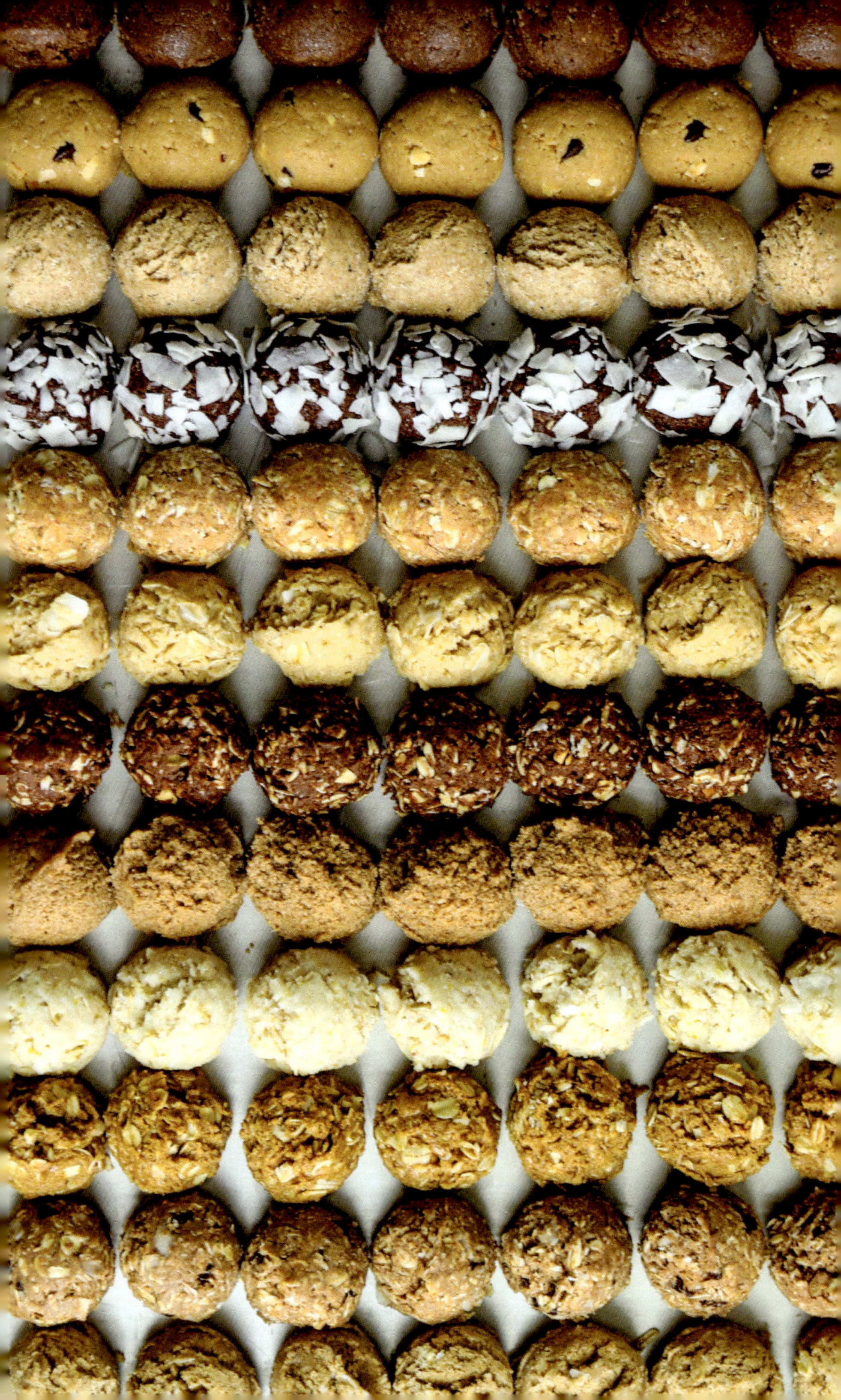

BUILD YOUR OWN OFFBEAT BITE
Makes 26 servings
90 calories / 4F/ 12C / 3P / per bite

---

1 cup OffBeat Butter, any flavor
½ cup raw honey
1 serving CSE Protein Powder, any flavor
1 ½ cups old-fashioned rolled oats
Dash sea salt
1 tsp. vanilla
Optional Add-Ins:
Chocolate chips
Unsweetened shredded coconut
Flaxseed meal
Rice Krispies
Chia seeds

1. Place all ingredients into a mixing bowl. Mix well.

2. Scoop with small cookie scoop and store in the fridge or freezer.

*Optional add-ins not included in macros.

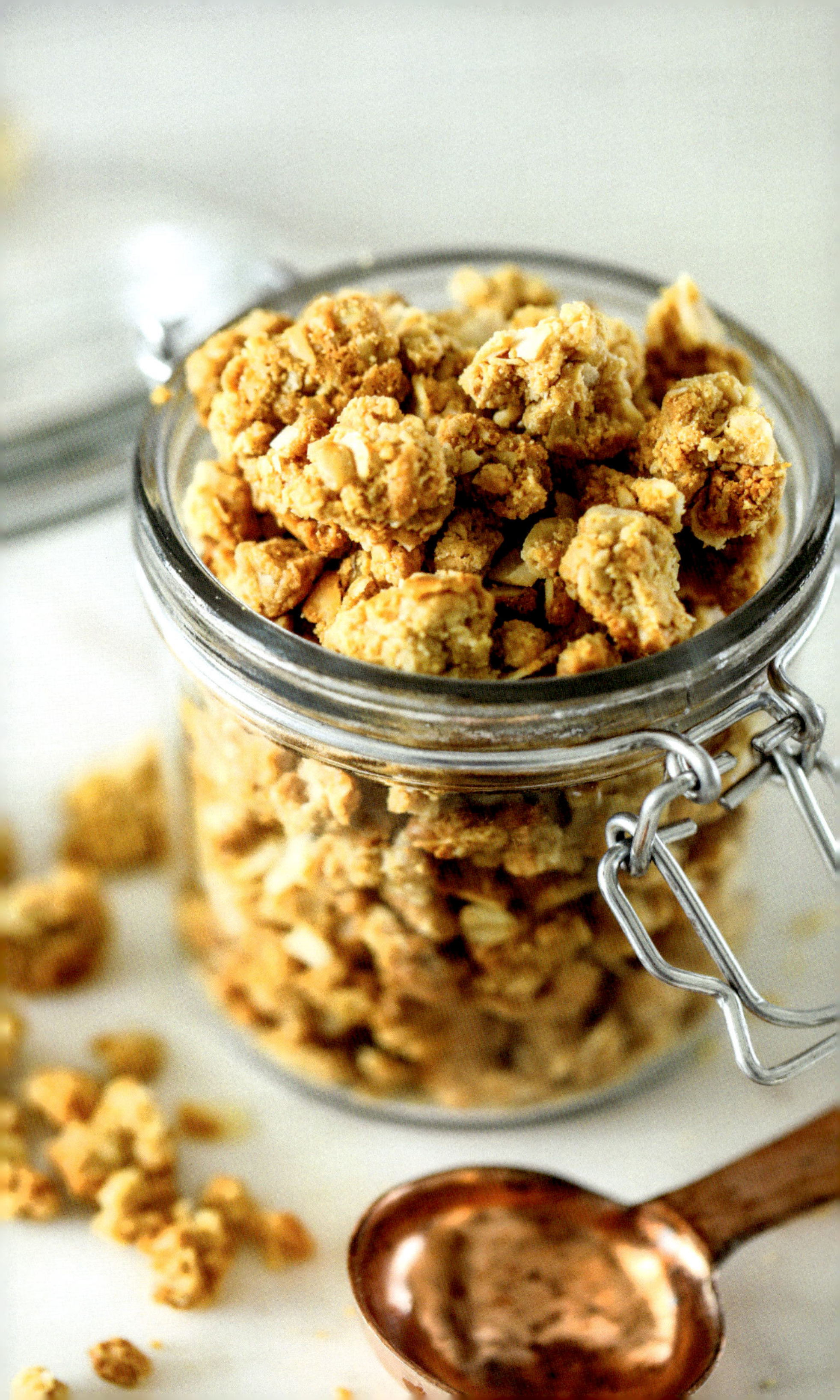

BUILD YOUR OWN OFFBEAT GRANOLA

Makes 26 servings / 30g per serving
115 calories / 5F / 14C / 4P

---

1 ¼ cups OffBeat Butter, any flavor
½ cup raw honey
2 servings CSE Protein Powder, any flavor
¼ tsp. sea salt
2 cups old-fashioned rolled oats
Optional Add-Ins:
Chocolate chips
Unsweetened shredded coconut
Flaxseed meal
Chia seeds
Cashews
Macadamia nuts

1. Preheat the oven to 375 degrees.

2. Add the OffBeat Butter, honey, protein powder and sea salt to a bowl. Mix well. Stir in the rolled oats and flaked coconut.

3. Pour the mixture out onto a baking sheet lined with parchment paper. Spread out into a single layer.

4. Bake for 5 minutes. Flip granola and bake another 4-5 minutes for soft granola or 6-7 minutes for crunchy granola.

5. Let cool, then transfer to a large jar and store in the fridge. Swap this in for any Clean Simple Eats recipe that calls for granola.

*Optional add-ins not included in macros.

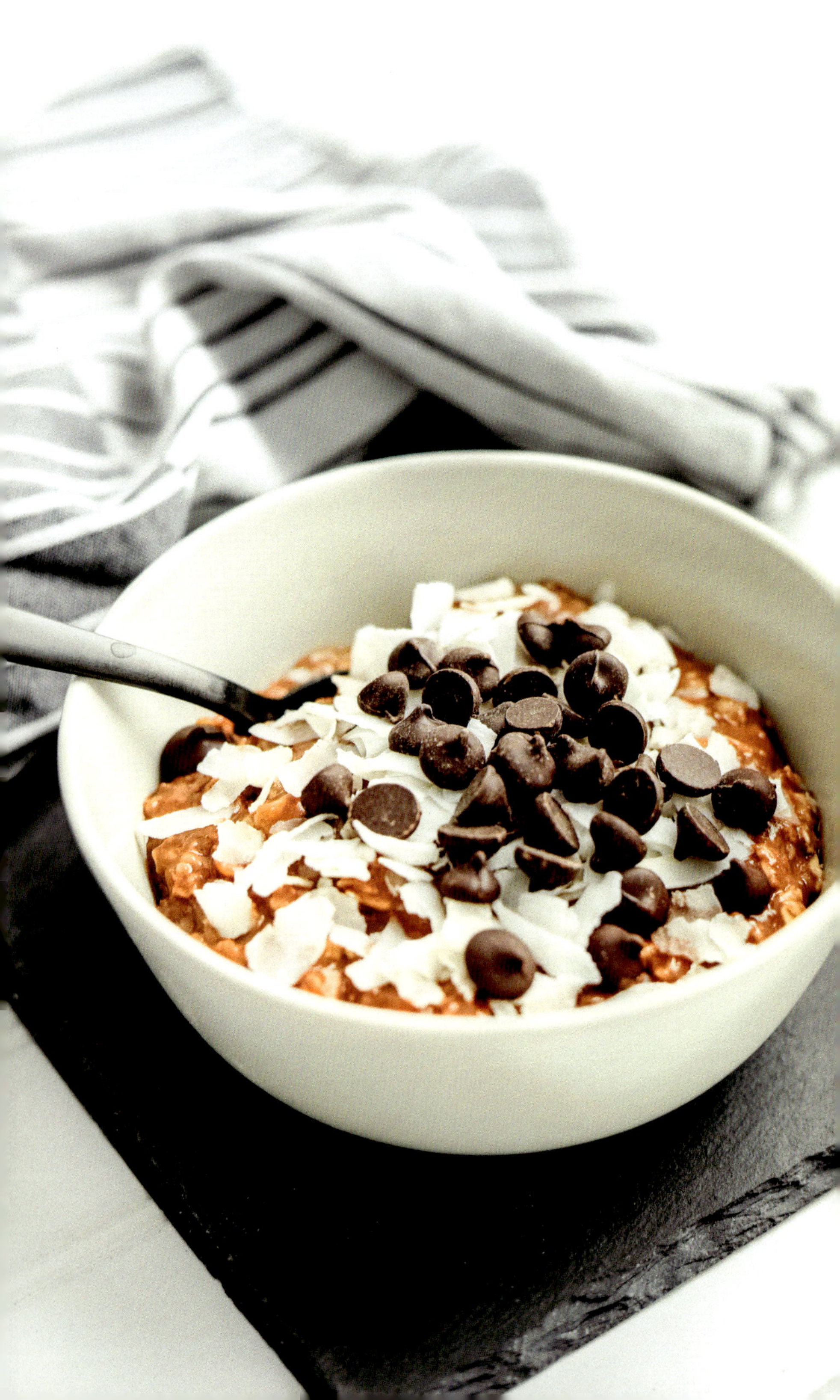

BUILD YOUR OWN OFFBEAT OATMEAL

Makes 1 serving
290 calories / 8F / 30C / 26P

⅓ cup oats
½ cup water
46 grams liquid egg whites
1 Tbs. OffBeat Butter, any flavor
¾ serving CSE Protein Powder, any flavor
Optional Toppings:
Chocolate chips
Unsweetened shredded coconut
Bananas
Berries
Powdered peanut butter
Greek yogurt
Spray whipped cream
Honey
Cinnamon
Brown sugar
Nuts

1. Add the oats, water and egg whites to a bowl. Microwave for 1-2 minutes.

2. Stir in the OffBeat Butter. Let cool for a couple minutes, then stir in the protein powder.

3. Top with any optional toppings (not included in macros). Enjoy!

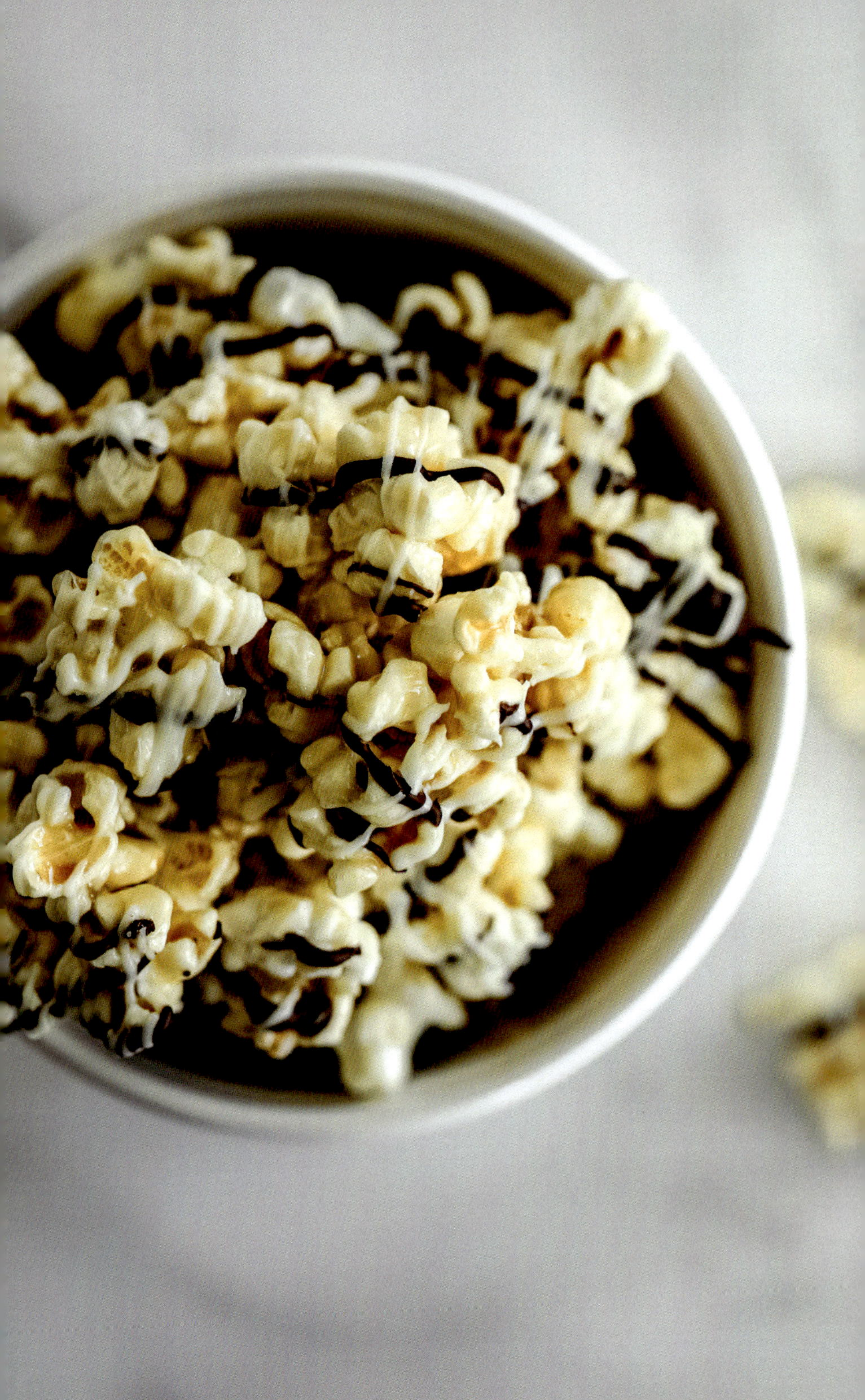

BUILD YOUR OWN OFFBEAT POPCORN
Makes 8 servings
180 calories / 10F / 20C / 6P / per serving

80g popcorn kernels
½ cup chocolate chips, any variety
¼ cup OffBeat Butter, any flavor
2 Tbs. grass-fed butter
1 tsp. vanilla extract
1 serving CSE Protein Powder, any flavor
Optional Toppings:
Melted chocolate drizzle
Chocolate chips
Powdered peanut butter
M&M's
Unsweetened coconut flakes

1. Use an air popper to pop the kernels in a large bowl and set aside.

2. Add the chocolate chips, OffBeat Butter and butter to a small saucepan. Melt over low heat until smooth. Remove from heat and whisk in the vanilla extract.

3. Pour the melted chocolate mixture over the popcorn and mix gently until the popcorn is well coated. Immediately add the protein powder and toss until the popcorn is well coated.

4. Add in any optional toppings (not included in macros). Divide into eight servings (approximately 1.25 oz. per serving) and enjoy!

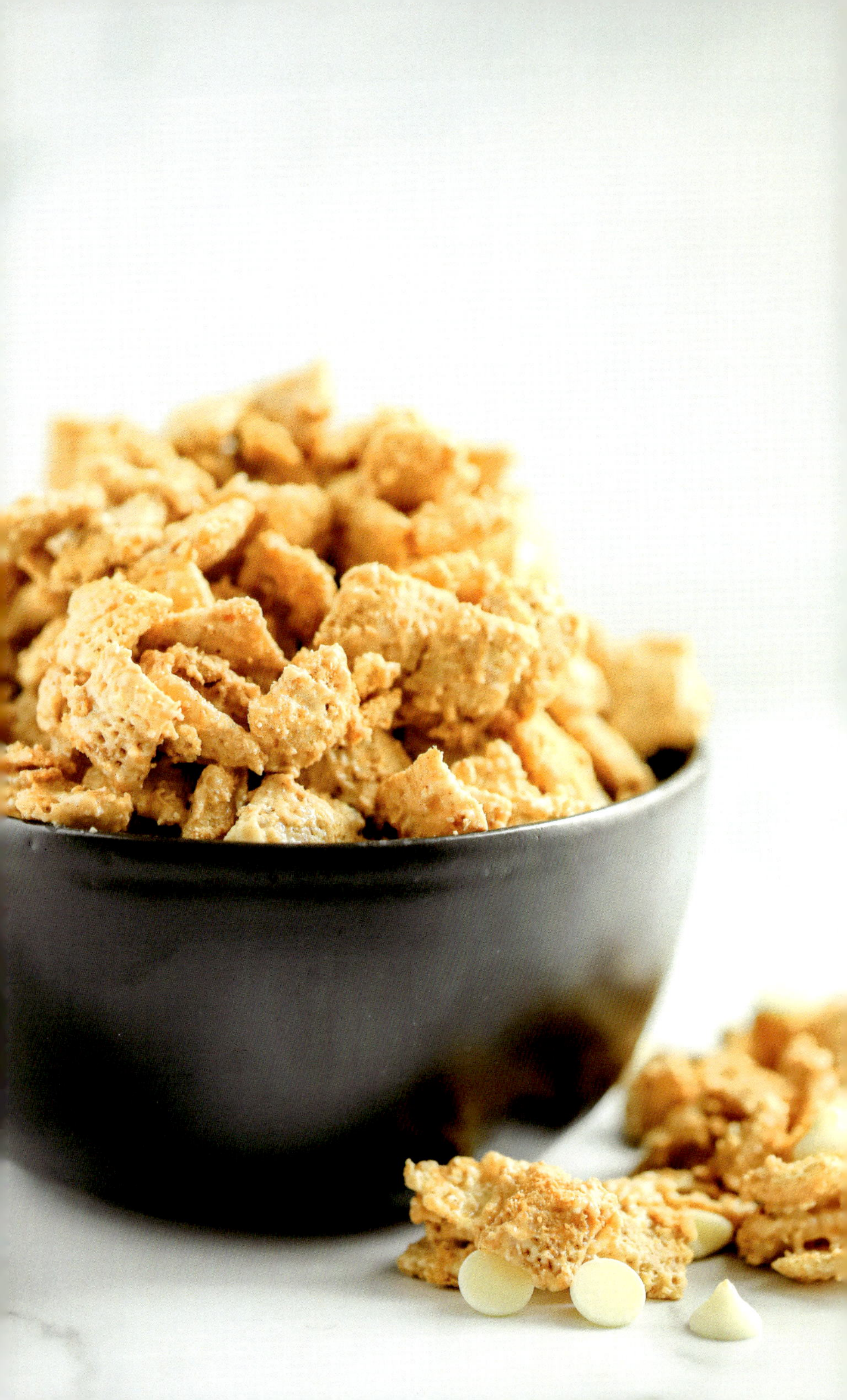

BUILD YOUR OWN OFFBEAT PUPPY CHOW
Makes 12 servings
250 calories / 11F / 32C / 7P / per serving

¼ cup grass-fed butter
½ cup chocolate chips, any variety
½ cup OffBeat Butter, any flavor
¼ cup raw honey
2 serving CSE Protein Powder, any flavor
8 cups Chex cereal, any variety
Optional Add-Ins:
Powdered peanut butter
Marshmallows
Graham cracker crumbs
Unsweetened coconut flakes
M&M's
Chocolate chips

1. In a small saucepan, melt the butter, chocolate chips, OffBeat Butter, and honey over low heat. Stir until melted together and smooth, then remove from heat. Stir in one serving of protein powder.

2. Place Chex cereal into a large bowl. Pour the hot mixture over the top and gently stir until the cereal is well coated.

3. Sprinkle with an additional serving of protein powder. Add in any optional add-ins (not included in macros). Stir and serve. Enjoy!

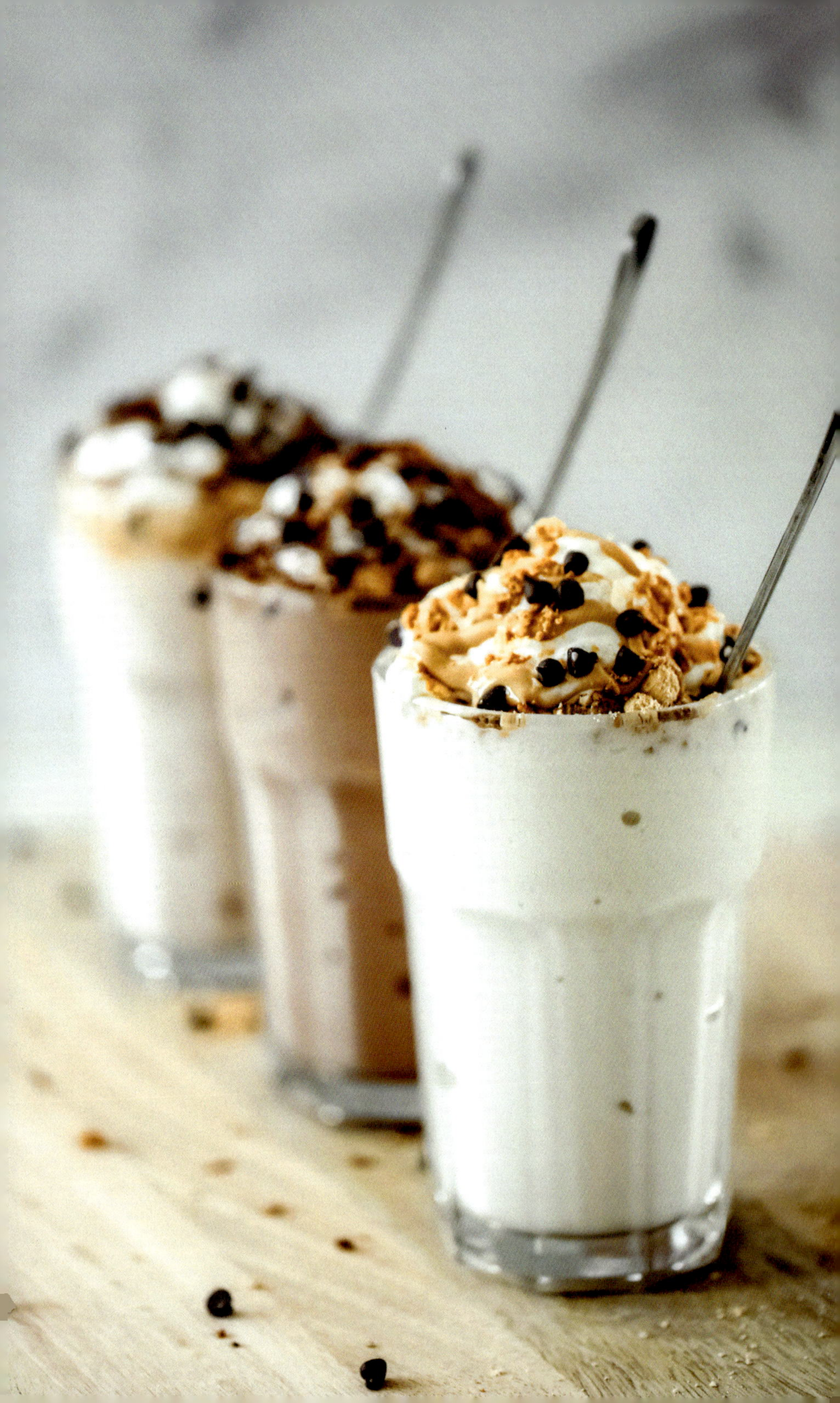

BUILD YOUR OWN OFFBEAT SHAKE
Makes 1 serving
310 calories / 9F / 34C / 24P

---

1 cup unsweetened almond milk
1 serving CSE Protein Powder, any flavor
1 Tbs. OffBeat Butter, any flavor
80g frozen banana slices
120g ice cubes
Optional Add-Ins:
Swap banana for any fruit
Cottage cheese
Optional Toppings:
Powdered peanut butter
Cocoa powder
Chocolate chips
Spray whipped cream
Granola

1. Add all of the ingredients to a high-powered blender. Blend on high until smooth.

2. Add any optional toppings (not included in macros). Pour into a cup. Enjoy!

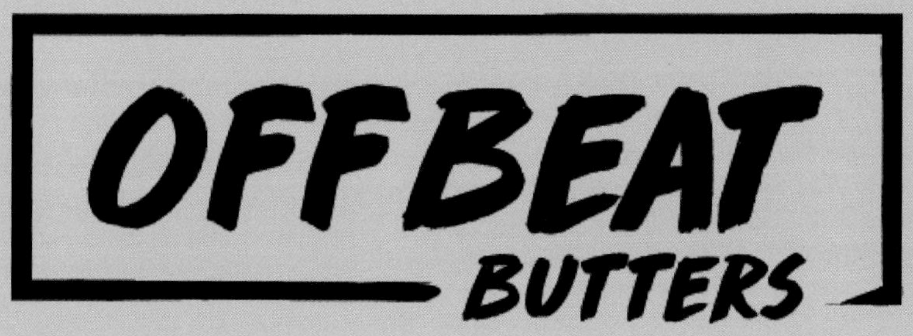

WWW.CLEANSIMPLEEATS.COM